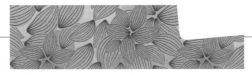

What Every Mental Health Professional Needs to Know About Sex

Stephanie Buehler, MPW, PsyD, CST, is a licensed psychologist and sex therapist. Dr. Buehler is the author of *Sex, Love, and Mental Illness: A Couple's Guide to Staying Connected* and multiple articles for professionals and the lay public on sexuality and relationships. She is a graduate of University of California at Los Angeles, University of Southern California, Pepperdine University, and Alliant/California School of Professional Psychology. Dr. Buehler has worked in settings that range from San Diego Children's Hospital to the Marine Corps Air Station at El Toro. She is Director of The Buehler Institute in Newport Beach, California, providing sex therapy to men, women, and couples, and continuing education opportunities for professionals. She resides in Orange County, California, with her husband of more than 25 years; together they have an adult daughter Anneka.

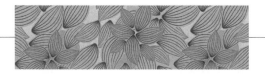

What Every Mental Health Professional Needs to Know About Sex

Stephanie Buehler, MPW, PsyD, CST

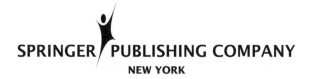

SPRINGER PUBLISHING COMPANY
NEW YORK

Springer Publishing Company, LLC
11 West 42nd Street
New York, NY 10036
www.springerpub.com

Acquisitions Editor: Nancy Hale
Production Editor: Dana Bigelow
Composition: diacriTech

ISBN: 978-0-8261-7121-4
e-book ISBN: 978-0-8261-7122-1

Practitioner Resources are available from springerpub.com/buehler-ancillary
978-0-8261-7123-8

13 14 15 16 17 / 5 4 3 2 1

The author and the publisher of this Work have made every effort to use sources believed to be reliable to provide information that is accurate and compatible with the standards generally accepted at the time of publication. The author and publisher shall not be liable for any special, consequential, or exemplary damages resulting, in whole or in part, from the readers' use of, or reliance on, the information contained in this book. The publisher has no responsibility for the persistence or accuracy of URLs for external or third-party Internet websites referred to in this publication and does not guarantee that any content on such websites is, or will remain, accurate or appropriate.

Library of Congress Cataloging-in-Publication Data
Buehler, Stephanie (Stephanie J.)
  What every mental health professional needs to know about sex / Stephanie Buehler, MPW, PsyD, CST.
    pages cm
  Includes bibliographical references and index.
  ISBN 978-0-8261-7121-4 (alk. paper)
  1. Sexual health. 2. Sex therapy. 3. Sexual abuse victims—Rehabilitation. 4. Older people—Sexual behavior. I. Title.
  RA788.B84 2014
  613.9—dc23
                        2013020630

Special discounts on bulk quantities of our books are available to corporations, professional associations, pharmaceutical companies, health care organizations, and other qualifying groups. If you are interested in a custom book, including chapters from more than one of our titles, we can provide that service as well.

For details, please contact:
Special Sales Department, Springer Publishing Company, LLC
11 West 42nd Street, 15th Floor, New York, NY 10036-8002
Phone: 877-687-7476 or 212-431-4370; Fax: 212-941-7842
E-mail: sales@springerpub.com

Printed in the United States of America by Edwards Brothers.

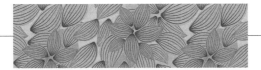

Contents

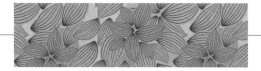

Foreword

When I speak at colleges about sex, I often start by asking students in the audience "How many of your parents told you what a clitoris is when you were growing up?" In an audience of 300 students, perhaps five will raise their hands. When I ask "How many of your parents explained to you what masturbation is or told you what orgasms are?" Ten or fifteen hands will go up. These are students at some of the top colleges who were raised by some of the smartest parents on the planet during the 1990s—not the 1950s.

When parents are not comfortable giving their children words for some of the most powerful physical and emotional experiences they will have in life, a veil of secrecy is created around the subject of sex that children carry with them into adulthood. This is why there is such a great need for a book like *What Every Mental Health Professional Needs to Know About Sex*. It doesn't matter if the therapy we do is cognitively based, psychodynamic, interpersonal, or experiential, this book explores aspects of sex that are essential for therapists of all orientations to know.

Sex is an important part of most people's lives, yet few mental health professionals receive any instruction about sex other than learning how to report suspected abuse. As a result, we aren't always comfortable talking about sex and sexual pleasure with our patients. While reading this book won't turn us into Kinseys or Masters and Johnsons, it will help us to relax more and to listen better. And that, in itself, is an important accomplishment regardless of how much or how little familiarity we have with sex education and sex research.

I have written a 1,200-page book on sex that is used in dozens of college and medical school sex-education classes. I have also read countless studies on sexual orientation, gender, pornography, paraphilias, sexual pain, low sex drive, high sex drive, casual sex, pedophilia, and the physiology and neurology of sexual response. Yet when I am with a patient or when a fellow mental health professional is consulting with me about a patient's sexual issues, the most important thing I can do, besides being kind and caring, is to listen without making judgments. This is not always easy when you are raised in a culture with no shortage of shame-based messages about sex.

For example, consider our perceptions about women versus men when it comes to casual sex. Few of us would haul out our *DSM-5*s when a male informs us he has had 10 or 15 lifetime sexual partners. But if a woman has had 10 or 15 partners, or 20 or more, many of us would assume she was abused as a child, or she's bipolar or borderline, or she's a "sex addict." And what if she enjoys having threesomes, or she asks her partner to spank her or to act out rape fantasies? What if she wants sex way more than her partner does?

This book was written by a highly experienced and sensible mental health professional who encourages readers to listen and think rather than to automatically pathologize or apply assumptions about sexual behavior that are 50 years out of date. It reminds us that sexual behaviors that could reflect a psychological struggle for one person might reflect psychological health for another. One of our jobs is to evaluate which is which.

One of the biggest challenges we face in evaluating sexual behaviors is how multifaced sex can be. Sexual feelings often begin as an erotic tension somewhere within our psyche or soma. They are then sifted through the labyrinth of our cognitive, cultural, and religious beliefs. When something is going wrong sexually, there are multiple layers where the problem can reside. I can't imagine trying to help a patient sort through sexual issues without knowing what Dr. Buehler explains in the pages that follow.

And finally, I want to caution you about the current state of sexual knowledge and sexual research: Our knowledge of human sexuality remains elementary. Researchers are still struggling to define what women's sexual orientation is and how it develops over the life span. Several of the top researchers are questioning the validity of the state-of-the-art fMRI brain studies about sexual behavior that the media loves to sensationalize and therapists love to quote. And it's difficult to know if studies about sex and relationships apply to anyone besides the students in college psychology courses who are getting extra credit for participating in them.

Fortunately, we have Dr. Stephanie Buehler's very thoughtful, approachable, and well-written book to help us with this process.

Paul Joannides, PsyD
Author of *Guide to Getting It On!*, Seventh Edition

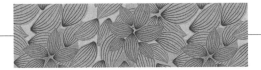

Preface

An endocrinologist with whom I once ran an integrated wellness center encouraged me to become a sex therapist, explaining that many of her patients request hormone testing because they had no sex drive. "But," she said, "It is hardly ever their hormones that need adjusting." I already had a background in treating people with chronic illness, and I understood right away that sexual problems were, perhaps, the ultimate expression of mind/body symptoms. But how, I wondered, did one become a sex therapist?

One thing I knew for certain, the 10 hours in human sexuality that I was required to take to become a psychologist wasn't anywhere near what I needed to know to talk to our shared clients about sex. I hadn't learned much of anything in those 10 hours, except that there existed some mighty peculiar old sex education films and that many therapists in the audience were squeamish about sex. I wasn't squeamish at all. I grew up in a liberal household in Los Angeles during the sexual revolution. Nothing offended me. But if I was going to truly hang out my shingle as treating sexual problems, I was in sore need of education and training.

Like many psychotherapists—who tend to be an introverted bunch—my first stop was to do some background reading. I chose a book online and as soon as it arrived I sat down to read, highlighter in hand. It wasn't long before I closed the book, my mind reeling. It wasn't because there was anything wrong with the writing itself. All of the contributing authors appeared to know their topic well. However, I still had no sense of "This is how to do sex therapy." I felt rudderless, adrift in a sea of technical language, with bits and pieces of various theories floating past like flotsam and jetsam.

Perhaps joining an appropriate organization might help me, I reasoned. I joined the American Association of Educators, Counselors, and Therapists and learned they had a certification process that included education and supervision. I chose Stephen Braveman, MFT, as my supervisor, and through his patient guidance and generous spirit (he sent me away with a duffle bag of materials on human sexuality), I began the 2-year trek to learn all I could to be an effective sex therapist.

Along the way, I received an entirely different education. First, colleagues and other professionals questioned my choice to become a sex therapist. Wouldn't I be dealing with pedophiles and other pariahs? Second, some confused me with a sexual surrogate, a type of person who operates under the legal radar to teach people about their sexuality in a way that a professional license prohibited, for example, touching clients or having them examine bodies, both their own and that of the surrogate. Third, it struck me again and again how ludicrous it was, with all my education, that none of my college professors at the graduate level had ever really talked about sex. Why didn't I know anything about the connection between eating disorders and sexual problems? How come I had never heard of painful sex and what to do about it? Didn't I need to know how to assess persons who had been sexually abused about their current ability to function normally in their adult relationships?

Additionally, I began to pay attention to what clients said when they found my services. If they were referred by another therapist, it was often because the therapists "didn't 'do' sex." If they had been in therapy but were self-referred, it might be that they felt the *therapist* would be uncomfortable if they brought up the topic. Others were in therapy for years, but since the topic never came up, they never said anything. It was only when they realized that all the time and money they were spending had zero effect on their sexual pleasure that they searched for someone who would help them with the "real" problem.

I held two feelings about this. On one hand, I was happy that I received appropriate referrals. On the other, I was upset that other therapists added to the client's shame about sex. By refusing or neglecting to ask about the client's sex life, therapists reinforced the cultural message that "nice people don't talk about sex." But if people (nice or not) can't talk about sex in the therapist's office, where can they talk about it? Clearly something needed to change.

Back I went to thinking about my own evolution as a therapist. Information about treating sexual problems, I knew, was difficult reading. Few of the books take the therapist by the hand and lead them through the entire process of assessment and treatment from the moment of the intake call through termination. None of them deal with one of the most important issues of all: the sexuality of the therapist. Unless the therapist is comfortable with sex, there would be no discussion of the topic in the therapy office. That fact alerted me that if I were to write a book on how to do sex therapy, I needed to start there, with helping the reader to make sense of what sexuality is and how to understand one's own development, experiences, thoughts, attitudes, and beliefs about sex.

In your hand or on your screen, you have the text I envisioned for every therapist to have as a reference on his or her bookshelf. Whether you want to embrace sex therapy as a niche for your practice, or you want to be a therapist who "does" sex, my hope is that *What Every Mental Health Professional Needs to Know About Sex* will be a clear, pragmatic entrance into helping clients of all kinds resolve sexual concerns—a boat of sorts to help you navigate what can be a confusing area of human experience. I also hope that it will become a book you can turn to again and again when a client presents with a sexual concern to remind yourself that there exists an approach and information to calmly tackle common, and uncommon, sexual problems.

Human sexuality is perhaps one of the most complicated on the planet. Shrouded in secrecy, regulated by religion and law, and assigned meanings from original sin to the ultimate expression of sacred joy, sexuality can perplex even the wisest therapists. Sexuality is often a topic ignored in graduate programs in psychology, marriage and family therapy, and social work. In California where I practice, a psychologist is required to merely complete 12 hours (not course hours, *hours*) of instruction in sex therapy. This training was disembodied, that is, it had no connection to the 4 to 5 years of coursework learning about all other aspects of the human mind.

What Every Mental Health Professional Needs to Know About Sex is a straightforward, plain-language book designed to take the therapist who knows very little or who might be uncomfortable about sex, to a place of knowledge and competence. To accomplish this, Part I: The Courage to Treat Sexual Problems begins in Chapter 1 with a rationale regarding the reasons why all mental health professionals need to be able to address clients' sexual concerns, especially the fact that our current social climate has raised clients' expectations about pleasure. In Chapter 2, the reader will find topics concerning one's own sexuality, including overcoming any associated shame and guilt related to sexual behavior, improving attitudes toward sexual pleasure, and embracing sexual diversity—not only the LGBTQ community, but sexuality in those who are ill or aging, or who engage in alternative sexual practices, for example, fetish behavior. Psychosexual development and the physiology of sex are covered in Chapter 3, while Chapter 4 is an examination of definitions of sexual health generated by various experts and organizations.

Part II: Assessing and Treating Sexual Concerns begins with an introduction to the thorough assessment of sexual problems that relies on two models and that forms a core part of the book. The first is Annon's PLISSIT model, described in detail in Chapter 5; the second is an ecosystemic framework for understanding and solving a client's symptoms across different contexts. The PLISSIT model is ideal for a mental health professional at the early stages of treating sexual problems, as it guides the professional in deciding whether the presenting problem will benefit from psychoeducation and recommendations, or if more intensive, long-term therapy will be required. The ecosystemic framework, based on the work of Bronfenbrenner (1977), is an expansion of the biopsychosocial model as it includes interactions between two systems, which in the case of sex therapy relates to the frequency that couples present for treatment. A thorough sexual assessment is included, to use when it is determined that the presenting problem will require more intensive work.

The next two chapters cover women's and then men's common sexual complaints as they pertain to the individual, their biological make-up, development, relationship, and culture. Chapter 5 on women's sexual problems covers sexual aversion, which occurs in both men and women. Chapter 6 includes delayed ejaculation, a problem once considered rare but is on the upswing as some men desensitize their arousal levels by viewing pornography, as well as the fact that people's expectations of men as they age have increased. Both chapters include informational worksheets for the client's—and therapist's—benefit.

Addressing common sexual problems in couples explodes the myth that by fixing the couple's relationship, their sex life will automatically improve. In fact, even couples that get along sometimes have sexual problems. As the therapist will learn in Chapter 8, whether the relationship is blissful or chaotic, most couples benefit from good sexual information; improved communication about sex; encouragement to explore the boundaries of their sexuality; and suggestions to help them. The most common problem is a discrepancy in sexual desire, which requires the therapist's problem-solving skills to help the couple to stop blaming one another and learn how to derive solutions when the problem is sex.

Chapter 9 includes material I have not yet seen in any other book for therapists on the topic of treating sexual complaints: helping parents address their concerns about their children's sexual development and answering their children's questions about sex. The chapter also provides a framework as to when to refer to a specialist for evaluation of atypical sexual behavior or development. The entirety of Chapter 10 is devoted to understanding the needs of LGBTQ clients who may, ironically, have suffered because of their parents' lack of information about sexual orientation.

Good mental health is essential to good sexual health, while mental illness can contribute to sexual dysfunction. In turn, feelings of guilt, shame, and sexual inadequacy can sometimes lead to mental health problems. In 2010, I wrote a ground-breaking book entitled *Sex, Love, and Mental Illness: A Couple's Guide to Staying Connected* in which I addressed the effects of depression, anxiety, substance abuse, eating disorders, AD/HD, and other disorders on the individual's ability to function sexually and in a relationship. Chapter 11 is a broad summary of this review of the literature, while Chapter 12 provides an in-depth guide to understanding and treating sexual problems in adults related to sexual abuse experienced as a child or teen.

Chapters 13 to 16 are related in that they each cover an aspect of sexuality that is intimately tied to biology. Chapter 13 covers the effects of pelvic and genital pain on sexuality in men and women, which affects large numbers of people who sometimes have great difficulty finding appropriate treatment, lending to their suffering. In Chapter 14, therapists will learn what happens when recreation meets procreation, or how sexuality is affected by infertility. Sexuality can also be affected by all kinds of medical conditions, from diabetes to spinal lesions and paralysis, which is the topic of Chapter 15. The effects of aging on sexuality and relationships are the focus of Chapter 16.

Rounding up Part II, Chapters 17 and 18 explore what happens when people traverse conventional or expected boundaries, with Chapter 17 focusing on sex and the Internet, and Chapter 18 on paraphilias, also known as "alt sex" (as in "alternative"). Though sexual images have seemingly been in existence since ancient cultures constructed phallic and other fertility-related symbols, there has been an explosion in sexual imagery of all kinds since the dawn of the Internet. The enormous availability and variety of pornography has both helped (people can indulge in fantasy material in private, such as looking at people having sex while wearing latex or furs) and hurt in that viewing pornography may drain sexual energy away from a primary relationship. Meanwhile, those who practice alt sex need all kinds of care and support from therapists, from absolution from shame to helping them accept and perhaps participate in their partner's erotic life.

Part III: Ethics and Practice of Sex Therapy wraps up the book with Chapter 19 on the ethical challenges of working with people who have sexual concerns, including respecting boundaries regarding touch; managing romantic or sexual transference and countertransference; managing secrets in conjoint therapy; and considering special topics such as treating people whose sexuality differs from one's own and the effects of the field of sexual medicine on sex therapy. Finally, Chapter 20 completes the book with a look forward toward the future of sex therapy and the integration of sex therapy into one's practice.

As with any book, there were some challenges presented. One challenge was the unwieldy term "mental health professional" used in the book's title. Rather than shortening the term to "MHP," which seemed impersonal, I most frequently use the term "therapist" to refer to the variety of people working in the helping profession. Both "mental health professional" and "therapist" refer to psychiatrists, psychologists, psychiatric nurses, social workers, marriage and family therapists, and professional counselors, including those medical providers who discuss sexual problems with their patients.

Another challenge was the use of gendered pronouns. As much as possible, I have used the word "partner" rather than "man," "woman," "husband," "wife," and so forth. Although gay, lesbian, bisexual, transgender, and queer (those individuals who do not identify strictly as male or female, or who question their orientation) roles and relationships are not strictly analogous to traditional heterosexual experiences, I have drawn from my clinical observation in classifying some components of all erotic relationships as being universal. Sexual desire, arousal, and orgasm are not exclusive to any group of people, and when two people hold one another as special and dear, it is nearly always called love.

A third challenge is culture as it relates to sexuality. In some areas, as with infertility, there exists a decent body of literature about the effect of culture on sexual beliefs or behaviors. In others, such as paraphilias, almost nothing has been written, although it can be assumed that an individual from a conservative family and culture may have different feelings about having a fetish than one from a more open and permissive culture. Fortunately, there exists online a tremendous resource, *The Continuum Complete International Encyclopedia of Sexuality* (Francoeur & Noonan, 2004), which any therapist can access to learn about the sexual practices of over 50 cultures.

Lastly, my hope is that the reader will find *What Every Mental Health Professional Needs to Know About Sex* to be a jumping off point for addressing the sexual concerns of clients and not the definitive or final word on how to do sex therapy. My own understanding of human sexuality continues to evolve, as does the field as experts research the multiple biopsychosocial factors that make us think and act as we do between the sheets. If I have done my job, your own interest in sexuality will be piqued and you will continue to deepen your knowledge and ability to be a therapist who "does sex."

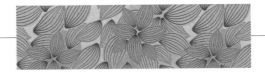

Acknowledgments

This book would not be possible without the support of my family, friends, and colleagues.

First, I'd like to thank my small but mighty family. To my wonderful husband Mark, thank you for providing love and support, and those life-preserving weekend beach walks. To my daughter Anneka, thank you for sending humorous material from afar; a true demonstration of Buehler affection. Also, thanks to Bodhi, my "therapy parrot," for distracting me with squawks and squeaks during long hours at the keyboard.

Thank you to my dear friend Jacqueline Richard, who supplied much-needed cheerleading from the sidelines whenever my will to write flagged. To my friends Barbara and Stuart Bloom, Piet and Judi Dwinger, and Christauria Welland, I appreciate your encouraging words, hugs, and humor. While I appreciate all my interns, I want to especially thank Liz Dubé for her patience with me as I wrote this book.

Finally, I have an amazing network of colleagues who have inspired me and enabled me to become the professional I am today. Stephen Braveman, my sex therapy supervisor, I thank you for your incredible generosity; I carry your words of wisdom with me into the pages of this book. I also have too many wonderful professional friends to thank to list them all individually. Therefore, I want to express tremendous appreciation to fellow members of the following organizations whom I consider friends too numerous to count: American Association of Sexuality Educators, Counselors, and Therapists; Society for Sex Therapy and Research; International Society for the Study of Women's Sexual Health; Society for the Scientific Study of Sexuality; Orange County Psychological Association; and California Psychological Association. Your knowledge and support have been invaluable to me.

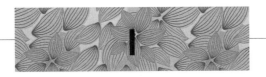

The Courage to Treat
Sexual Problems

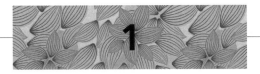

Sexuality and the Mental Health Profession

When I decided to become certified in sex therapy, my supervisor Stephen Braveman early on stated, "In our culture, no one escapes having some form of sexual damage." Unfortunately, this statement also describes the influence of culture on mental health professionals across the lifespan. Consider how other systems, such as family, school, or peers, influenced your own sexual development. Perhaps you experienced being sexually harassed on the schoolyard or the workplace. You may be the one in four women or one in six men who were molested as children and who did not feel supported enough by parents or school to tell. You may have engaged in sex when you didn't want to—or you even coerced someone into having sex with you—which changed your cognitive framework and your approach to sex, even in safe relationships. Or perhaps you were educated as a therapist in a setting influenced by the larger culture, where sexuality was a marginalized topic of study.

With any luck, you grew up to be a sexually functioning adult capable of emotional and physical intimacy with a partner of your choosing, but there is a strong likelihood that you have had struggles with your sexuality, as do surprisingly large numbers of men and women in the population at large (Laumann, Paik, & Rosen, 1999). It is in regard to our sexuality that we are perhaps most like our clients, kept in the dark about its nature and discouraged from opening the door to understanding. Insight and knowledge into sexuality requires that therapists pay attention to their own development, but our training reflects the reluctance of our culture as a whole to "go there." For most therapists, learning how to address sexual topics requires specialized training that may be difficult to access, requiring travel and other expense.

What happens to our clients if we, ourselves, don't have or make the opportunity to understand our own sexuality? Can we call ourselves competent if we don't assess or treat the entire spectrum of human experience, including those that are baffling or taboo? As self-appointed healers of mental health, I believe we must take responsibility to heal the *whole person*, including the sexual part of the self. Otherwise, we may inadvertently sustain or contribute to a client's struggle with sexuality. Mental health and medical professions have yet to fully recognize that sexual problems can contribute to depression, anxiety, trauma, eating disorders, substance abuse, pain disorders, and so on; conversely, such problems can affect a person's sexuality, yet remain unaddressed in the therapist's office. Yet if we don't "do sex" as part of our practice, we may miss out on an essential part of what is troubling our clients.

Consider Len, a client in his mid-60s who was so guilt ridden after his first attempt at intercourse that he struggled with erectile dysfunction for all the years that followed. Len became depressed after a divorce and sought relief through therapy, medications, and, at times, alcohol. In all his years of counseling, no one had asked him about his sex life—until he mentioned a urology appointment. Concerned he might be ill, the therapist asked more about the appointment. The question prompted Len to cry as he told her about his impotence. Fortunately, the therapist soon realized this was a long-standing, complex issue for Len and a referral was made for my help. After months of treatment with Len and his partner, he was, at last, able to resolve his sexual concerns.

But how different might Len's life have been if someone had earlier inquired, "How's your sex life?" Len's treatment was influenced by a culture in which nonspecialized therapists lack training or comfort discussing sexual topics. He also needed a therapist who could use a systemic approach to understand why his struggle was so long-standing and intense, which had to do with his development in an extremely restrictive family, church, and community environment. The restrictive environment caused Len undue shame about his sexual needs, which in turn caused him to lose his erection in his first sexual encounter. Later in life, changes in Len's biological system made attaining any kind of erection almost impossible, adding further frustration. Only when Len's frustration was more painful than his secret could he break out of his shell and reach out for help.

Clients come to us to help them solve all kinds of problems, which may include sexual concerns. The Laumann survey (Laumann, Paik & Rosen, 1999) of male and female sexual problems—the largest of its kind—reported that about 60% of women and 30% of men have had some type of sexual dysfunction. With numbers like these, it is safe to assume that a good portion of your current clients have a sexual problem. If you do not ask, however, you may never hear about these issues. But clients sometimes do tell me, as an identified sex therapist, some of the reasons why they left a former therapist who didn't talk about sex:

- One woman found the courage to seek help for the fact that she was still a virgin 7 years after her wedding night due to *vaginismus* (spasm of the vagina that prevents penetration), but she could not bring herself to tell the therapist about her problem. Since the therapist never asked about sex, the client got the message loud and clear: Sex is not spoken here.
- A couple trying to get past an affair that nearly destroyed their marriage couldn't bring themselves to tell their "uptight" therapist that they had enjoyed swinging early in their relationship. The couple's history added to their confusion about boundaries and rules in the marriage, but their weeks in therapy were useless because they feared the therapist would judge them if they disclosed their early history.
- Sam and Cynthia sought a therapist's help for Cynthia, who believed she had a low sex drive as a result of being molested as a child. Because the couple had difficulty talking about sex, the therapist changed the topic from sex to finances because, explained Sam, "the therapist thought if we made more money, we'd be happier." Two years later, Cynthia still had a low sex drive; fortunately, the couple sought appropriate help.

No one, least of all our clients, wants to be judged as defective, naive, or perverse. People want reassurance that they are essentially normal, or that they can become more what they think normal is for them. When therapists don't talk about sex, they may convey a belief that the client is weird for wondering about their own sexuality. Of course, some therapists *do* ask about sex. In one survey, about half of therapists reported that they "always" ask about sex (Miller & Byers, 2009). But people in general (including therapists) over-report when it comes to sexuality, as they want to appear normal or current. What about the other half of therapists? There is an adage that we are always communicating, even if we say nothing. Therapists' silence about sex in the therapy room sends many messages, but perhaps the loudest is *please don't talk about sex!*

WHY THE SILENCE ABOUT SEXUALITY?

Almost everyone is raised in an atmosphere of secrecy when it comes to emotional and psychological aspects of sex. The reasons are complex. Depending on one's religious perspective, a person's very conception can be shrouded with mystery. As we grow, we covertly observe romantic and sexual behaviors between adults of which we are told little. We experience our own biological urges, such as a desire to masturbate, but are given neither tacit nor explicit permission to ask questions. When we do ask, we may not get an answer—or we may get a lecture on why some sexual topic is naughty or dirty, something good girls and boys avoid. Although many of today's parents talk openly with their children about sex, there are still households where sex is a forbidden topic. People still bar their children from attending formal sex education classes in school, and people from other countries, for example, Saudi Arabia, may not have been offered any sex education opportunities at all.

Our physical and psychological sexual development takes place on entirely different planes, and interactions between systems reflect this. Secondary sexual characteristics signal to adults around us that we must be protected from such risks as unwanted pregnancy or diease. Meanwhile, we are left to privately grapple with sexual dreams and fantasies, curiosity, and desire. Reflecting what is still often a Puritanical culture, we aren't given information about giving and receiving sexual pleasure. The complexities of a sexual relationship are explained away with myths like, "All men are interested in is sex," or "Once you get married, your sex life will disappear."

We certainly aren't told how to manage feelings of sexual inadequacy, so if a problem comes up like difficulty having an orgasm or getting an erection, we may keep it under wraps for *decades*. As a society, we also may act as if sexual problems appear suddenly in adulthood. However, as I have learned from my clients, teens (who on average in the United States begin having intercourse at 15) have sexual problems that plague them, sometimes leading to depression, eating disorders, alcoholism, and other mental illness. As therapists know all too well, secrecy and silence are associated with feelings of shame and guilt that can contribute to overall poor mental health. Nowhere, perhaps, is this truer than when it affects our sexual development.

It doesn't help that sex does have a murky side. Subjects like sexual abuse, assault, and rape tend to be hushed by the victim and, if they learn about it, family members or friends. If the media gets hold of such a story, it is sensationalized, which may cause victims to further retreat, away from possible unwanted attention. Meanwhile, media attention on cases such as Jerry Sandusky, the Penn State football coach convicted of molesting children, do little to address underlying problems such as the need to educate children at an early age about appropriate physical boundaries, the right to say no to unwanted touch, and permission to tell if someone harms them.

Our culture also has done a poor job of acknowledging that pedophiles and people with other difficult sex and social problems do exist and frequently deserve compassionate treatment (Cantor, 2012).

For teens and young adults, date rape is distressingly common on college campuses; many young women have shared with me that the reputed response of campus security was so lukewarm that they made a decision not to report. Yet, its effects can linger well into adulthood. Today's young adults are also the first to grow up in the digital age. Many have spent so much time viewing Internet pornography that they neglected to develop the social and sexual skills to have a real partner. How might things be different if they were raised in a culture that acknowledged sexual needs, made it easy to attain contraception, and talked openly about what it means to be in a healthy sexual relationship?

Therapists are not immune to such sexual negativity. Pope and Feldman-Summers (1992) report that about two-thirds of female and one-third of male therapists responding to a survey regarding sexual abuse among therapists had experienced molestation, the majority of incidents with a close relative. It isn't difficult to surmise that one reason therapists may avoid the topic of sex may be that they have been victims of sexual abuse or exposed to other types of negative sexual experiences, from mild harassment to outright assault. Although therapists may be drawn to the field to help other victims become survivors, they may be disappointed with how little attention their graduate training gives to the sexual late effects of abuse.

The negative effects of such experiences may intensify what Saakvitne & Pearlman (1996) called *vicarious traumatization*. Vicarious traumatization is defined as "the therapist's inner experience as a result of his or her empathic engagement with and responsibility for a traumatized client." Listening to sexual material can be difficult for therapists if they have their own sexual struggles. Like our clients, we may have trouble setting appropriate sexual boundaries; struggle with questions about the morality of sexual practices (anything from casual "hook-ups" to looking at—or even engaging in the making of—hardcore pornography); be dealing with our own sexual inhibitions; be worrying about a partner's sexual function after cancer or other illness; or simply have basic concerns about our own physical appearance and sexual attractiveness. Discussing such matters may create such distress for the therapist that they are simply avoided.

Another reason for many therapists' silence about sex is the fear of becoming isolated or being ostracized by colleagues. Not only do therapists fear being judged by clients for expressing interest in their sex life, but also by other therapists who find dealing with sexual problems too uncomfortable or distasteful. For example, I recently lucked upon an opportunity to share space in a pretty office with a psychoanalyst. My deposit was promptly returned because, on reflection, the analyst decided that my sex therapy practice was not a good fit for her office, presumably since she and her clients might happen upon my (drooling?) clients in the waiting room. Working with sexual problems can also feel unsafe in certain communities because of the social and political climate. Where I live in Southern California, condoms and lubricants are sold over the counter at the drugstore, but there are still parts of the country where such items are difficult to procure. Designating oneself as a sex therapist in such areas can mean opening one's self up to ridicule or harassment.

Therapists may also be quiet about sex due to strict training in laws and ethics concerning sexual contact with clients, a topic covered in detail in Chapter 19. Therapists are rightly warned that because there is an inherent power differential in relationship with the client—who is dependent on us for emotional support—the potential for doing serious emotional damage by acting out sexual urges comes with enormous risk. Little is said, however, about reconciling the need to manage one's sexual attraction or arousal while discussing sex in a therapeutic manner with the client. In any case, stern warnings about curbing one's sexual feelings may send the message that it's best not to deal with sex in the treatment room.

A final reason for therapist reticence about sex concerns diversity. While learning to tolerate cultural differences has been a priority in training programs, tolerance of a wide range of gender, orientation, and sexual behaviors has not. In my area of California, for example, human sexuality credits for marriage and family therapists have been cut to the minimum requirement in several schools. If therapists are to properly address client sexuality, then they must not only have appropriate training, but they also must become sexually sensitive—a tall order for those raised in an American society that lags in tolerance behind many developed countries, including neighboring Canada.

On the other hand, perhaps none of these concerns about being silent about sex applies to you! You might be a therapist like my intern Liz Dube, who, upon reading this chapter for a requested critique, quipped that the only thing that held her back from talking to clients about sex was lack of knowledge. Speaking for herself, she has had a long abiding passion to help people have satisfying sex lives. If that describes you, then you're in luck, because this book will give you information that will help you fulfill a desire to help clients with their sexual struggles.

Otherwise, consider that you are about to become at least one step ahead of your clients as you learn more about sexuality. You won't be a therapist who "doesn't 'do' sex." You will be able to help clients overcome their deepest fears so that they can enjoy one of life's pleasures without undue shame or guilt. Increasing a client's capacity to love and be loved often has a ripple effect in the client's life, giving them the optimism, confidence, and freedom to tackle other developmental milestones such as finding a healthy relationship or even making a much-feared job change. Our sexuality is such a core part of who we are, and as therapists we are fortunate to be in a position to help our clients achieve health in this critical area of human existence.

ACTIVITIES

1. Whether you have refrained from talking about sex with your clients or do so on a regular basis, it can be fruitful to examine your own attitudes about human sexuality. In a "sexological journal," write about influences have you had at each of the five levels: microsystemic, mesosystemic, macrosystemic, exosystemic, and chronosystemic.
2. What steps have you taken or will you take to increase your comfort in talking with clients about sex? List them in your journal.
3. Locate a colleague with whom you can consult or from whom you can receive formal supervision of cases that present with sexual issues. Keep notes on your consultations in your journal.

RESOURCES

The Kinsey Institute website has produced a page of resources for professionals interested in the field of sexology entitled Kinsey Confidential. Kinsey Confidential can be found at http://kinseyconfidential.org/resources/sex-research-sex-therapy

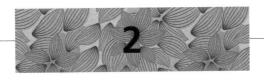

2

Making the Shift: Comfort With Sexuality

One of the things I treasure most about the mental health profession is its optimism and emphasis on growth and change. When it comes to sexuality, we have the ability to adopt new beliefs, modify our role with clients, and change the rules about talking about sex in the therapy room. Knowledge is an imperative in helping clients make those changes, and can be acquired by following a 4-stage model (Harris & Hays, 2008):

Stage 1: Self-examination

Stage 2: Awareness of the problem from the client's point of view

Stage 3: Increased freedom and comfort in discussing sexual topics

Stage 4: Awareness of a new level of comfort with clients' sexual issues

STAGE 1: SELF-EXAMINATION

The first step requires the therapist to examine his or her *sexological world-view* (Sitron & Dyson, 2012). Sexological worldview is defined as "the result of the socialization process that is comprised of values, beliefs, opinions, attitudes, and concepts specific to sexuality, including any and all sexual behavior and identities." These values, beliefs, and so forth come from many sources, including one's family, school, religion, peers, and media, as well as through sexual relationships and experiences. In order to be nonjudgmental, empathic, and effective in helping clients with sexual problems, the therapist must set aside biases and deal with the client's matter at hand, though they may differ in sexological worldview.

As a whole, therapists tend to be more liberal than their clients, but there are areas where this isn't true. Since premarital sex has become more prevalent in our society, many young sexually active adults are likely to have had multiple partners. Ford and Hendrick (2003) report that both male and female therapists tend to view clients who have had multiple sexual encounters as having more pathology than monogamous clients, reflecting a more conservative sexological worldview on the part of therapists. In such instances, therapist and client must together explore the meaning of sex with multiple partners. The therapist may discover that the client believes that sexual experimentation is a requirement in order to find a suitable partner, or that they were exposed to one or both parents in the wake of divorce who had active sex lives with subsequent partners. In any case, the therapists would be mistaken in undervaluing present mores and overvaluing his or her personal opinion.

There are additional issues that may create a conundrum for a therapist trained in traditional psychodynamic or systemic theories. Therapists are less likely to condone lifestyles such as swinging (married or committed couples switching sexual partners) or *polyamorous* relationships (couples who simultaneously have sexual and romantic partnerships with other adults, with everyone's mutual knowledge and consent). While such "consensual nonmonogamy" (Barker & Langridge, 2010) is rare (about 1%–3% of the population), therapists cannot automatically assume that participants possess underlying pathology, such as viewing one partner as so depressed or fragile that they give in to the wishes of the other. Therapists may be interested to know that couples with these arrangements will sometimes seek help from a sex therapist even when the problem isn't sexual, because they fear judgment by "vanilla" therapists. By developing an attitude of acceptance and flexibility, most therapists will find they can establish rapport and conduct an earnest assessment of the presenting couple's issues without condemning personal choices.

Another unfortunate bias that some therapists hold is toward variations in sexual orientation. While having improved in recent years, one study of social work students found that 11% of those surveyed had homophobic attitudes toward gays and lesbians (Ahmad & Bhugra, 2010). Although homosexuality was removed from the *Diagnostic and Statistical Manual* in 1986, there is still a contingent of psychotherapists who practice conversion or "reorientation" therapy for clients who believe they can change their sexual orientation.* There is also confusion about the wide range of orientation, as well as its fluid nature. A woman may change orientation more than once over the course of her life (Diamond, 2009), while a man may have sex with men but not identify as gay (Nichols, 2006). In the LGBTQ community there is a faction of people who identify as Q, which is understood as being "questioning" or "queer" and not of any one orientation. Understanding and affirming that an individual can have a bisexual physical orientation but a heterosexual romantic orientation can reduce a client's confusion and shame while he or she explores a definition of sexuality.

Unlike their mature clients, therapists may hold the view that sex is for the young. They may be ignorant that people continue to have vital sex lives into age 60, 70, and beyond if they are in good health and have a partner available. (I recall that while teaching a course on human sexuality, the mere mention of people in their 70s still having intercourse elicited "Ew!" from a young student at the back of the room.) Stereotypes of "dirty old men" and "cougars" (older women who "prey" on younger men, as Mrs. Robinson seduced Benjamin in *The Graduate*) add to the prejudice. Additionally, the misunderstanding that "sex" means "intercourse" precludes therapists and clients from imagining an intimate physical connection between partners even when intercourse is no longer possible, thus maintaining a damaging stereotype.

Additional sexual stereotypes also persist. Wiederman (2001) reports specifically on the dangers of myths, such as the belief that men "always" have more interest in sex than women, or that men and women reach a "sexual peak" at different times. People can be harmed by such myths, since the expectation is that they will experience frustration if they remain in a long-term relationship. In his article, Wiederman demonstrates that this myth has persisted despite faulty empirical data. Therapists need to be aware of myths about gender differences as well as other phenomena so that they can educate clients and create an understanding of the diversity within human sexual experience.

STAGE 2: SEX FROM THE CLIENT'S POINT OF VIEW

The way in which clients present sexual problems may differ from presentation of other common problems such as grief over the loss of a loved one or a behavioral problem in a child. Although not all clients feel embarrassed by their sexual behavior, many are fearful of being judged. Clients may not use the same language as the therapist to describe sexual problems or activities. Just the word *sex* may mean many things, from penetrative penis-vagina intercourse to any sort of sexual contact. While the therapist can model the use of appropriate language ("You used the word 'va-jay-jay,' I say *vagina*"),

---

*As of this writing, a bill has been introduced into the California State Senate to ban the use of so-called reparative therapy to convert orientation from gay to straight.

acceptance of the client's language, whether describing symptoms or sexual acts, is important and is covered in depth in Chapter 3.

Clients also may have limited knowledge about the complexities of sexuality. Like therapists, their sexual education may be based on what they learned in school or from peers. They also have expectations about sexual performance from the media that may be all out of proportion to what most people experience in their day-to-day relationship, such as believing that all women have orgasm from intercourse, or that acquiescing to anal sex is a woman's ultimate expression of love for her man. Much of the therapist's task is to disassemble myths and impart appropriate knowledge to help the client realistically overcome challenges.

STAGE 3: FREEDOM AND COMFORT IN TALKING ABOUT SEX

Sex is funny in that most partners think it's something they do with each other without any discussion. It is difficult to imagine another human activity that is so shrouded in silence. Hence, one of the major causes of both therapist and client discomfort with sex is lack of communication. Clearly, if a goal of therapy is to improve communication about all topics, clients need to be more at ease both talking to the therapist and to their partners.

One way to become more fluent in talking about sex is to become familiar with the chapters in this book on sexual health and history taking. These chapters will give you a road map on how to start a conversation about sex and where to guide it. To increase comfort, you can role play with colleagues to practice asking questions or simply permit yourself to say words aloud that aren't part of your everyday vocabulary. Supervision or consultation, discussed below, is also a place to speak comfortably about sex.

STAGE 4: A NEW LEVEL OF COMFORT WITH CLIENTS' ISSUES

As you learn more about sex from all aspects, you will feel less inhibited and more confident in your ability to talk to clients about sex. Your clients will grow, too; in my practice, clients often express appreciation for having a safe place to learn to talk about sex, and they are visibly more relaxed after several sessions. The only way to reach this stage is to talk about sex with your clients at every appropriate opportunity. The more you talk about sex, the more you will understand why it is such a critical topic if you want to promote true mental health in your clients.

SUPERVISION AND CONSULTATION

These are the other requirements for becoming competent in treating clients' sexual concerns. Before addressing this need, it may help to clarify differences between "supervision" and "consultation," which are sometimes used synonymously, though they are not necessarily the same. *Supervision* occurs prior to becoming licensed in most states, but is also the term used when one's cases are supervised for certification in a type of therapy or technique, such as sex therapy or eye movement desensitization reprocessing (EMDR). In some settings, licensed clinicians may continue to work under the direction of a *supervisor*, who continues to hold ultimate responsibility for the care of patients or clients within the clinical setting, though this person often holds the title of "director." Consultation occurs in diverse contexts and with a variety of appropriate consultants, including former instructors and supervisors, colleagues, and paid experts. Peer consultation groups, either lead by someone in a consulting position or leaderless, are also a possibility.

Whether seeking supervision or consultation, either is essential when first planning and treating clients with sexual complaints. For all the reasons that therapists avoid the topic of sex in the first place, countertransference—in the form of anxiety, embarrassment, or moral judgment—may cloud potential solutions. For example, consider what a newly minted therapist might think if presented with the following situation:

> In the intake call, Julian, age 68, described having a difficult time with delayed ejaculation, and the therapist assumed he meant with his wife. Thus, the therapist felt shocked when Julian revealed that he was having sex with massage therapists in order to resolve the problem he was having with his wife. Knowing that such activity was illegal and, in her eyes, immoral, the therapist choked and muttered some thoughts about aging and sexuality, including the bias that sexuality activity among elderly people is unseemly. Julian left the office without any help for the frustrating situation with his wife.

Cases such as this often occur in the context of problematic relationships, so it is helpful to have a seasoned and objective supervisor or consultant for guidance and to examine the source of negative countertransference. Supervisors and consultants can be found in various ways. One way is to inquire in one's local professional organizations regarding experts in sexuality who might be available. There also are several organizations listed in *Resources* at the end of the chapter that provide support in various ways to therapists in their quest for understanding and treating sexual concerns, including certification, conferences, journals, and so forth.

ACTIVITIES

1. Nearly everyone carries stereotypes about sex. Some of these are relatively harmless or even amusing (the horny middle school student) while others are destructive ("all men want sex all the time"). Examine some stereotypes you have observed, considering at what systemic level they may have been generated or perpetuated.

Examples include "religious women don't enjoy sex" or "passion always dies in a long-term relationship." Write your observations in your sexological journal.

2. What stereotypes about sex do you hold? As you think about your own sexual development, think about what messages you were given, implicitly or explicitly, about gender, orientation, reproduction, sexually transmitted disease, and sexual activity. Write in your journal.

3. The *Online Slang Dictionary* (www.onlineslangdictionary.com) lists 164 words for "sexual intercourse" including *boff, boink, horizontal bop, go all the way, make the beast with two backs, shtupp* (Yiddish), and *knock it out*. Either make a list or discuss some of the words you have read or used to describe other sexual acts, body parts, or people (e.g., virgins, gays, or the elderly). Are these words reflective of your own personal values about sex?

4. In what ways do you think your values and beliefs about sex might differ from those held in the population with which you work? How might you begin the work of being nonjudgmental about people's sexuality? Would supervision help? Identify someone who can help you with issues of treatment and/or countertransference.

5. Read widely about sexuality. Visit some of the following sites. Write about your impressions.
   - Advocates for Youth: *www.advocatesforyouth.org*
   - International Society for the Study of Women's Sexual Health: *www.isswsh.org*
   - New View on Women's Sexual Problems: *www.newviewcampaign.org*
   - Religious Institute on Sexuality, Moral Justice, and Healing: *www.religiousinstitute.org*
   - Sexuality and Information and Education Council of the United States: *www.siecus.org*
   - Society for the Scientific Study of Sexuality: *www.sexscience.org*
   - World Association for Sexology: *www.worldsexology.org*

RESOURCES

Joannides, P. (2009). *The guide to getting it on.* Waldport, OR: Goofy Foot Press.

Taverner, W., & McKee, R. (2011). *Taking sides: Clashing views in human sexuality.* Columbus, OH: McGraw-Hill/Dushkin.

Yarber, W., Sayad, B., & Strong, B. (2012). *Human sexuality: Diversity in contemporary America.* Columbus, OH: McGraw-Hill Humanities/Social Sciences/Languages.

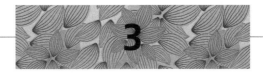

Sexual Anatomy and Psychosexual Development

In order to talk proficiently about sex with clients, therapists need to have a basic understanding of sexual anatomy and psychosexual development. Whether the population being served is rich or poor, young or old, high or low functioning, doesn't matter when it comes to anatomy and development. For most American adults, sex education takes place in sixth grade and stops there. People forget the details of how their bodies function or how hormones affect them. Conversely, people sometimes believe they are sexually sophisticated, either because they have had multiple sexual experiences or they consider themselves to be open-minded about sexual matters. However, I have found little correlation between sexual experience or attitudes toward sex and knowledge of sexual anatomy and development. In addition, many therapists treat a diverse population, such as clients who grew up in other cultures who had no sex education at all, but perhaps have been too embarrassed to ask or read about such things.

In writing about sexual anatomy, I address more than simply a catalog of body parts and labels; I also include information potentially about the client's viewpoint of their anatomy and social myths that can affect perception. The information in this chapter is also important because therapists generally treat people of all genders and cannot simply rely on information about their own gender. In the second part of the chapter, I paint the stages of sexual development in broad strokes, in part because very little has been written about them. Still, it is helpful to have such a framework so that the therapist can determine whether a client's complaints are typical or out of the norm for cohorts. Such information can inform the therapist's initial assessment and become part of the decision-making process as to how much education the client may need to move forward in his or her development.

SEXUAL ANATOMY

Female External Structures

Female genitalia (see page 29) consist of the *mons pubis,* or fatty pad below the abdomen, the *vulva* that consists of the *labia majora* (larger "lips") and *labia minora* (smaller lips), the *clitoris,* and the entrance to the *vagina,* called the *introitus.* The *perineum* is the strip of skin between the vagina and the anus.

The *clitoris* is the only organ in either the male or the female body that is designed for one purpose: sexual pleasure. Only recently was the clitoris discovered to be much larger in size than believed, as it has two leg-like extensions that are contained within a woman's pelvis. The clitoris is sensitive and so is covered by a "hood" of skin.

The labia are also filled with sensitive nerve endings that help with sexual arousal. This tissue swells and deepens in color with stimulation. Some women are self-conscious about the appearance of the labia, and recently there has been controversy over the surgical trimming of this tissue to neaten its appearance. The American College of Obstetricians and Gynecologists (ACOG) has taken the position that surgeries known as "vaginal rejuvenation," "designer vaginoplasty," "revirgination," and "G-spot amplification procedures" are not recommended, as they are not medically indicated, may cause scarring and adhesions, and interfere with a woman's sexual function and pleasure (ACOG website, 2007; http://www.acog.org/About_ACOG/News_Room/News_Releases/2007/ACOG_Advises_Against_Cosmetic_Vaginal_Procedures).

The breasts are considered to be part of the reproductive system. Their appearance at puberty depends on changes in sex-related hormones such as estrogen. The breasts consist of fat, connective tissue, lobes, lobules, ducts, and lymph nodes. *Lobules* are the glands that create milk after a woman delivers a baby, while ducts carry the milk to the nipple. The small dark area around the nipple is the *areola,* which contains sweat glands that moisturize the nipple during breastfeeding. Most, though certainly not all, women find stimulation of the nipple, areola, and breast sexually arousing.

Female Internal Structures

The basic internal structures (see page 30) include the *introitus* or entrance to the vagina, the vagina, the *Grafenberg* or *G-spot*, the *cervix*, the *uterus*, the *fallopian tubes*, and the *ovaries* that release an egg during the menstrual cycle. The *pelvic floor muscles* are responsible for holding up the uterus as well as other organs in the abdomen, as well as *continence* or the ability to retain or evacuate urine and feces. In addition, the bladder and the *urethra*, or tube from which urine is released from the body, are located between the clitoris and the vagina. The *hymen* is a very thin piece of tissue that in most women nearly covers the vagina. Over the course of human history, much has been made of a woman's purity as evidenced by the presence or absence of the hymen at first intercourse. However, the hymen can break or wear away due to vigorous exercise or injury. Conversely, in some women the hymen is very thick, necessitating surgery in order to allow penetration.

The vagina may seem like an empty passage, but it is actually a special environment with a *pH*-level that must be maintained for comfortable and pleasurable intercourse. When healthy, the lining of the vagina is filled with pores like sweat glands that emit a lubricating discharge. The lubrication increases with sexual arousal, which can occur in as little as 30 seconds. This can be deceptive, causing a couple to believe that a woman is fully prepared for intercourse when lubrication appears and leading to disappointing sexual encounters. However, with continued foreplay, the shape and size of the vagina change, causing it to lengthen and balloon at the top to accommodate a penis to make intercourse more comfortable.

Within the vagina, most women have a Grafenberg spot, or what three writers famously renamed as the G-spot in a book that was considered controversial at the time, *The G-Spot and Other Recent Discoveries About Human Sexuality* (Ladas, Whipple, & Perry, 1982). Arguments regarding the existence of the G-spot still occur between doubters and believers, who report that the G-spot was identified by Graffenberg as a bit of tissue on the anterior side of the vagina, about 2 inches from the introitus. When the G-spot is stimulated directly—with the penis during intercourse or manually with a finger or use of a sex toy—it can lead to orgasm in some women. Also, stimulation of the G-spot during intercourse is thought to facilitate so-called vaginal orgasm. (So-called because it can be difficult to discern whether an orgasm is from clitoral or vaginal penetration—and also because it makes little difference how a woman achieves orgasm as long as she feels satisfaction.) Some women, however, experience stimulation to the G-spot as painful or as causing an urge to urinate.

During a normal menstrual cycle, an ovary releases an egg. The egg is carried through the Fallopian tube to the uterus or womb, which has been prepared for possible pregnancy with a lining of tissue. If the egg is fertilized, a pregnancy develops; if not, the lining of the uterus is shed as menstrual fluid. When a woman develops certain medical problems in the uterus, such as the development of fibroid tumors, it can result in a hysterectomy, or surgery to remove the uterus (partial hysterectomy) and sometimes the fallopian tubes and ovaries as well (complete hysterectomy). A complete hysterectomy can put a woman into instant menopause, which is managed with hormones during the woman's lifetime. Some women find that they enjoy sex less after a hysterectomy because certain sensations they found enjoyable during intercourse have been eliminated.

A woman's pelvic floor muscles essentially hold up the internal organs within the abdomen. They form a looping, criss-cross path around the clitoris, urethra, vagina, and anus. For optimal sexual health, the pelvic floor muscles must be in good tone. Muscles that are too tight, or *hypertonic*, can contribute to a variety of medical problems, including painful intercourse. Muscles that are loose, or *hypotonic*, can make it difficult for a woman to experience appropriate stimulation during intercourse, which can lead to an inability to climax. If a woman's partner is male, he can also sometimes tell if the pelvic floor muscles are not properly toned, reporting that the woman's vagina is "too loose." (Sometimes, though, the problem is that the man's erection isn't firm enough, an important distinction to make when you hear this complaint.)

Female Sexual Hormones

Emitted by glands in the body such as the thyroid, hormones are substances that direct cellular activity. There are several hormones that are involved in sexual health, but for our purposes the most important ones are estrogen, progesterone, and testosterone. In women, the primary hormones responsible for the function of the reproductive system are estrogen and progesterone. The initial release of estrogen directs a girl's body into puberty and menstruation while progesterone is responsible for initial development of the breasts. Both estrogen and progesterone have a role in creating and sustaining a pregnancy. Women also have a miniscule amount of testosterone. This tiny amount contributes to the ability for a woman to have sexual fantasies, arousal, especially of the nipples and clitoris, and drive. When testosterone is low, a woman may complain of low drive; however, several studies have demonstrated that there is a poor correlation between the two.

Male External Structures

The main anatomical structures include the penis, the scrotum, and the perineum. The penis consists of three main parts: the root, which is contained within a man's body and is not visible to the eye; the shaft, which is the main part of the penis; and the *glans penis*, which is the top or "head" of the penis. Most commonly, the penis does not include the foreskin, as circumcision is the most common surgery worldwide (Payne, Thaler, Kukkonen, Carrier, & Binik, 2007). The opening of the urethra, or internal tube that carries either urine or semen external to the body, is visible at the tip of the glans penis. On the underside of the nonerect or flaccid penis, the corona (which means "crown" in Spanish) appears as a ridge. The frenulum is a cordlike structure also on the underside of the penis that connects the corona to the shaft. The entire glans penis is the most sensitive part of the penis, filled with nerve endings that help with arousal and orgasm.

The scrotum is the saclike structure that contains the testicles, the organs that manufacture sperm. The scrotum changes in appearance depending on temperature and level of arousal. When temperatures are cool, the scrotum pulls close to the body to keep the testicles warm, and when warm, the scrotum hangs away from the body. The perineum is the strip of skin that is visible from behind the scrotum to the anus. Most men enjoy stimulation to the scrotum and perineum, though they may complain if their partner doesn't appreciate the type of touch that is enjoyable. Such complaints can lead to a discussion of good communication or ways a man can show a partner how he likes to be touched.

Internal Male Anatomy

Within the penis are three chambers, two called the *corpus cavernosum* and one the corpus spongiosum. The corpus cavernosum are like parallel tubes in the penis that fill with blood during an erection, causing the penis to become rigid. The corpus spongiosum is a structure of spongy tissue that runs the length of the front of the penis. It also fills with blood during an erection. When a man becomes aroused, nerves cause blood vessels in a healthy penis to expand. Other chemical changes take place that cause more blood to flow into the penis than out, and then to retain the blood in the penis until either stimulation ceases or a man ejaculates. Damage to the structures of the penis can cause erectile dysfunction, as can cholesterol-caused blockage in the arteries that lead to the penis.

The testicles or testes are contained within the scrotum, suspended by a spermatic cord. This is the manufacturing plant for sperm. The testes contain seminiferous tubules, structures that would stretch to many feet if laid end to end. The epididymous and the vans deferens carry sperm from the testicles to the urethra, the tube that carries sperm or urine from within the body to its exit at the tip of the penis.

The seminal vesicles are glands that lie at the back of the bladder and create about 60% of the fluid that is ejaculated along with sperm. The prostate is another gland that produces about remaining 30% to 35% of ejaculate. The prostate can be a source of pleasure; both heterosexual and gay men may enjoy anal play or penetration that includes stimulation of the prostate. The prostate is also, unfortunately, the source of some male diseases, including prostatitis and prostate cancer.

The Cowper's or bulbourethral glands connect to the urethra through tiny ducts. They emit a thick fluid prior to orgasm and ejaculation that some people call "pre cum." In private practice, I have had one or two men who have confused this fluid with ejaculate, which made them believe they had early ejaculation, so education may be needed regarding this stage of sexual arousal. Also, this fluid may contain some sperm, and caution needs to be used to prevent unwanted pregnancy from rubbing this fluid onto a female partner's vulva.

Male Sexual Hormones

Testosterone is a steroid hormone produced in large amounts in the testicles. It is the hormone that begins the development of male sexual characteristics, including the growth of the penis, creation of sperm, and sexual drive and fantasy. It also contributes to larger muscle mass, overall energy, and healthy erections. Normally, levels of testosterone remain about the same until a man reaches 35, then decrease slowly over time.

Sometimes men experience abnormally low levels of testosterone, which can result in low drive, loss of muscle mass, weight gain, fatigue, and difficulty attaining or maintaining an erection. As a mental health professional, you may have noticed that some of these symptoms overlap with depression; that is why it is important to encourage a man with these complaints to get a physical that includes testosterone testing.

SEXUAL DEVELOPMENT

Sexuality begins in the womb, as ultrasound pictures of a male fetus masturbating have shown. Sexual development continues throughout our lives; even people in their 70s are sexually active if they are in good health and have an available partner.

Despite the importance of sexual development, there is a dearth of research on what is considered to be normal. Freud's psychosexual stages of development are now out of favor (oral, anal, phallic/oedipal, latency, and genital), but nothing has replaced them. Also, much current research about childhood sexuality comes from literature about child maltreatment. As a former elementary school teacher, I can tell you that children are definitely interested in sex and romance—certainly not in the same way adults are, but in their own way. Children have curiosity about bodies, experience "crushes," and observe adults in real life and in the media engaged in physical and romantic intimacy. Thus, our sexual development is influenced from a very young age.

Sexuality 0 to 2

From birth until 2, infants learn about the pleasure of touch not just on the genitals as caregivers attend to diapering, but all over the body. Infants and young toddlers discover their genitals on their own and may fondle themselves for soothing. Attachment takes place between caregiver and child through bonding behaviors, including caressing, kisses, eye gazing, smiling, cooing, and playing. Initial gender identity begins to form as parents make choices in activities, clothing, and toys based on expectations of male and female temperament and behavior.

Sexuality 2 to 5

Toddlers and preschoolers develop curiosity about their own bodies and those of their peers, sometimes asking questions about the bodies that they view. Such behavior indicates normal curiosity, not a desire to be "naughty" or "dirty." Children may also touch their genitals or rub them against objects or people. This type of behavior is also normal and is not to be shamed (Coleman & Charles, 2009); if the behavior is exhibited at an inappropriate time, the child can be distracted with a toy or activity or gently told to go to a private place if they want to touch their own body (Brown, Keller, & Stern, 2009). Curiosity about pregnancy is also common.

Tots begin to identify themselves as male or female and generally engage in stereotypical behavior and dress. When sexual orientation begins to develop is still unclear. There is evidence that it may have a biological basis, but both heterosexual and homosexual adults will report having attraction to members of the same sex. Sometimes if a person later identifies as gay or transgender, they may report having the very first inkling about their gender or orientation at this young age.

Sexuality 6 to 11

Freud described this time as "latency," when a child's sexual curiosity is subsumed to academic pursuits. However, anyone who has watched an elementary school playground knows that boys chase girls and girls chase boys as part of rudimentary social and sexual awareness. Children develop "crushes" and continue to be curious about bodies, going beyond looking to touching and exploring one another. As long as the play is between same and nearly the same age, it is considered normal and can also be used as an opportunity to teach a child about privacy, physical boundaries, and permission.

Some boys may discover masturbation and may masturbate to orgasm without ejaculation, which doesn't occur until puberty. Girls also discover genital pleasure, but usually later than do boys. For many people, having a parent or other adult discover evidence of masturbation or being caught in the act itself is a moment of embarrassment and shame. Often this is the beginning of carrying on one's sexual activity under a cloak of secrecy and guilt.

Sexuality in Adolescence

Adolescence is when sexuality begins to flower, and accurate information is needed by preteens starting at age 8 or 9 to prepare them for the changes to come. In both sexes, the hypothalamus gland, located deep within the brain, sends a gonadotropic-releasing hormone to the pituitary gland, which in turn stimulates other glands in the body to prepare the body for reproduction.

Menarche, or the onset of the menstrual cycle in females, is a sign that the ovaries are releasing luteinizing hormone (LH) and follicle-stimulating hormone (FSH), which stimulate the ovaries to produce estrogen. In girls, this process currently takes place at younger age than in past decades, with girls as young as 8 displaying physical signs such as the appearance of pubic hair.

In males, signals to the pituitary gland stimulate the testes into producing testosterone and sperm. At this stage, orgasm is accompanied by ejaculation or emission of the sticky fluid carrying the sperm. Boys generally start puberty later than girls, beginning at age 10 through 15.

The age at which puberty occurs can have an effect on a teen's feelings about their bodies and sexuality. When girls experience significant breast development at a young age, they can be exposed to unwanted attention and teasing. Boys, on the other hand, can feel sexually inadequate if they begin puberty later than their peers.

Though perhaps surprising to some therapists, the average age of intercourse for American teens is 15. By age 19, seven out of ten adolescents have experienced sexual intercourse, with 72% of females and 56% of males having intercourse with a steady partner (Mosher, Chandra, & Jones, 2005). When teens choose to abstain from sex, religion or moral reasons are most commonly given, with fear of pregnancy and not having found the right partner yet listed second and third, respectively.

Because people are becoming sexually active at younger ages and marrying later in life, most have had a nearly decade-long period where they are at risk for unwanted pregnancy and sexually transmitted disease.

For this reason, many communities and organizations put a great deal of emphasis on transmitting appropriate contraceptive and disease prevention information.

Such efforts have caused the pregnancy rates for teens to drop to a rate of about 7%, but the numbers are still sobering, as one study estimated that in 2008 there were 733,000 pregnancies among teenage girls ages 15 to 19 (Kost & Henshaw, 2012).

Teenagers also often begin to experience more feelings and behaviors related to sexual orientation, such as romantic and sexual attraction, erotic fantasies, sexual behaviors, and romantic and sexual relationships. While those who report a heterosexual orientation largely remain stable over time, those who identify as homosexual or bisexual may have a more fluid orientation. Females, in particular, may change orientation from lesbian to heterosexual as they develop (Savin-Williams & Ream, 2007).

Sexuality 21 to 45

Adults are marrying at lower rate and an older age than prior generations. For this reason, most adults have experimented sexually, with heterosexual men having an average of 6 to 8 female partners and heterosexual women 3 to 4 male partners (CDC, 2011). Despite delay in marriage, most people—whether straight or gay, male or female—report that they want to be part of a committed relationship. Negotiating a long-term sexual relationship can be a challenge when adults enter the bedroom with different sexual and relationship histories, as well as personal sexual tastes and preferences, sexual interest, and drive.

Before contraception was readily available, sex was seen as more for procreation than for recreation; marriage and pregnancy were essentially mandated for a couple that wanted a sexual relationship. With more birth control as well as lifestyle options available, many American adults are marrying at an older age, thus delaying childbearing, leading to problems with infertility. The strain of fertility treatment and the disappointment treatment brings when it doesn't work can put a huge strain on a couple's sexual intimacy, including feelings of sexual inadequacy.

As much as couples may state they want a family, the fact is that childless couples tend to be happier (Twenge, Campbell, & Foster, 2003). Raising children puts a strain on a couple's emotional, physical, and financial resources. The researchers' data suggest that while women become somewhat happier as children age, as compared to childless women, for men the decline in marital satisfaction remains similar across ages. Role conflicts and restriction of freedom seem to have the strongest impact on low levels of satisfaction in higher socioeconomic groups.

Divorce is also a common experience, and it brings its own sexual challenges. According to the Pew Foundation:

> *About 2.3 million men reported that they wed within the previous year, and 1.2 million said they divorced. About 2.2 million women said they wed and 1.3 million said they divorced. About one-in-twenty Americans who ever have been married said they had been married three or more times.* (Pew Research, 2009)

People who divorce sometimes complain of feeling awkward or unprepared to date, let alone experience a new sexual partner. Some adults who divorce were virgins at marriage and never experimented sexually; they fear social pressures to quickly engage in sexual relationships. Therapists need to be prepared to help divorced men and women sort out their current sexual values and boundaries as they search for a new partner.

Sexuality 46 to 65

People experience aging in different ways, with varying effects on sexual function. In women, the hormone estrogen diminishes over time, sometimes starting as young as 35. This decrease heralds the cluster of symptoms known as *perimenopause* (Cobia & Harper, 2005). Along with annoying or uncomfortable symptoms such as hot flashes and night sweats, many women also experience lower sex drive. As estrogen dips, so does testosterone, which contributes to lower sexual interest and less sensation in erogenous zones including the nipples and clitoris.

At an average age of 53, women enter *menopause*, which is marked by 1 year without any menstrual cycle. At one time women were routinely treated with hormone replacement therapy (HRT), but in 2002 the Women's Health Initiative study was stopped when women in the experimental group taking estrogen plus progestin were diagnosed with breast cancer and cardiovascular disease at a significant rate (National Institutes of Health, 2002). In women who do not use HRT, because of personal choice or a family history of breast or gynecological cancers (e.g., cervical cancer), women sometimes experience vaginal dryness and thinning of the vaginal and vulvar tissues, which can lead to painful sex. Because many women are embarrassed by this symptom, they will sometimes tolerate painful intercourse; in counseling women in their late 40s and 50s, you may need to ask to learn if this is a problem.

In men levels of testosterone decrease more slowly. When testosterone becomes too low, men have symptoms such as fatigue, loss of muscle mass, weight gain, low sex drive, and less firm erections or difficult attaining or maintaining an erection altogether. This condition has recently been called *andropause* to suggest that it is analogous to menopause (Pines, 2011). However, unlike women, men are readily treated with testosterone after ruling out other conditions that may cause the condition, such as a pituitary tumor. Men on testosterone replacement—which can be given as a shot, spread on the skin as a gel, or inserted anally as a pellet—must be carefully monitored, as prostate cancer is a risk for high levels of testosterone.

In addition to normal hormonal changes caused by aging, as people age they are more at risk for all types of disease, which can impede on a couple's romantic relationship and sex life. Pain and fatigue, as well as side effects from medications and treatment, contribute to a loss of interest in sex. Of course, some diseases directly affect sexual function, such as testicular cancer, breast cancer, and vulvar cancer. Physicians, nurses, and the patients themselves are often so focused on the illness that they put sex and relationship needs at the bottom of the list, sometimes to their detriment.

Sexuality 66 to 90 (And Up)

These days, 65 is considered to be "young old." People are living longer and are in better health than past generations. In addition, Viagra™ and other medications designed to help with erections has made it possible for men to continue to function well into their 70s and even 80s. Unfortunately (or fortunately, depending upon your view of medical treatment of sexual desire), women are sometimes hard-pressed to keep up with their male partners if they are heterosexual.

Senior communities, assisted living settings, nursing homes, and the like can be very hopping places. As long as mature adults are healthy enough and have an available partner, they will continue to be sexually active. They may be unable to have vigorous intercourse, refractory periods between ejaculations may have increased for males, and orgasm may be elusive for females, but they are still able to cuddle, kiss, fondle, and croon over one another. Most recently, a medical ethicist appeared on video on the *Medscape* website to make the case that seniors in nursing homes should be permitted to engage in sexual behavior (Caplan, 2012).

ACTIVITIES

1. Understanding your own anatomy: use diagram and mirror to identify your own anatomy. Women, use this as a guideline from *Our Bodies, Ourselves*: http://www.ourbodiesourselves.org/book/companion .asp?id=13&compID=37. Men, use this guideline from GoofyFoot Press: http://www.goofyfootpress.com/blogs/anatomy/male-anatomy/
2. Are there any parts of your sexual anatomy that you find distasteful? Why? Are there any parts of people of other genders that you find distasteful? Why? Are there any you especially like? How do you know, that is, what is your response?

3. Sexual timeline: In your journal create two timelines. On one time-line, note major developmental milestones and the year they occurred. On the other timeline, note your sexuality milestones, e.g., noticing secondary sexual characteristics or exploring someone else's body. Write about any patterns or observations you have about your sexual development.

RESOURCES

For Parents

American College of Obstetricians and Gynecologists. (2007). Retrieved from http://www.acog.org/About_ACOG/News_Room/News_Releases/2007/ACOG_Advises_Against_Cosmetic_Vaginal_Procedures

Berman, L. (2009). *Talking to your kids about sex: Turning "the talk" into a conversation for life.* New York, NY: DK Publishing.

Ladas, A. K., Whipple, B., and Perry, J. D. (1982). The G spot: And Other Discoveries About Human Sexuality. New York, NY: Holt, Rinehart, and Winston.

Gossart, M. & Sequoia, J. *No place like home.* Retrieved from http://www.noplacelikehome.org.

Payne, K., Thaler, L., Kukkonen, T., Carrier, S., and Binik, Y. (2007). Sensation and sexual arousal in circumcised and uncircumcised men. Journal of Sexual Medicine 4, 667–674.

Schwartz, P., & Capello, D. (2000). *Ten talks parents must have with their children about sex and character.* New York, NY: Hyperion.

For Teens

American Girl. (1998). *The care and keeping of you: The body book for girls.* Middleton, WI: Pleasant Company Publications.

Dunham, K., & Bjorkman, S. (2007). *The boys body book: Everything you need to know for growing up YOU.* New York, NY: Applesauce Press.

Harris, R. H., & Emberley, M. (2009). *It's perfectly normal: Changing bodies, growing up, sex, and sexual health.* Somerville, MA: Candlewick.

Loulan, L., Worthen, B., & Quackenbush, M. (Illustrator). (2001). *Period: A girl's guide.* Minnetonka, MN: The Book Peddlers.

FEMALE SEXUAL ANATOMY: EXTERNAL STRUCTURES

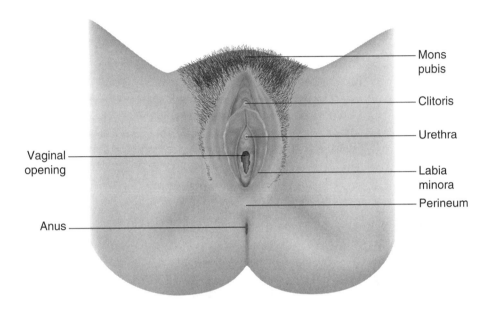

FEMALE SEXUAL ANATOMY: INTERNAL STRUCTURES

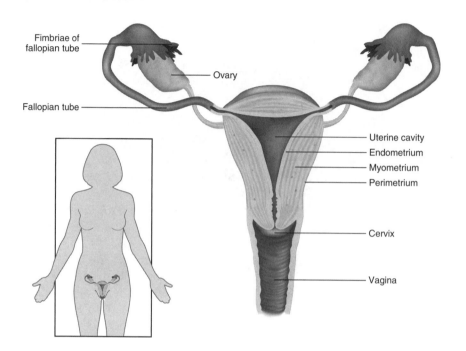

MALE SEXUAL ANATOMY: EXTERNAL STRUCTURES

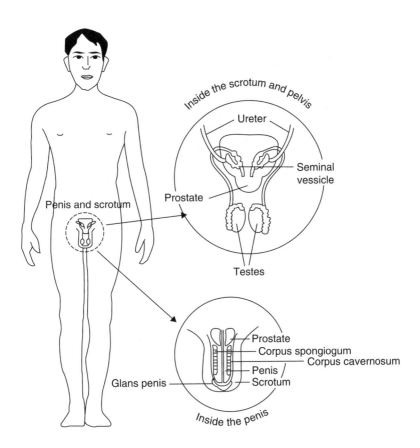

MALE SEXUAL ANATOMY: INTERNAL STRUCTURES

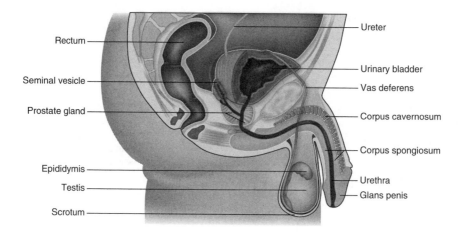

Rectum

Seminal vesicle

Prostate gland

Epididymis

Testis

Scrotum

Ureter

Urinary bladder

Vas deferens

Corpus cavernosum

Corpus spongiosum

Urethra

Glans penis

KEGELS FOR EVERYONE

Kegel exercises, named for Dr. Arnold Kegel, can help improve sexual function. When the pubococcygeus (PC) muscle is exercised, women report greater awareness of sexual sensation and arousal, as well as improved capacity for orgasm. It also has the added benefit of helping with childbirth and continence, or bladder control. Men can also perform Kegel exercises to improve quality of erection and increase ejaculatory timing.

Finding the PC Muscle

For women: Sit on the toilet with legs parted. Start a stream of urine and then try to stop the flow. The muscle you feel tightening when you stop the flow is your PC muscle. If you don't feel it the first time, try the next time you urinate.

For men: Pretend you are trying to keep from emitting intestinal gas or that you are trying to retract the penis by lifting the scrotum or testicles.

How to Exercise the Pelvic Floor

There are two types of Kegel exercises helpful for sexual function.

Slow Kegels: Tighten the PC muscle and hold for a count of three, then release it.
Quick Kegels: Quickly tighten and relax the PC muscle.

A "set" of exercises is to do 10 of each type. Aim for doing a set five times a day. You can do the exercises any time; no one will notice! Try doing them while you are on the telephone, waiting at a red light, reading, or watching TV.

Some women have a hard time identifying just how to tighten and relax the PC muscle and end up making the muscle too tight. If you aren't sure if you are doing the exercises correctly, you should contact a physical therapist who specializes in the pelvic floor; consult the International Pelvic Pain Society for a referral (www.pelvicpain.org).

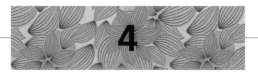

4

Defining Sexual Health

If one purpose of psychotherapy is to treat *all* mental illness, including sexual problems, then the therapist needs a definition of sexual health, a concept that may be fuzzy for all the aforementioned reasons in Chapters 1 and 2. Besides being a vague concept, sexual health is also complex, more than the recognition that sex should be enjoyed without undue inhibition. It also does not simply mean an absence of symptoms such as early ejaculation. Sexual health entails attitudes, behaviors, and beliefs that foster increased feelings of self-esteem, the ability to explore erotic dimensions of human experience, and enhancement of adult attachment. Sexologists' understanding of sexual health also continues to evolve with increased research and knowledge about sexual behavior and the body. While the term "sexual health" may seem a quaint concept from hygiene class, it is actually one that addresses part of the core of what it means to be human.

HISTORICAL VIEW OF SEXUAL HEALTH

Early to Mid-20th Century

A little over 100 years ago, Freud penned *Three Essays on Sexuality*, in which sexual problems were said to have stemmed from unconscious conflicts in early development, for example, the Oedipal complex in which a boy was thought to develop taboo romantic and sexual fantasies for his mother that needed to be resolved in order to make a later appropriate adult relationship.

From Freud we get mythical ideas about female orgasm that unfortunately persist today, as he labeled "mature" women as having vaginal orgasms, "immature" women as having clitoral orgasms, and women who did not have orgasm at all as "frigid" or emotionally cold. Freud also used the term *libido* to describe sexual drive or appetite, which was a force located within the id, or instinctual part of the self. What we now call erectile dysfunction (ED)* Freud called "impotence," reflecting a man's lack initiative or power; Freud and his cohorts were unaware that a number of physiological factors can cause or contribute to ED. Sexual health was obtained by eliminating neurosis through Freud's "talking cure," or years of psychoanalysis. The psychoanalytic approach prevailed for decades, in part because there was very little research on sexual behavior due to social mores. For example, when former APA President O. H. Mowrer was a student at the University of Missouri, the questionnaire he created for conducting research regarding attitudes of college men and women toward illicit sex created a scandal that cost two faculty members their jobs.

Much of that changed when zoologist Alfred Kinsey and his colleagues at Indiana University sought to quantify human sexual behavior in the so-called "Kinsey reports." Kinsey pushed the boundaries of public opinion as he and his team directly observed people during sexual activity. He became an instant celebrity when he published *Sexual Behavior of the Male* in 1948, followed by *Sexual Behavior of the Female* in 1953. Kinsey understood sexual problems as emanating from two root causes: behavioral variation from expected norms and ignorance about physiology. At a time when many mental health professionals viewed homosexuality as a mental disorder, Kinsey did not rigidly define sexual orientation. He developed what is now known as the *Kinsey Scale* which ranged from 0 or completely heterosexual to 6 as completely homosexual. He refrained from judging sexual behavior and encouraged others to do likewise, famously stating, "The only unnatural sex act is that which you cannot perform."

Mid-20th Century to 1980

Kinsey's work laid the foundation for gynecologist William Howell Masters and researcher Virginia Eshelman Johnson, who sought to understand sexual health as uninhibited sexual pleasure. Masters and Johnson gained their knowledge by developing unique tools for studying sexual pleasure, famously creating a model that they published in *The Human Sexual Response* in 1966. Their model included four stages:

- Excitement (initial arousal)
- Plateau phase (full arousal but not yet at orgasm)

---

*The term *erectile dysfunction* was actually coined by pharmaceutical companies.

- Orgasm
- Resolution (period after orgasm)

Sexual problems occurred because of disruptions in any one of these stages. But instead of using psychoanalysis to address symptoms, Masters and Johnson employed intensive behavioral therapy and prescribed activities. One such activity known as *sensate focus* directed a couple, in the privacy of their hotel, room to take turns touching one another without the goal of intercourse. They would report on their experience the following day in conjoint therapy sessions, a novel idea at the time. Treatment generally took place over the course of a week, and Masters and Johnson claimed a 90% success rate. Though the high success rate has been questioned, their treatment represented a nonpathological approach to sexual health.

One of Masters and Johnson's prodigies, physician and psychoanalyst Helen Singer Kaplan, found that her treatment success rates were not as high as those proffered by her mentors, and she decided to try something different. She would first try a behavioral approach, like sensate focus activities, to reduce symptoms. If she found the behavioral approach insufficient, she would then add a course of psychodynamic therapy to address underlying issues. Thus, Kaplan is credited with creating one of the first integrative therapies. Kaplan also modified Masters and Johnson's four-phase model to a tri-phase model:

- Desire
- Arousal
- Orgasm

Without desire, there would be no arousal; without arousal, there would be no orgasm. Reflecting the insight of a seasoned analyst, Kaplan felt that desire was the most difficult phase to treat, the one most likely rooted in deeper psychological conflict. While still a linear model, it demonstrated that sexual health was not simply behavioral, but encompassed sound mental health. Kaplan was the author of several books that specifically helped sex therapists to treat a variety of problems, including *The Evaluation of Sexual Disorders: Psychological and Medical Aspects* (1983) and *The Illustrated Manual of Sex Therapy* (1988).

As treatment of sexual problems evolved, so did American society. In the bright aftermath of World War II, the emphasis was on pleasure of all kinds, followed by interest in the 1960s in personal growth and life satisfaction. The new oral contraceptive pill was introduced, drastically reducing fears of unwanted pregnancy and increasing the incidence of premarital sexual experimentation. The media exploded with sexual information, including books such as *Everything You Always Wanted to Know About Sex but Were Afraid to Ask* (Reuben, 1969/1999) and *The Joy of Sex* (1972). The "sexual revolution" was born, and people were interested in increasing sexual performance and having "peak" sexual experiences, perhaps best summed up with the slogan of the era, "If it feels good, do it." During that era, the sex therapist's office became a place where people could privately get information and reassurance on how to have a better sex life.

1980s to Present Day

If the sun rose during the Sexual Revolution of the 60s and 70s, then it set with the discovery of HIV/AIDS in the early 1980s. Suddenly, attention was drawn to the risks of casual sex in a way that hadn't been seen in decades. While syphilis and gonorrhea could be treated with penicillin, scientists struggled to find a treatment for a disease that was killing thousands of people. Because the first reports of spread of the disease came from the gay community, some people attributed the origin and spread of the illness to homosexual behaviors, bringing further strain and humiliation to sufferers. Health officials closed down bathhouses frequented by gay men and first responders to medical emergencies worried about contracting HIV from bleeding trauma victims. When the disease was also discovered to be rampant in heterosexual people, some of the initial hysteria faded. But the effects lingered, and abstinence-only sex education for teens gained in popularity. In some circles, sexual health was being defined as an absence of venereal disease and retaining virginity until marriage. What happened after marriage, however, remained—and still remains—a mystery for many of those who took vows of chastity.

Medicine also began to delve more and more into treatments and cures for sexual problems, making sexual health attainable through a physician's prescription. Approved by the FDA in 1998, over 35 million prescriptions have been filled for Viagra™ (a PDE5 inhibitor) worldwide (Stout, 2011). Aiming to piggyback on Pfizer's success, Procter & Gamble (P&G) attempted to get FDA approval for Intrinsa™, a micro-dose testosterone patch designed for women complaining of low sexual desire. P&G's efforts to find a "female Viagra™" backfired, however, as Tiefer (2001) lead a vocal campaign against the medicalization of sexual problems. Ultimately, the FDA rejected the medication and similar ones that followed. Whatever one believes about the role of medications in the treatment of sexual problems, the field benefited from increased interest by researchers, the media, and the public in the biological aspects of sexual health. For some physicians and sex therapists, there has grown to be more collaboration in treating difficult cases of low sexual desire, sexual pain disorders, sexual dysfunction related to chronic illness and cancer, and other complex issues.

The Internet has also had a role in forming attitudes and beliefs about sexual health. For better or worse, some users find their definition in pornography, where participants freely experiment with sexual behaviors—but where exploitation may be the rule rather than the exception. Others find it on websites that make empty promises ("Extend your penis 2 inches today!"), motivated by a belief that sexual health is defined by optimized genitalia. Others follow the advice of celebrity sex experts, for whom sexual health may be defined as what sells books. What is a therapist to do? Clearly, therapists need a working definition if they are to help clients discern bad information from good and develop a more satisfying sex life.

SCHOLARLY DEFINITIONS OF SEXUAL HEALTH

The definition of sexual health is dependent on a variety of factors, including the field of study from which a definition is derived. Physicians view sexual health as a state to be attained through assessment and treatment of physical symptoms of sexual dysfunction. Sex educators might relate sexual health to the prevention of unwanted pregnancy or sexually transmitted illness. The consumer may think of sexual health in terms of low sexual desire or libido. How, then, to define sexual health?

There are many contemporary definitions of sexual health, especially within the eclectic psychotherapy environment. Such definitions reflect a particular researcher's or writer's own sexological worldview. For example, Ogden (2006) writes about the Integrating Sexuality and Spirituality (ISIS) model, in which she focuses on four elements of sexual health: mind, body, heart, and spirit. Resnick bases her definition on attachment (2012) and pleasure (2003). Rosenbaum (2013), a physical therapist as well as psychotherapist, views the role of the pelvic floor muscle as playing a large role in a person's ability to have sexual health, while Kort (2007) who identifies as a gay therapist, sees coming to terms with one's orientation as a having a part. Metz and McCarthy (2010) created their "good enough sex" model, which emphasizes that couples content with their sex life have realistic expectations about the range of sexual experiences they may have, from boom to bust.

Based in good measure on the recommendations of Edwards & Coleman (2004), I have chosen the following definitions as examples because they are positive in outlook, as well as broad enough to cover most points while staying succinct. Definitions such as these can inform the therapist in the employment of various theoretical frameworks as they guide clients to a place of enjoying optimal sexual health.

Surgeon General's Report (2001)

Sexual health is inextricably bound to both physical and mental health. Just as physical and mental health problems can contribute to sexual dysfunction and disease, those dysfunctions and diseases can contribute to physical and mental health problems. Sexual health is not limited to the absence of disease or dysfunction, nor is its important (sic) confined to just the reproductive years. . . . It includes freedom from sexual abuse and discrimination and the ability to integrate their sexuality into their lives, derive pleasure from it, and to reproduce.

Robinson, Bockting, Rosser, Miner, & Coleman (2002)

Sexual health is defined as an approach to sexuality founded in accurate knowledge, personal awareness, and self-acceptance, where one's behavior, values, and emotions are congruent and integrated within a person's wider personality structure and self-definition. Sexual health involves an ability to be intimate with a partner, to communicate explicitly about sexual needs and desires, to be sexually functional (to have desire, become aroused, and obtain sexual fulfillment), to act intentionally and responsibly, and to set appropriate sexual boundaries. . . . Sexual health includes a sense of self-esteem, personal attractiveness and competence, as well as freedom from sexual dysfunction, sexually transmitted diseases, and sexual assault/coercion. Sexual health affirms sexuality as a positive force, enhancing other dimensions of one's life.

World Health Organization (2006a)

Sexual health is a state of physical, emotional, mental, and social well-being related to sexuality; it is not merely the absence of disease, dysfunction, or infirmity. Sexual health requires a positive and respectful approach to sexuality and sexual relationships, as well as the possibility of having pleasurable and safe sexual experiences, free of coercion, discrimination and violence. For sexual health to be attained and maintained, the sexual rights of all persons must be respected, protected and fulfilled.

All three definitions suggest that people have a right to accurate information about sex, a right to sexual pleasure, and a right to freedom from sexual coercion or violence. Sexual well-being is more than having a functional physiological system; it is also the ability to have satisfying sexual encounters. Pleasure can be derived in many ways and as long as activity is consensual (and noncommercial) between two adults, all is good.

An important concept is that sexual health doesn't necessarily mean man-woman penis-vagina intercourse. People can have good sexual health whether they are enjoying autoerotic or partnered activity; with a partner of the same or opposite sex; using any and all of their senses to enjoy the experience; employing hands, fingers, toes, tongue, genitals, and any other body part to induce arousal and climax. This understanding becomes important when a person's sexual function is severely impaired, as when a woman has a sexual pain disorder or a man is having difficulty recovering erectile function after prostate cancer. It is also important for couples to broaden their ideas of what constitutes "sex" if they are tired or stressed, as after the birth of a child, or as they grow older. It can be liberating to be told that a foot-rub or an old-fashioned make-out session can be seen as sexual activity.

Speaking of sexual practices, as a therapist you may wonder if you will be comfortable knowing the details of a client's sexual practices. It is interesting to consider that you might listen to the details of a woman's gruesome, botched labor and delivery, a soldier's description of a battle, or even (as I was surprised to learn as a therapist) about a client's bowel habits without judgment, but the thought of someone admitting that they enjoy oral sex more than intercourse can make you shudder. Just as clients struggle with their sexuality, a therapist's struggle may come from a variety of complex feelings about sex based on one's family of origin experience, religious upbringing, culture, peer cohort behavior, and so forth. That is why it is imperative for therapists to define healthy sexuality for themselves, with the understanding that someone can sexually engage with partners in very different ways, and still be practicing good sexual health.

Though sexual health may be portrayed as a basic human right, it is not necessarily an innate human state. The next section examines some common factors that undermine sexual health.

BASIC RISKS TO SEXUAL HEALTH

Sexual problems can occur at any time in the course of someone's development. People can be born with ambiguous genitals (also described as being born *intersex*), have gender or orientation confusion, or experience a disease or surgery that compromises one's sexuality. Adult sexual health, however, may depend on the absence of some of the following risk factors (Lue et al., 2004).

- Overall good health
- Diabetes and cardiovascular disease
- Urinary tract disease
- Pelvic floor dysfunction
- Cancer
- Psychiatric/psychological factors
- Medications and recreational drugs, including tobacco
- Infertility
- Phase of life issues such as the birth of a child or retirement
- Vocational problems

The risk factors that apply to your own client population will be a unique amalgam. Consider such populations as female survivors of domestic violence; unemployed veteran soldiers; lower class minorities without access to appropriate birth control; new fathers; male survivors of prostate cancer; and so forth. Each group faces its own risks to sexual health. However, armed with a definition of such, therapists are in a position to optimize a client's sexual relationship and pleasure, no matter what the challenge.

Your ideas about sexual happiness may change over time as you work with people whose definitions may differ from your own, but indicate a healthy point of view nonetheless. The way in which you help individuals and couples meet their goals of a more satisfying sex life may also evolve as you gain knowledge and experience. What may perhaps be the most surprising thing is that you will realize how deeply people are affected when their sex life is a source of shame, sadness, worry, or embarrassment. You will come to see that helping people become more sexually fulfilled is indeed a worthwhile goal, that sex is not a frill, but an essential factor in achieving good quality of life.

SEXUALLY TRANSMITTED DISEASE

Sexual health includes prevention of sexually transmitted disease. According to the Center on Disease Control (2010), there are 19 million new infections every year in the United States, with a cost of $17 billion every year, not to mention the cost to health and quality of life. For example, untreated gonorrhea and chlamydia—diseases that can be harbored in a woman's body undetected—causes about 24,000 women in the United States to become infertile. Untreated syphilis can lead to serious problems including brain, cardiovascular, and organ damage. Additionally, people with gonorrhea, chlamydia, or syphilis are at increased risk for HIV.

Although therapists are not medical doctors, there may be a moral as well as common sense imperative to talk about safe sex practices with clients. Aside from abstinence, clients can be encouraged to limit partners to people whom they know; agree to mutual testing before engaging in sex; consistent and correct use latex condoms; and seek immediate treatment if there are any signs or symptoms of a sexually transmitted disease, for example, pain with urination or rash. Condoms, however, cannot completely prevent disease, as some diseases such as genital herpes can be spread through contact on the unprotected areas of the skin and mucosa of the genitals.

PSYCHOLOGICAL AND RELATIONAL FACTORS CONTRIBUTING TO SEXUAL HEALTH

In the end, the most valuable definition of sexual health may come from clients wishing to have "great sex" with their partner. While the pharmaceutical companies might have people believing that a fully functioning penis or a hormonally moisturized vagina create the best sex worth having, the truth is that there are multiple factors. Kleinplatz (2007), a psychologist and sex therapist, created a conceptual model of optimal sexuality that includes six building blocks of pleasure, including (1) being fully present, (2) authenticity, (3) intense emotional connection, (4) sexual and erotic intimacy, (5) communication, and (6) transcendence. The fact is that in the therapy room, clients often learn much more about themselves and their own sexuality than they ever imagined based on being presented with such concepts.

Being Fully Present

What Kleinplatz calls "being fully present" has also been called "eyes wide open sex" (Schnarch, 2009), securely attached (Johnson & Zuccarini, 2010), and "mindful" (Brotto, 2011). The essential concept is that both partners show up not just physically, but prepared to give and receive pleasure in the context of a safe and trusting relationship. Each individual maintains self-awareness of the sensual experience of having sex, while being attuned to their partner's experience through observation and their partner's responses. People who are not fully present for sex may complain of sex as being "mechanical," "a duty," or "something I check off the list."

When people *cannot* show up for sex, they may have an affliction that needs to be addressed. For example, a survivor of trauma may enter into a disassociative state during sex; partners may state that "it's like no one is there" and the survivor may report little or no arousal. Other types of mental health problems, including mood and anxiety disorders, substance abuse, difficulties with attention, and Asperger's syndrome can also interfere with one's ability to be fully present to a sexual experience.

Authenticity

Being authentic is predicated on each participant feeling free to express his or her sexual wants, wishes, and desires. Authenticity is what creates an experience of intimate connection, an erotic knowing of one another's mind, body, and spirit. In individuals and couples who come to the therapy office, this is sometimes the most difficult quality to achieve because of shame and guilt associated with the admission that one wants, needs, or (perhaps scariest of all) likes sex.

Intense Emotional Connection

While the myth persists that the most exciting sex takes place early in a relationship—or even with a stranger—the truth is that partners who experience an emotional connection during sex may report the best sexual experiences. Couples expressed this as, "Sex is the time when I feel closest to my partner," or "I feel most in love with my partner after we've had sex." Sexual experiences also activate a variety of neurochemical events that create an emotional attachment (Fisher, 2004a; Resnick, 2012).

Sexual and Erotic Intimacy

Great sex requires each individual be willing to explore the capacity for pleasure. Being able to identify and tell one's partner what might feel pleasurable—what behavior, what attitude, what role—might move them from the mundane to the sensual. This is where sexual technique comes into play—and it is critical to the continuation of a couple's sex life.

For many couples, I have observed the initial rush of sexual and emotional intimacy carries them forward and helps to solidify their emotional bond. Once that rush has receded, some couples, perhaps instinctually, perhaps by agreement, agree that they must now enter a period of exploration. Others couples flounder, however, uncertain how to proceed.

The fact that one partner is more sexually experienced doesn't necessarily help, as the experienced partner is sometimes embarrassed or ashamed to let their partner know what they know about sex. The more experienced partner sometimes will become frustrated with the less experienced partner if the latter is reticent to move outside the boundaries of their original explorations. This is one area where the media such as *Cosmopolitan* or *Men's Health* excel in terms of sexual information with articles such as "10 Ways to Heighten Your Partner's Orgasm." But in the end, it takes the next element to make a couple's sex life satisfactory.

Communication

The ability to be able to talk about all the myriad facets of a couple's sex life is crucial to great sex. Couples need to be able to talk about what they like and don't like in terms of sensual experience. They also need to negotiate when, where, and how they'd like to have sex. McCarthy and Thestrup (2008) have written of "bridges to desire," in which couples need to create and communicate the type of scenario that is most likely to seduce them into the desire for sex. Communication also takes place nonverbally as couples express their feelings through various types of touch.

Couples I have treated sometimes share with me that they have literally never shared a single word about or during sex. They may need permission to speak up about what they enjoy or dislike about their sexual experiences in order to have a more gratifying interlude.

Transcendence

For some people, sex is a sacred act, the closest a being can get to experiencing God or spirit through the connection with a beloved partner. Ogden (2006) has studied this transcendent experience and created the ISIS model in which participants are invited to think about mind, body, heart, and spirit in relationship to their sexuality. In the past decade or so, there has been increased interest in the practice of tantric sex, a type of sexual yoga in which partners participate in activities that are used purposefully to create a sense of spiritual connection, such as eye gazing, chanting, and playing with sexual energy.

THE SEXUALITY OF THE THERAPIST

As you read through this chapter, you may have thought about your own sexual health. Perhaps you are finding that you have had an overall positive experience. Perhaps it hasn't been an area of your life that has been especially fulfilling. Yet, therapists often help clients in areas in which they, themselves, have experienced conflict or ambiguity. A therapist may have been unlucky in love, but that doesn't mean he or she can't help someone else navigate a relationship—unless, of course, the therapist is in the throes of a high conflict divorce. As with all the human problems therapists treat, if the therapist doesn't have a sound grasp or his or her sexual health, then time must be spent developing such.

Notice, also, that the definitions of sexual health are relatively value free. One therapist may be repulsed by a particular sexual act, while another barely blinks an eye at its mention. Therapists are raised in homes that fall along the spectrum, in which some parents advocate abstinence, while others freely talk about sex and its mores. Developing one's own opinions, while respecting those of the client, is always part of learning to be nonjudgmental of clients. If thoughts and behaviors do no harm, then the therapist has no duty to prelude clients from participating in any activity. This theme of the self of the therapist in relationship to client's sexuality is one that will be revisited throughout the chapters that follow.

ACTIVITIES

The following activities are meant to be discussed with a colleague, in a small group, or written about in your sexological journal.

1. How might you define sexual health?
   a. Using this chapter or the "Declaration of Sexual Rights" (page 47) as a guide, write a response in your journal.
   b. Clients also benefit from discussion of the "Declaration of Sexual Rights," especially when there has been a history of coercion/being coerced or other negativity surrounding the topic of sex.

2. Do you find yourself in agreement regarding the building blocks of good sex that Kleinplatz described? Would you subtract and/or add other building blocks? What would they be? Does sexual health differ between an individual and a couple? Is it possible for an individual to have a healthy autoerotic sex life?
3. How does culture impact definitions of sexual health? Can you compare sexual beliefs with one or two other cultures with which you are familiar?
4. How does each situation fit or not fit the definition of sexual health in this chapter? Your own definition?
   a. A husband and wife agree that he can enjoy cross-dressing when she travels out of town on business. When she is home, they agree they have an enjoyable sex life.
   b. Two male partners agree that they wish to have sex with a third male partner simultaneously. The third male partner agrees to join them.
   c. A transsexual female (a male who lives as female) decides that her orientation is to female partners.
   d. A couple that feels themselves to be best friends admits to one another that they aren't and have never really been interested in sex. They decide to live together as husband and wife in an asexual arrangement.

RESOURCES

Centers for Disease Control and Prevention—Sexual Health: *www.cdc.gov/sexualhealth*
Fact Sheets on Sexually Transmitted Disease: *www.cdc.gov/std/healthcomm/fact_sheets.htm*
Medline: Sexual Health: *www.nlm.nih.gov/medlineplus/sexualhealth.html*
U.S. Surgeon General's Call to Action to Support Sexual Health and Responsible Sexual Behavior: *www.surgeongeneral.gov/library/calls/sexualhealth/index.html*
World Association for Sexual Health: *www.worldsexology.org*
World Health Organization—Sexual Health: *www.who.int/topics/sexual_health/en*

DECLARATION OF SEXUAL RIGHTS

The World Association for Sexual Health (WAS) created the "Declaration of Sexual Rights" to serve as guidance for the work of sexologists, but also guidance in creating government policies regarding sexual health. The WAS declaration reads, in part, that "[sexual] development depends upon the satisfaction of basic human needs such as the desire for contact, intimacy, emotional expression, pleasure, tenderness and love." The rights include:

1. The right to sexual freedom

2. The right to sexual autonomy, sexual integrity, and safety of the sexual body

3. The right to sexual privacy

4. The right to sexual equity

5. The right to sexual pleasure

6. The right to emotional sexual expression

7. The right to sexually associate freely

8. The right to make free and responsible reproductive choices

9. The right to sexual information based upon scientific inquiry

10. The right to comprehensive sexuality education

11. The right to sexual health care

HOW TO USE A CONDOM CONSISTENTLY AND CORRECTLY

- Use a new condom for every act of vaginal, anal, and oral sex throughout the *entire* sex act (from start to finish).

- Before any genital contact, put the condom on the tip of the erect penis with the rolled side out.

- If the condom does not have a reservoir tip, pinch the tip enough to leave a half-inch space for semen to collect. Holding the tip, unroll the condom all the way to the base of the erect penis.

- After ejaculation and before the penis gets soft, grip the rim of the condom and carefully withdraw. Then gently pull the condom off the penis, making sure that semen doesn't spill out.

- Wrap the condom in a tissue and throw it in the trash where others won't handle it.

- If you feel the condom break at any point during sexual activity, stop immediately, withdraw, remove the broken condom, and put on a new condom.

- Ensure that adequate lubrication is used during vaginal and anal sex, which might require water-based lubricants. Oil-based lubricants (e.g., petroleum jelly, shortening, mineral oil, massage oils, body lotions, and cooking oil) should not be used because they can weaken latex, causing breakage.

Source: www.cdc.gov/condomeffectiveness/brief.html

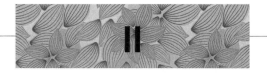

Assessing and Treating
Sexual Concerns

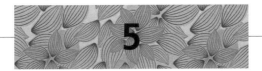

Assessing Sexual Problems

Clients' sexual complaints vary greatly, from those that arise from the simple need for information to those that may require weekly visits for 6 months to a year or more. As with all presenting problems, the therapist needs to determine what, exactly, are the client's symptoms, when they appeared, and what has been tried to resolve them. The therapist also needs a framework to guide inquiry and treatment planning. In my observation, most sex therapists use an all-encompassing theoretical approach because of the need to sort out the biological from the psychological factors, as well as the effect of the client's relationship and social environment on symptoms.

Before commencing any assessment, therapists may do well to hold in mind the PLISSIT model (Annon, 1976) of assessment. PLISSIT is an acronym for *Permission, Limited Information, Specific Suggestions*, and *Intensive Therapy*. As an assessment, PLISSIT is more a decision tree that guides the work the therapist needs to do. PLISSIT begins with the idea that the mental health professional must first ask permission to speak to the client about sex. One way to go about this task is to include a simple yes/no question on the intake form such as: Do you have any sexual concerns you would like to discuss today? Another implicit way to normalize assessing a client's sexual health is to make mention of it on one's website and to openly display sexual health materials, such as books and pamphlets. Therapists may also explicitly tell a client that they can ask questions about virtually anything, including sex.

The PLISSIT assessment also helps the therapist keep in mind that not all clients with sexual problems will present them in a setting that permits time to conduct a long assessment. Clients also sometimes are highly functioning, but because sexual development typically lags behind other development (e.g., due to little or no sex education) they may simply have questions. In such cases, the therapist can provide information and suggestions. If the presenting problem is longstanding or complex and there is time, or if information and suggestions were not enough to solve the problem, then more intensive therapy may be required, which is dependent on a thorough assessment.

In my own sex therapy practice, I use an *ecosystemic* approach to assessment, meaning that I look at each individual or couple I treat within a broad context. I originally used this approach in writing my dissertation on families of children with cancer (Buehler, 1999), but found it served me well when I moved into treating adults with chronic illness and later, adults with sexual problems. Ecological systems theory is not new, but its application to understanding sexual problems has only recently been published in research journals (Jones, 2011). Working in the 1940s, anthropologist Gregory Bateson is credited with applying ideas about how mechanical systems intersect with the social sciences. Child development specialist Urie Bronfenbrenner used Bateson's ideas to develop ecological systems theory or ecosystems theory in 1979.

With its emphasis on understanding the context in which an individual develops and interacts with others, ecosystems theory seems ideal for analyzing not only what factors are causing or exacerbating a sexual problem, but also designing an effective treatment plan. The ecosystem consists of several subsystems, which range from those containing institutions most involved with the individual's development, to the element of time, the most abstract system. The five subsystems—microsystem, mesosystem, exosystem, macrosystem, and chronosystem—are described in detail below. The sexual history taking form at the end of this chapter is based on ecosystemic theory.

MICROSYSTEM

The microsystem consists of those subsystems and institutions closest to and most influential upon an individual's development, including family and peers, as well as one's biological and psychological makeup.

Biology

Individual differences in anatomical features as well as hormones have an influence on sexual development. People reach puberty at different ages, which can have an effect on peer relationships. They also have different levels of sexual curiosity and drive, so that some people are motivated to express their sexuality while others experience it as a quieter component. One's sexual orientation may also be considered as biologically determined and certainly must be assessed; in fact, people sometimes seek sex therapy because they are confused about their orientation. A person's health status also has an effect on their sexual development. In one case, a man in my office had had a kidney transplant as he entered puberty. Because his activities were restricted and he missed a great deal of school, he had difficulty understanding how to negotiate a romantic relationship, let along a sexual one.

Biology also includes a person's lifestyle. In conducting an assessment, care must be taken to ask about diet, exercise, sleep hygiene, and alcohol and drug intake. Many people are unaware that their physical well-being has an impact on their sex drive.

Psychology

Comorbid psychiatric and sexual issues are common (Buehler, 2011). People often do not seek treatment until they have a sexual problem and can no longer enjoy one of life's pleasures, but they do not realize that depression, anxiety, obsessive compulsive disorder (OCD), posttraumatic stress disorder (PTSD), attention deficit hyperactivity disorder (ADHD), and other disorders can all disrupt sexual response. Substance abuse or dependence also needs to be ruled out. Many people depend on substances to help them function sexually, but there can be unwanted effects. Unfortunately, prescribed psychotropic and other medications can also cause sexual side effects. A later chapter is devoted to mental health and sexuality.

STEP INTO MY OFFICE...

Margaret and Leo had been married 5 years. They rarely had sex unless they had been out drinking at a bar. Leo also had a history of depression as well as problems with explosive anger. Margaret eventually insisted that Leo get treatment; he was referred to an anger management group, prescribed an antidepressant, and also advised not to drink. To show support, Margaret also cut back on drinking. Without alcohol, however, they both felt inhibited. Margaret sensed that Leo was uncomfortable and she responded with her own inhibitions. Eventually, they contacted a therapist because their sex life had come to a halt, never realizing they were abusing alcohol to cover up fears about sex and intimacy.

Family of Origin

A person's family of origin provides the foundation for the development of sexuality. Parental messages about sex are extremely varied, ranging from extreme taboo and silence on the subject, to acting out sexually in inappropriate ways. Children do learn about sex by observing their parents' relationship, noticing whether parents are affectionate, if they sleep in the same bed or in separate rooms, and even their reactions to sexy scenes on

TV. Children and teens may also intuit or know about their parents' sexual problems, such as a parent engaging in extramarital affairs, possible history of molestation, or complete lack of sexual activity.

How parents react to evidence of a child's sexual knowledge and activity can also be important. One client told me that when her parents discovered that, at age 16, she had had sex with her boyfriend they installed an alarm system. When that didn't satisfy their need for control, they moved away altogether and sent her to a different school. The client believed that the extreme reaction interfered with her ability to enjoy sex and have orgasm even now with her husband.

Peers

For better or worse, most people learn about sex from peers on the playground and in the locker and dorm rooms. Peers create a fount of misinformation, but they also offer opportunities for discussing one's ideas and fears about sex. Peers tease one another, sometimes mercilessly, about sexual characteristics, which can create lifelong problems with self-esteem. Girls who develop early are more likely to feel self-conscious, while boys who develop later in their teens have lower self-esteem. However challenging the topic of sexuality can be among peers, peers are also the appropriate choice for early sexual experimentation, such as kissing and fondling, that are integral to development.

MESOSYTEM

The mesosystem encompasses interactions between institutions within the microsystem. For example, a person raised in a conservative home may be exposed to progressive ideas about sexual choices in college, thus developing a different sexological worldview than their parents. The mesosystem also contains the interactions between individuals; this is especially pertinent for sexual problems that occur mostly within the context of a relationship. Much as when a therapist is assessing couples of differing religions and culture, sexual problems can also be understood in terms of differences in development. When a woman who began sexual experimentation in her teens—with her mother's blessing of appropriate contraception—marries a virgin man from a traditional background, it has the potential to create misunderstandings in communication, rules, and roles.

EXOSYSTEM

The exosystem includes those institutions that exert an influence on one's development, but are not intimately involved with one's daily life in the way that parents or peers may be.

School

Most schools offer a sex education program in fifth or sixth grade, which is considered to be prior to the onset of puberty, although today girls on average are entering puberty at age 8 or 9. In general children need permission to attend the program, but not every parent allows their child to attend. Programs tend to emphasize "prevention and plumbing"; I have never met a woman who learned about the clitoris and orgasm from this instruction. School is also an unfortunate source of lots of misinformation about conception, sex, and love as peers share their observations and myths.

Religion

Religions notably vary in their views of sexuality and its expression, especially regarding premarital sex, sexual orientation, and masturbation. Some religions, such as the United Church of Christ, are liberal in their approaches, believing that individuals must decide for themselves how to express their sexual nature. Others, such as the Church of Jesus Christ of Latter Day Saints (Mormonism) and Catholicism, take an austere view of premarital experimentation and masturbation. Stereotypes are to be avoided; I recall, for example, one young man, a Jehovah's Witness, telling me that sex was discussed openly in their home, while another man from the same religion stated that when his grandmother caught him masturbating, his grandmother beat him and called him terrible names.

In a country where freedom of religion is a basic right, clients are all over the map in terms of their adherence to religious beliefs about sex. Some leave their religion because they feel it doesn't support their view, while others embrace and practice their religion's beliefs about sex; moving even slightly away can precipitate strong inhibitions and feelings of guilt. Developing different religious beliefs than one's parents can lead to feelings of guilt and family rifts that are sometimes never repaired.

Media

Individuals are highly influenced by the media, which includes the Internet. Messages are sent regarding idealized physical attributes, sexual behaviors, relationship formation, gender roles, and so forth. Increasingly, young teens are exposed to pornographic material, often unbeknownst to parents. Attitudes among sex therapists about teen exposure to pornography varies from seeing it as a teaching tool to concern that it sends the wrong message about sexual relationships as well as sexual exploitation.

Health Care System

Health care can influence sexual behaviors in that the field of medicine controls much of what we know about contraception, sexually transmitted disease, and reproduction. Some people have physicians who are proactive in this area, advising teens and their parents to have the teen vaccinated against human papilloma virus (HPV), while others are silent on the subject. Concerns about infertility, creating an unwanted pregnancy, witnessing childbirth or being exposed to (sometimes gruesome) stories about childbirth, and so forth are also part of the influence of health care on an individual.

MACROSYSTEM

Broadly held attitudes and beliefs constitute this level of the ecosystem, such as those found in a particular culture.

Culture

The culture includes influences such as socioeconomic status, ethnicity, heritage, and values. A man who grows up in a culture that values a man's right to sexual expression may take a "boys will be boys" view of extramarital affairs, for example. Individuals within the same culture may also vary, so that a woman growing up in the same culture but who is highly educated may have a more democratic view of the sexes.

Other cultures, both Western and Eastern, vary in their outlook on sex. European countries may seem more liberal or permissive because of more relaxed attitudes toward the body and sex, but in countries where the majority of the population is Catholic (e.g., Spain and Portugal) there are still traditional expectations about refraining from intercourse before marriage. In countries where Islamic religion dominates, sexuality is largely repressed, though there exists an accepted double standard that men will be sexual before marriage, while women stay chaste. Asian cultures vary widely depending on how Westernized the area where the client or the client's family immigrated from.

STEP INTO MY OFFICE...

Lawrence, a 32-year-old heterosexual, second-generation Chinese-American man who grew up in a small farming town in central California, met his 23-year-old Chinese-born future wife, Mei Ying, on an extended business trip to Hong Kong. They fell in love and maintained a long distance relationship, but Mei Ying complained, "We had very little sex." Thinking that sex would improve if they married, Mei Ying agreed to come to the United States to marry Lawrence. Mei Ying was soon disappointed, while Lawrence was overwhelmed with Mei Ying's high sex drive.

I needed to put aside my preconceptions about members of Chinese culture and conduct an ecosystemic assessment. Lawrence reported that he never saw his parents touch, nor did they ever speak to him about sex. In fact, Lawrence thought that marrying a Chinese woman from what he believed was a more traditional culture would be perfect, since he didn't understand the "big deal" about sex. However, Mei Ying was from cosmopolitan Hong Kong and not very traditional at all. Her parents had divorced after her father had an affair, and both parents then openly dated new partners. This was clearly a case where family of origin issues superseded cultural issues, but all factors needed to be accounted for in the assessment in order to understand the systemic influences.

Gender

Most people hold the belief that one's gender is biologically determined by the appearance of one's genitals at birth. In fact, much of what we call *gender* is socially determined. Additionally, for some individuals who are *transgender* (having the feeling and belief that there is a mismatch between one's biological gender and one's psychological gender) or *intersex* (an individual born with genitals that are ambiguous in appearance), gender is not a black or white, either/or construct. Many myths that people hold about gender and sexuality can, in fact, be quite damaging. For example, comedians often joke about women's lower sex drive. However, men are almost equally found to have a lower drive than their female partner. When this occurs, both men and women struggle with its meaning, with women often shaming or embarrassing their male partner because they have less sexual interest.

CHRONOSYSTEM

The chronosystem is the influence of time on all other institutions and interactions as a person develops. The chronosystem involves both changes in institutions (such as the popularization of the Internet in the 1990s) as well as the experience of various developmental milestones. For example, the median age in the United States for beginning intercourse is currently 15. Individuals who begin intercourse earlier have often been at risk for having been sexually abused and/or commenced using drugs and alcohol, while those who fail to begin intercourse after entering their 20s, 30s, or beyond may either feel ostracized or be at risk for disorders such as social anxiety or Asperger's syndrome.

CONDUCTING AN ECOSYSTEMIC ASSESSMENT

In my sex therapy practice, I begin with a fairly standard psychiatric intake form that the client fills out online through an electronic medical records system. From this standard form, I formulate questions about the client's sexual development that I will ask when we meet. I note the age of the client to determine normative expectations. For example, I know that men in their 40s sometimes are surprised to experience the normal effects of declining testosterone at a time when they may have recently divorced and are on the dating market again. I look at the medications they are taking, whether or not they have a healthy lifestyle, and their alcohol and drug intake. I see what religion, if any, they adhere to and whether or not they were born in the United States. I review what they have said about their family of origin, if anything. Has there been divorce? Abuse? Has either parent had a mental illness? Has the client ever been in therapy? If so, what for? In other words, I form an impression about the person's ecosystem. If I am seeing a couple, I begin to note potential differences in development prior to meeting.

The questions included in the ecosystemic assessment are meant to be guidelines. The questions are designed to prompt answers that will determine whether or not further exploration will be necessary or fruitful. Some questions focus on factual information, others on interactions. Questions are also broad, but can be tailored to a specific presenting problem, for example, if a woman presents with sexual complaints after breast cancer, then inquiry can be focused initially on the biological level, then moved to the mesosystem where a woman's interactions with her partner can be understood.

Sample questions are provided for conducting a thorough ecosystemic assessment are provided on the pages that follow. Therapists who work in private practice and offer long-term treatment generally will want to conduct a more thorough assessment than those who work in settings with time limits or other constrictions on treatment. Nevertheless, keeping in mind the different levels of assessment can be helpful if aspects of a person's sexual history are confusing, or even later, if and when treatment stalls. Clients don't always remember their own development, but discussion of issues may create memory cues. If possible, the therapist can conduct several very thorough assessments to get a feel of the type of information various questions elicit, then develop a more personal or flexible style with experience.

ACTIVITIES

1. Assess your own sexual ecosystem at each level to gain a better understanding of your own sexuality. What systems had the greatest impact on you? How has your sexuality developed or changed as you matured?

2. Write down a few ways to introduce the topic of a client's sexual health in the context of the setting in which you practice. Discuss with a supervisor or colleague.

3. If possible, take turns with a trusted colleague to take an ecosystemic assessment of sexuality. Decide in advance how much detail the person playing the client will share. Alternatively, agree with a trusted colleague

that you will each take an ecosystemic assessment of an actual client. Reflect on the process of taking and giving information in this way.

4. How might you modify the assessment to fit into your setting or your theoretical approach? What levels of the model might you emphasize or perhaps eliminate?

RESOURCES

Visit the following websites for articles containing additional information on taking a sexual history, or to get a different perspective.

Downey, J. I., & Friedman, R. C. (2009, September 1). Psychiatry online: Clinical synthesis. Taking a sexual history: The adult psychiatric patient. *Focus, 7,* 435–440. Retrieved from http://focus.psychiatryonline.org/article.aspx?articleid=52988

Nusbaum, M. R. H., & Hamilton, C. D. (2002, November 1). The proactive sexual health history. *American Family Physicians, 66*(9), 1705–1713. Retrieved from www .aafp.org/afp/2002/1101/p1705.html

Royal College of Nursing. *Taking a sexual history.* Retrieved from www.rcn.org.uk/ development/practice/cpd_online_learning/sexual_health_for_non-experts/ taking_a_sexual_history

SEXUAL ECOSYSTEM QUESTIONNAIRE

Microsystem

Developmental Experiences/Family of Origin

Early Childhood

- Can you remember first knowing that you had a gender?
- Did you feel happy knowing your gender?
- Did you sense that your parents were or were not happy about your gender?
- Do you remember first recognizing your genitals?
- Do you have any positive or negative experiences about sex early in your life?

Middle Childhood

- Did your parents talk to you about sex?
- If so, what did they say?
- Did you experience any sexual abuse at any age?
- Were you prepared for puberty?
- Did you have normal sex play with your friends?
- If your parents discovered you involved in sex play or sexual self-exploration/masturbation, how did they respond?
- At what age do you remember beginning to masturbate?
- Were you exposed to inappropriate sexual material at any age?

Preteen

- What were your feelings about puberty? How did you feel about the changes in your body?
- What, if anything, did parents or other caregivers say anything about puberty?
- Was there any sexual teasing or harassment you'd like to talk about?
- Tell me about having crushes or romantic fantasies. Were they satisfying, or was there anything disturbing about them?
- At what age did you learn about sex and sexual intercourse? How and what did you learn about sex?
- Did you question your gender or orientation at any age? If so, were you able to talk to anyone about it?

Adolescence

- If you started experimenting sexually during adolescence, was it in the context of a relationship? Was the relationship a healthy one?

- Were early experiences pleasurable, or was there something about any of them that bother you?

- If you were discovered to be experimenting sexually, how did your parents or caregivers react?

- Were you truthful with yourself and others about sexual knowledge and/or experiences? How did you relate to peers and their sexuality?

- How regularly did you masturbate? How did you feel about it?

- Did you have access to pornography? Did you use it frequently? How did you feel about it?

Biological Issues

- Did you ever have an illness that affected your sexual or social development?

- Do you now have an illness that affects your sexuality and/or your relationships?

- Are you taking any medications?

- Tell me about your alcohol and drug history.

- Have you ever been treated for a psychiatric illness? Tell me if you think it is having an effect on your sexuality.

Mesosystem

Relationships

Late Adolescence and Adulthood

- Did you have any relationships lasting more than a few months? Did they include sexual activity, and if so, was it pleasurable?

- Did you feel comfortable or insecure about your sexuality?

- Did you have anyone you could get information from as a teen?

- Was there ever, at any age, an unwanted pregnancy?

- Did you have many/a few/no sexual partners before your current relationship?

- Have you had any relationships that included satisfying sex? What made them satisfying?

- Have you had any relationships in which you were dissatisfied? What made them unsatisfactory?

- Do you have believe in your relationship that one of you has a problem with drive (wanting to have sex)?
- What about arousal (getting turned on)?
- For men: Problems with erections and/or early ejaculation?
- For men: Does it ever take longer than you'd like or expect to ejaculate?
- For women: Problems with orgasm?
- Is sex ever painful? When? Does it prevent you from having sex?
- Do you have sexual fantasies? Do you enjoy them, or not? Do you share them?
- Do you have any sexual behaviors (e.g., a fetish) that interferes with sexual enjoyment with yourself or your partner?
- Does your partner have any behaviors that you have difficulty accepting or getting aroused by?
- What questions about your gender or orientation would you like to explore?
- Are any of your sexual problems possibly related to stress, like change in job, moving, birth of a child, death of a loved one, and so on?

Exosystem

Indirect Influence of Other Systems on Sexuality

- If you have a spiritual life, does it or does it not support your exploration of your sexuality?
- Have you left or changed religion because of differences in ideas about sexuality? How has that been for you?
- Does your workplace support work/life balance? How does this affect your sexual expression?
- Tell me about any interactions with health care providers regarding sexual concerns. Did they go well?

Macrosystem

Socio-Cultural Influences on Sexuality

- Tell me about attitudes toward sex in your culture/culture of your family of origin.

- In what ways was your family more or less permissive?

- What attitudes do you have about how people of any gender are supposed to act in a sexual relationship? For example, are men supposed to be the initiators?

- How do you think your sexual development has been influenced by ideas you have read about or learned of in the media?

- What are your beliefs about the place of sexuality in a person's life? In a person's relationships?

- How do you feel about sexual experimentation?

- Do you consider yourself to have a more or less permissive attitude about sexuality?

DIAGRAM OF AN ECOSYSTEM

Make one copy for each participant. Write on the diagram or use it as a guide for interviewing. For couples, compare diagrams to see areas of similarity and difference.

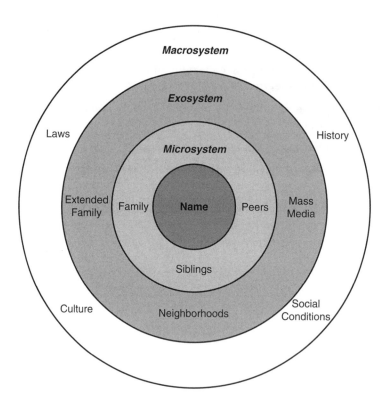

6

Women's Sexual Health Problems

For many women, sexual problems may be solved with information and suggestions. But even when women are given adequate education and tools, sometimes they come back to report that such remedies had little effect, signaling that something deeper may be wrong, something of which they were initially unaware. In part due to socialization, women often suppress sexual thoughts and feelings; it may be only through a trusted therapist's exploration that a woman recognizes blocks to enjoying her sexual potential. Therapeutic exploration may reveal almost any type of obstacle, from seemingly minor problems such as constant skirmishes regarding chores, to major issues such as growing up in a restrictive home environment where sex was a taboo topic or having a very demanding sexual partner, replicating a victim-perpetrator relationship if the woman has experienced molestation.

Reflecting significant change from the *DSM-IV-TR* (2000), the following sexual dysfunctions are listed in the *Diagnostic and Statistical Manual, 5th ed. (DSM-5)*:

- Female Sexual Interest/Arousal Disorder
- Female Orgasmic Disorder
- Other Specified Sexual Dysfunction

There are a few differences between diagnostic categories in the *DSM-IV* and *DSM-5*. In the *DSM-IV*, Sexual Arousal and Hypoactive Sexual Desire were distinct from one another, while in the *DSM-5* they are unified as one disorder. Sexual Aversion has been eliminated from the *DSM-5*; it can be diagnosed as Other Specified Sexual Dysfunction, with "sexual aversion" as the specified reason for treatment. It is good reminder, however, that the *DSM-5* is primarily a psychiatric text that is used for forensic purposes (First & Zucker, 2013). Aside from psychiatric disorders, psychological problems do exist and deserve treatment.

The *DSM-IV* had criticized by sexologists because low desire and arousal reflected Masters and Johnson's linear model which has been criticized as being linear and more descriptive of the male experience of sex. Basson (2005) created a *circular* model to reflect the experience of women, especially in long-term relationships. She proposes that women may not fantasize about sex or feel turned on enough to initiate, but will *respond* to their partner's initiation with increased arousal and, potentially, orgasm. Basson's model also isn't without critics, as it suggests female passivity and neglects sexuality in lesbian relationships. A recent article (Meana, 2010) questions whether it is the quality of relationship that always drives desire; elements such as eroticism and the feeling of being desired may play an equal, or perhaps larger, role. Also, different models may describe people at different times in their lives, with women in menopause sometimes describing that they feel no desire at all. However, in clinical experience many couples resonate with Basson's model; the reframing seems to ease any feelings of guilt that a woman may bear because she doesn't feel much desire for her partner.

Another perspective of sexual dysfunction is the "New View" (Tiefer, Hall, & Tavris, 2002), in which is the authors postulated that problems like hypoactive sexual desire are mainly the product of disease mongering by pharmaceutical companies. As with depression, the debate rages on about the appropriateness of medical interventions for problems that may be mainly psychological. In the meantime, a percentage of women do report true suffering when they lose the emotional and physical sensation of desire, and should not be denied a collaborative ecosystemic approach to treatment.

The main point is, if a client complains about one disorder, then it is important to assess for overlapping or multiple contributing factors. If a woman has no desire, is it because she does not have orgasm and therefore finds sex unrewarding? If she complains she never has orgasm, is it because she hasn't communicated to her partner what arouses her? Help the client make the connection between different aspects of her sexual experience.

KEY TO PLEASURABLE SEX: AROUSAL

For most women, sex without arousal is an emotionless and unfulfilling event. Sexual arousal is largely a subjective state of excitement in anticipation of or during a desired sexual act. Sexual arousal disorder is diagnosed when there is a persistent or recurring inability to attain or maintain sexual excitement, leading to personal distress. In women, arousal is variously signaled with visible changes such as vaginal lubrication, swelling labia, erect nipples, flushing, and quickened respiration, as well as internal changes such as feelings described as excitement, passion, or increasing pleasure.

Lack of arousal is subjective and can have many presentations. One woman may enjoy being caressed by her partner, yet she may be distressed by lack of lubrication. This condition can occur because of hormonal changes during a woman's menstrual cycle, use of oral contraceptives, or stress. A woman could also display signs of excitement, yet report she doesn't really feel excited. This state may indicate a more psychological problem such as mood disorder or anxiety. In one study (Bradford & Meston, 2006), women diagnosed with Generalized Anxiety Disorder (GAD) and women in a control group were both shown erotic films while blood flow to the vagina and lubrication were measured. Women in the control group were physically aroused and able to report psychological arousal; measurements confirmed women with GAD were physically aroused, but denied the psychological feeling of arousal.

Thus, coexisting medical and psychological disorders must be ruled out (Buehler, 2011). Although as a mental health professional you cannot make a medical diagnosis, you need to know enough about biological factors to make an appropriate referral. All types of medical conditions can interfere with nerve signals and/or blood flow to erogenous areas of the body and genitals (Katz, 2007), including:

- Neurological conditions such as Parkinson's disease or multiple sclerosis
- Cardiovascular conditions such as high blood pressure or atherosclerosis (hardening of the arteries)
- Endocrine disorders including diabetes and thyroid conditions
- Pelvic surgery or trauma of any kind to the reproductive system

Hormone imbalances, particularly related to estrogen and testosterone levels, can affect sensitivity of tissues such as nipples and clitoris. Hormonal changes can occur due to stress, pregnancy and the postpartum period, hysterectomy, or the process of aging and menopause. Hormonal changes also regulate mood and behavior, which can also have an impact on a woman's ability to enjoy sex.

Varied psychological problems can intrude on a woman's experience of pleasure (Buehler, 2011), including major depression and dysthymia (mild, unrelenting depression); anxiety disorders such as GAD, Obsessive Compulsive Disorder (OCD), and Posttraumatic Stress Disorder (PTSD); Attention Deficit Disorder (ADD); substance abuse; eating disorders; and somatic disorders. The impact of each disorder on sexuality is more thoroughly addressed in Chapter 11. Stress due to work and family responsibilities and an oft-mentioned inability to relax are also psychological contributors.

Family of origin issues can also impede arousal. Women raised in homes where sex is taboo or associated with conservative religious upbringing may suppress physical and emotional feelings and fantasies before (Ahrold, Farmer, Trapnell, & Meston, 2011) or during sex (Penner & Penner, 2003). When women either decide to enter into a premarital sexual relationship (generally in their early 20s) or wait until marriage, they have often described to me the difficulty of "flipping the switch" from being a "good girl" to a fully sexually responsive woman (Penner & Penner, 2003). In terms of role models, many clients have awareness that parents may have had a sexless relationship. Sometimes, divorced parents model the same when they never date or remarry after the split.

There exists little research regarding the effects of relationship problems on arousal, but it isn't too difficult to imagine their effects, with lack of communication being perhaps the most common issue. Women may not tell or show their partner what they enjoy, often because they hold the belief that a good lover is so intuitive they can just figure it out, or embarrassment over admitting what they would really like to do. A related issue is sexual boredom, which can be painful to admit to a partner. Suggestions about assertive communication and role play may be necessary to help a woman tell her partner about her sexual needs at a given point in time.

Understanding messages a woman may have received from institutions involved in her development may be fruitful in assessing lack of arousal, such as:

- *Religion:* Sex is for procreation, not recreation.
- *School:* Sex is a reproductive event that involves particular organs of the body. It has nothing to do with the clitoris or orgasm (neither of which are ever mentioned in sex education class).
- *Media:* Bad girls have the most fun with sex; it's okay to fake orgasm.

Arousal levels may change with a woman's age and stage of life. When a woman is young and has high hormone levels, she may be just as desirous and aroused by sex as her suitors. After pregnancy, however, and especially while breastfeeding, hormone levels drop, as does sexual arousal. However, such broad statements may be damaging. Some women feel empowered and sexy after giving birth; some women, liberated from having menstrual periods and fear of unwanted pregnancy, find that menopause is one of the sexiest times they've experienced.

INTERVENTIONS FOR INCREASING AROUSAL

The initial suggestion is often a referral to the woman's gynecologist or, if available, a sexual medicine specialist to rule out or treat medical problems. In the meantime, you can make suggestions such as always applying a good quality lubricant to her own and her partner's genitals prior to intercourse. By making this a routine, it becomes incorporated into the couple's sexual script and eliminates pressure for a woman to demonstrate arousal, in the case that there are hormonal or other physical changes. Another suggestion is for the couple to incorporate sex toys such as vibrators, which can provide strong stimulation and enhance arousal. A third, for some couples, is to make use of erotica or fantasies to facilitate behaviors that are a turn-on.

Stress is readily addressed with relaxation techniques, assertiveness, and scheduling. Mild anxiety can also be addressed with brief cognitive and solution-focused interventions. If these do not suffice, then it is possible that you may want to refer the client for a psychiatric evaluation, more long-term psychological work, or make an agreement not to address sexual issues until the stress, anxiety, or other psychological problem has largely resolved.

Attention must be paid to communication. Simply giving a woman and/ or her partner permission to talk about sex in your office can be a helpful intervention. You can also assist the client with telling her partner under what conditions she is most likely to feel aroused, what activities she has enjoyed in the past or would like to try, or what type of setting she likes best (Sunday mornings in bed vs. Tuesday night after dance class).

Intensive therapy for problems with arousal is usually indicated when there is a comorbid sexual problem such as an aversion; a serious mental disorder such as PTSD; or when a woman and her partner are fighting about sex or involved in longstanding patterns of unresolved conflict (Buehler, 2011).

ANORGASMIA: PROBLEMS WITH EXPERIENCING ORGASM

An orgasm has been variously described as a peak experience, waves of pleasure, release of tension, or an ecstatic or even spiritual experience (Sayin, 2012). It occurs when arousal is so heightened that the body—especially the pelvic floor, genitals, and anus—tenses, then releases in a series of contractions that generally are felt as pleasure. Orgasm is also a psychological event in that pleasure-promoting neurochemicals including opioids are released. Orgasm encompasses a relational or bonding event in that the brain generates chemicals involved in attachment, such as oxytocin and prolactin (Sayin, 2012).

The capacity for orgasm falls along a normal distribution (Kingsberg & Althof, 2009), with anorgasmic women at one end, and women with Persistent Genital Arousal Disorder (PGAD) at the other (Facelle, Sadeghi-Nejad, & Goldmeier, 2013; Leiblum, Seehus, & Brown, 2007). (Women with PGAD have what they describe as being an unpleasant and frequent urge to have orgasm; more detail follows in Chapter 13.) Problems with having orgasm can be lifelong or acquired, and global or situational. While women who are truly anorgasmic may not be bothered by lack of orgasm, sometimes the partner may express dismay, interpreting anorgasmia as lack of sexual interest or even loving feelings. In such cases, partners must be counseled to accept and adapt to their partner's physical state.

Medical and physiological problems with orgasm include neurological disorders such as MS; chronic kidney disease; atherosclerosis and contributing factors that include smoking, diabetes, and hypertension; fibromyalgia; and pelvic conditions such as hypotonic (loose) pelvic floor or nerve damage (Finger, 2006; Ramage, 2006). Hormonal imbalances associated with menopause or disorders such as hypothyroid disease can cause a woman to be less sexually sensitive and responsive to pleasurable stimulation. Testosterone, in particular, is sometimes attributed to decreased sensation in the nipples and clitoris, while declining rates of estrogen and progesterone can contribute to lack of lubrication, atrophy and thinning of the vaginal walls, and uncomfortable sexual experiences. Declines in testosterone are not only associated with menopause; there is also a decline from ages 22 to 44, perhaps reflecting declining fertility as women age (Fooladi & Davis, 2012).

Mental illness can also interfere with orgasm. Depression causes not only a decrease in the perception of pleasure, but also a sense of isolation that can impede the emotional connection that can enhance arousal and orgasm (Baldwin, 2001; Baldwin & Mayers, 2003; Balon & Segraves; Clayton, 2007). Performance anxiety, whether self- or partner-induced (Elliott & O'Donohue, 1997), as well as concerns about body image are common complaints (Conner, Charlotte, & Grogan, 2004). Finally, while light consumption of alcohol may facilitate orgasmic response, heavy consumption of alcohol can suppress it (Johnson, Phelps, & Cottler, 2004), as can street drugs. In fact, sometimes women over-consume alcohol to avoid feeling sexual sensations, as might be the case in a woman molested as a child (Liebschutz et al., 2002).

Psychotropic medications, particularly selective serotonin reuptake inhibitors (SSRIs) such as fluoxetine (Prozac™), paroxetine (Paxil™), and sertraline (Zoloft™), as well as antipsychotics and mood stabilizers, can inhibit orgasm by elevating serotonin levels. An exception is nefazodone because its action in part counteracts the effects of elevated levels of serotonin. Buspirone, which is sometimes prescribed to facilitate orgasm and desire in women, also decreases the release of serotonin (Baldwin & Mayers, 2003; Balon & Segraves; Clayton, 2007).

A woman's lack of knowledge and familiarity with her own body is a major cause of anorgasmia. Women who are reticent to touch their own genitals with either hand or vibrator to masturbate are often uncomfortable with partner touch as well. This discomfort with one's body can lead to avoidance, which in turn can lead a woman to a lack sexual experience and development. Being unreceptive to a partner's attempts to excite can lead to feelings of guilt and increase performance anxiety.

In terms of the couple, a woman's lack of knowledge and inability to communicate to her partner what will arouse her and bring her to orgasm definitely contributes to problems. But partners are also sometimes ignorant and simply assume that all is well unless a woman complains. However, women can be too embarrassed to say anything or fearful that a complaint may make their partner feel inadequate.

STEP INTO MY OFFICE...

Referred to me by a couple's therapist, Felice complained that she had never had orgasm—not by herself, and not with her husband of 28 years. When I asked if her husband had ever checked in with her to see if she enjoyed their encounters, she looked at me with surprise and said, "No, and I never thought it was unusual that he didn't ask, but now that you mention it, it's kind of weird!" After several meetings geared toward developing rapport and educating Felice about the mechanism of orgasm, William came to the office with her. William explained that all these years he just thought Felice was enjoying herself. The couple admitted that they were both brought up in conservative households where no one talked about sex and that they were virgins when they married. Thus, neither one really had an idea of what was supposed to happen when a woman had orgasm, or how to get Felice to that point.

The first step toward helping Felice experience climax was getting the couple to overcome their shame and embarrassment so that they could simply talk to one another about sex. Fortunately, this couple was resilient in that they were able to compliment themselves on all the ways in which they had grown together and functioned well as a couple; other couples in the same circumstances do not always fare so well when a woman finally tells her partner that she has never had an orgasm.

Women are faced with overt and covert messages about female pleasure. If or when they attended a sex education class, women (and men) might be presented with an outline of the uterus, fallopian tubes, and ovaries—no mention of the vulva, clitoris, or vagina. They are sold products to freshen natural odors, sending the message that female genitals are "dirty." More recently, women are faced with physicians who are willing to provide "vaginal rejuvenation" and surgical reduction of the labia, with the implication that normal labia are unattractive. Finally, most women learn about orgasm from friends or the Internet, which can be a fount of misinformation, including Freud's misinformed idea that mature women have orgasm through intercourse. Even lesbian women sometimes need counseling to understand the importance of clitoral stimulation.

Maintaining control of one's sexual urges is a common cognition contributing to anorgasmia. Orgasm requires letting go of muscle tension as well as permitting the emotional experience of fun and pleasure. Many women raised with the message that "nice girls don't" or who have suppressed sexual fantasies and feelings in the service of religious beliefs often express that once they are in an appropriate relationship, it is difficult to "flip the switch." They have a hard time believing that they deserve pleasure and generally put much more energy into all other endeavors of a relationship than into sex.

INTERVENTIONS FOR FACILITATING ORGASM

Since there can be organic causes, you may need to refer a woman back to her gynecologist or appropriate specialist for evaluation and treatment, which can include hormonal testing and possible replacement unless counter indicated by her own and her family's health history. Bupropion (Wellbutrin) is sometimes recommended (Crenshaw, Goldberg, & Stern, 1987), while a small number of women benefit from sildenafil citrate (Viagra) which helps with blood flow and sensitivity of the labia and clitoris (Berman, Berman, Tolder, Gill, & Haughie, 2003). Topical applications such as Zestra, a botanical concoction that is rubbed into the labia and clitoris to encourage blood flow, may also be recommended (IsHak, Bokarius, Jeffrey, Davis, & Bakhta, 2010).* The Eros Clitoral Therapy Device™ is an FDA-approved device for the treatment of anorgasmia. It is a small vacuum pump that is applied over the clitoris for several minutes a day to provide blood flow and nerve repair (Wilson, Delk, & Billups, 2001). Clinically, women who have nerve damage, for example, due to diabetes, may find the Eros device a useful therapy (Billups, 2002).

You should have on hand a simple line drawing of female external genitals in order to review anatomy with your client, such as the worksheet found at the end of Chapter 3. Explain that most women need stimulation of the clitoris to achieve orgasm. In order to be able to tell a partner how to stimulate the clitoris in a way that is pleasing, a woman needs to be able to understand her own body. One common suggestion is to ask a woman to view her own genitals with a hand mirror if she has never seen them before so that she can identify—and admire—her own anatomy. There are also several good, contemporary books on female orgasm listed under *Resources*.

Strengthening the pelvic floor muscle can help increase the strength of sensation due to strengthening of nerves and improvement of blood flow to the genitals, as well as help a woman focus on feelings in the vulva and vagina as she tightens and relaxes the pubococcygeus muscle (IsHak et al., 2010). The exercises are described on page 33.

Everyone can benefit from learning deep breathing and other forms of relaxation, but women with anorgasmia need special encouragement to learn release of tension. While it may seem ironic that relaxation can help with arousal, if a woman is tense, no arousal or orgasm can occur. Deep breathing and progressive muscle relaxation-type activities can be helpful, as can scheduling time for rest and repair into a woman's schedule. For women who are entrenched in patterns of stress, more intensive cognitive work may be necessary to release them from the "musts" of life and to give themselves permission to take time for pleasure.

---

*If you are the one making the suggestion for this or any other over-the-counter botanical oil or warming lubricant, recommend that the woman check with her physician first before trying this or any other topical preparation in case of allergies or sensitivity.

Women might also be directed to masturbate. While this sounds clinical, in practice it is anything but. The idea is to help a woman become more comfortable with touching her own body and fantasizing about sex to increase arousal, which happens gradually at the woman's own pace (McCabe, 2009). She may start with familiar activities, such as bathing, during which she can allow herself to explore her erogenous areas while she is using soap or lotion. She can also touch her body a bit more while she is getting dressed, or touch herself over her clothing. Imagining times of physical and emotional pleasure can spur fantasies about sex. All of this prepares a woman for experimentation with actual masturbation, which can take place over many weeks. Telling a woman to use lubricant to make masturbation comfortable, giving herself permission to fantasize, and using different ways of stroking her clitoris and labia while staying relaxed will generally lead to orgasm. Once she is able to experience orgasm, she can transfer her understanding to her partner, either verbally directing his exploration and stimulation of her genitals, showing him what she does, or letting his hand "ride" on top of hers. The couple can also experiment with different sexual positions during intercourse to provide additional clitoral stimulation.

A woman and/or her partner may use vibrators of all types if manual stimulation seems not to provide enough "oomph" to get to climax (Ramage, 2006). This is as true in women who have primary anorgasmia as women who acquired the problem after menopause or other disruption. A vibrator can be instrumental in helping a woman who is frustrated experience orgasm more quickly. Once she learns the reward of orgasm and sees that none of her fears about losing control occurred, she may have an easier time with future attempts. Men (and in the case of lesbian relationships, sometimes women) find their partner's use of a vibrator threatening. This requires education on the part of the therapist, who can explain that anatomy differs from one woman to another or changes as we age, or that using a vibrator is akin to using a blender to make a smoothie—it simply does away with frustration. Vibrators that are smooth and less phallic in appearance may be more acceptable to both partners. Finally, there are also vibrators for men, who may enjoy them for stimulation during intercourse as with a vibrating ring, or during self-pleasure as with a prostate-stimulating device.

Many couples dispense with foreplay and go right to intercourse, with the expectation that they will experience simultaneous orgasm as an expression of love and passion. Sensate focus activities, described on the next page and on pages 81 to 82, allow a couple to decrease performance anxiety and approximate foreplay without the pressure of intercourse and orgasm (De Villers & Turgeon, 2005). It also allows a couple that has been struggling with sexual problems for a long time to establish or re-establish a foundation for future exploration. The activities are also a path to creating relaxation and arousal, two keys for experiencing the best sex.

ABOUT SENSATE FOCUS ACTIVITIES

Masters and Johnson's sensate focus activities have stood the test of time. Purists, such as those clinicians who were trained by the infamous pair, always give instructions in the same way. In my experience, by doing it in this way, I developed a good sense of the kinds of comments and concerns that come up with clients, such as not having enough time; feeling overwhelmed or detached during the activity; or not understanding the purpose. However, this lead me to a few modifications, including:

- Starting with something simpler and less intimate, such as a foot rub or hand massage
- Leaving clothing on for the first round of exercises, for example, for those with a sexual aversion or recovering from trauma
- Allowing clients to develop their own pace
- Permitting some clients to proceed to intercourse, if they both agree that they want to include this and if not contraindicated, for example, one or both partners do not have excessive performance anxiety

You can experiment and choose if you'd like to stay in the purist camp, or you'd like to be more flexible in your use of the activities with your clients.

In practice, most women who learn about orgasm are enthusiastic about trying out activities. Some women, however, have a history of trauma, relationship conflict or betrayal, or strong religious or cultural messages about women's sexuality. They are armored against their natural feelings, fearful of the chaos and the unknown, of punishment and shame. Those women who have been molested present a particular challenge in that they may have experienced physical pleasure during the abuse (Maltz, 2012). It is important to *normalize* that the body is made for pleasure and that the nervous system is not completely under conscious control. Cognitive behavioral therapy that addresses these fears, combined with a new understanding and perspective on one's sexual development, often helps women overcome barriers to pleasure.

SEXUAL AVERSION: OVERCOMING HATRED OF SEX

A woman (or man) is said to have a sexual aversion when she finds all or some aspects of sexual activity repulsive. Sexual aversion is associated with feelings of disgust, humiliation, shame, and low self-esteem (DSM IV-TR, 2000). The aversion can be to an act, such as oral sex or being penetrated; an odor, such as semen; a sensation, such as saliva during kissing or sweat; a body part, such as the woman's or partner's genitals; or even a sound, such as a partner's moan during orgasm. It can also be a thought or fantasy associated with sex. The aversion can be situational or generalized.

A woman may, for example, enjoy all aspects of sex except kissing, or she may avoid all sexual stimuli. The symptoms of sexual aversion include avoidance of sexual stimuli; physical symptoms typically associated with panic attacks; and nausea and vomiting. There is generally a disturbance in the woman's relationships, or she may never have been in a romantic or sexual relationship because of the aversion. Sometimes alcohol and drug use cover up a sexual aversion, as they allow a woman to numb herself for participation in sex even when the activity is unwanted.

The prevalence rate for sexual aversion is unknown, though it may develop early in life, perhaps due to negative sexual experiences. There has been some recent discussion about placing Sexual Aversion Disorder with Anxiety Disorders in the *DSM-5*, as it closely resembles a phobia (Brotto, 2010), but perhaps because it is so often associated with partner activity as well as learned social messages, it doesn't fit the criteria for that diagnostic category.

People usually drag a partner who has an aversion into therapy. Sometimes aversion initially looks like low desire, but aversion becomes apparent through statements such as, "I'd rather eat dirt than have sex," or developing somatic symptoms after sex, for example, migraine headaches. Someone with aversion may also hide their aversion, only confessing to a therapist when alone for fear of hurting their partner, who enjoys sex.

A differential diagnosis may also need to be made. For example, women with obsessive personality traits may participate in sex, but need to shower, change the sheets, execute rules about when sex will take place, spray the room with air freshener after sex, and so on, but may still enjoy the period when they are participating in the act with their partner. Painful sex, such as vaginismus, should also be ruled out. A woman who has vaginismus may actually enjoy other types of sexual activity, but be unable to relax enough to have intercourse. You also will need to assess for past sexual violation, as treatment for complex trauma differs from treatment for aversion due to sexual molestation or assault.

STEP INTO MY OFFICE...

Jo Ann developed a sexual aversion because her husband had pressured her since before marriage to have sex, coercing her by making her feel ashamed for having had sex a few times with other partners but not with him. Over time, giving in to her husband lead Jo Ann to feel repulsed when he touched her genitals or breasts. Thus, she avoided sex and they were active only once or twice a month, which led to escalating passive aggressive behavior by the husband, such as complaining and wheedling Jo Ann for sex, which was a further turn-off.

The prognosis for sexual aversion is generally guarded or poor, in part because treatment is long-term and intensive. The treatment plan consists of couples therapy if the woman is in a relationship; education; cognitive behavioral therapy; relaxation; and customized activities that are designed to help desensitize the woman to the unwanted sexual stimuli. It is highly individualized because of the variety of stimuli to which a woman can develop an aversion.

Cognitive work addresses maladaptive beliefs about sex, such as worry about getting pregnant by kissing, losing control during orgasm, or sex "always being for the man's benefit." Some exploration regarding where the myth originated can be helpful as the client may realize that what she heard as a child or teen doesn't fit the adult self's schema of sexuality.

To treat with systematic desensitization, employ the client's help in creating a hierarchy of activity from least to most noxious. In the case example above, the woman didn't mind if her husband stroked the tops of her thighs, but would start to feel nervous if he approached the inner thigh, so we identified a starting point for sensate-focus type activity. Choosing to do the touching activity with clothing on or off creates another step in the hierarchy, as from being touched on the inner thigh she thought she could manage being touched at the groin with clothing on as a next step. From there, she progressed to being touched on the *mons* with clothing on. She then repeated the sequence with clothing off and the couple next worked their way to the husband being able to touch her on her labia. The most important aspects are relaxation and building trust.

In couples therapy, the focus is often on issues of control. An aversion is a defense mechanism that controls either some aspect or nearly all of a person's sex life, including how emotionally close they can become to a partner. Creating an atmosphere of understanding and compassion between the couple helps them see that they are both part of the solution. As they work on the assignments together, they are strengthening their emotional bond as well as learning the elements of good sex: patience, knowledge, time, exploration, relaxation, arousal, and last but not least, love.

LOSING A NATURAL DRIVE: LOW DESIRE

Anecdotally, most every sex therapist reports that by far the most common female complaint is lack of interest in sex, perhaps because all other sexual problems interfere with desire. Additionally, people commonly have unrealistic beliefs about sex in their long-term relationships (Fisher, 2004a; McCarthy & McCarthy, 2003; Perel, 2007; Schnarch, 2009), particularly that while other aspects of their lives change, sex is somehow supposed to be static rather than an experience that grows and wanes in importance depending on the context of a woman's or a couple's life. However, one of the criteria for diagnosing low desire is that it is lower *than what would be expected* for a woman's age and stage of life. Most young women in good health feel a great deal of desire either to engage in a relationship or sexual activity, but few of them will have the same level of desire after the birth of a child or, even later in life, after menopause.

It can be either the woman or her partner who believes she should display all the signs of wanting and initiating passionate sex despite being stuck in a dull routine; failing to nurture compatibility; bickering; being uncooperative; or any number of relationship issues. No wonder various bloggers enjoy reporting that they would rather read a novel or eat chocolate than have sex, or that 25% of American marriages are what McCarthy & McCarthy called "sexless" in which sexual activity takes place less than a dozen times per year. Even though the stirrings of desire may naturally weaken, when they are completely absent—physically, mentally, and emotionally—a woman may feel that something is truly wrong.

Still, if a woman is distressed by her low desire or if it interferes with her relationship, then an assessment is warranted. It is critical to rule out any physical impediments, including conditions affecting the neurological, circulatory, or endocrine (hormone) system; pelvic surgery or trauma to the reproductive system; use of oral contraceptive pills (OCPs); hormonal changes resulting from pregnancy, the postpartum period, or breastfeeding; heavy smoking of nicotine or marijuana, which can restrict blood flow; or poor hygiene, for example, lack of sleep or exercise, eating a nonnutritious diet, and so on.

Low desire also needs to be differentiated from other psychiatric disorders, especially mood and anxiety disorders, including generalized anxiety, OCD, and PTSD (Buehler, 2011). Many women simply don't know the symptoms of mental illness, and even if they did, might not make a connection between the two. Other disorders that can affect desire include Bipolar Disorder, depressed phase; substance abuse; eating disorders; confusion about sexual orientation; adjustment disorder; and personality disorders, for example, avoidant personality.

Aside from psychiatric problems, any of the following may be present:

- Stress related to work and other responsibilities
- Conflicted relationships with immediate or extended family
- Inability to relax
- Religious or cultural beliefs that lead to suppressed sexual fantasies
- Traumatic sexual experiences

Finally, as with other sexual problems, you will need to ascertain whether the client is taking any psychotropic medications that are notorious for sexual side effects.

When it comes to desire, many therapists make the mistake of believing that if you fix a couple's problems outside the bedroom, the sexual problems will resolve on their own. The thinking is along the lines of, "No wonder this couple doesn't have sex, they fight all the time!" But I assure you, many couples that fight still have an active sex life. In fact, I would propose the reverse: Couples that have problems in the bedroom sometimes fight because they have never had a way to talk about sexual problems. When a woman cannot admit that she doesn't have orgasms or that sex is uncomfortable, she may begin to avoid sex, causing strife in the relationship.

Low desire is sometimes a play for power and control in the relationship. A woman who feels she has little to control except her body may deny her partner, ignoring the fact that she has needs, too. Problems with desire can also indicate a lack of differentiation, to the point that the low desire partner has felt engulfed during sex, or has "given in" so many times that a woman may no longer be in touch with her own urge for connection. If a woman has been coerced or manipulated into having sex through guilt or putdowns, she may also close the door to pleasure.

Myths about sexual desire also get in the way, such as:

- Men always have more desire.
- It is the man's place to initiate sex.
- Having sex is the ultimate sign of love.
- Sex is only good when it is spontaneous.

Finally, sometimes a woman lacks desire because her partner has a sexual dysfunction that he or she hasn't attended to. When a male partner, for example, has early ejaculation or erectile dysfunction, sex may become more of a drag than a pleasure. A partner may also have certain demands during sex, from requiring a woman to wear lingerie to asking, like one couple in my practice, for his partner to wear a skintight latex suit "because he didn't like to feel any roughness on my skin." Mental exhaustion from living with a partner who has alcoholism or drug dependence or other untreated mental illness will also play a role in low desire.

Mention must be made of the fact that in many cases of "low desire," couples actually have *mismatched* desire (McCarthy & McCarthy, 2003; Schnarch, 2009). When couples are mismatched in some other regard, say, the desire to cook or go dancing, they can frequently work these out through problem-solving and brainstorming. Because the topic of sex is so confusing and laden with emotion, couples can't work out their differences and avoid or fight about sex. Sex, like other aspects of a couple's life, can be negotiated—but some couples need a mediator to learn how to do so successfully.

TREATING HYPOACTIVE SEXUAL DESIRE

My observation is that many gynecologists have little interest in treating low desire, perhaps because there are very few medical treatments available. Though the correlation between testosterone and low desire is poorly correlated in women (Wierman et al., 2010), it occasionally is prescribed with some beneficial results. However, physicians are generally very cautious in prescribing testosterone for women because of unwanted side effects, including excessive hair, acne, irritability, and sexual hyperactivity. Testosterone is rarely recommended to women who have a family history of breast cancer because it is associated with overgrowth of cells. Thus, when possible, refer to a specialist in sexual medicine. Gynecologists will sometimes switch OCPs or change a woman's form of birth control if OCPs appear to be a culprit. Psychiatrists can be consulted regarding sexual side effects of psychotropic medications.

A safer and easier route is generally to help a woman manage her lifestyle. Whether working at a career or as a homemaker, many women need to learn how to manage stress, particularly in setting limits with others. Women also make unrealistic demands of themselves and must be persuaded to give up overly high standards to create time for relaxation and pleasure, both sexual and nonsexual. Other lifestyle changes include exercise to improve mood, body image, and body awareness. Many psychotherapists recommend yoga as a form of relaxation; meditation at the end of a yoga session can help a woman tune in to her feelings. Eating a healthful diet and getting adequate rest also provide energy and stamina for sexual activity.

Because so many couples complain of infrequent sex, most sex therapists will recommend that couples schedule sex, putting it on the calendar just as they would anything else of critical importance. Many couples balk at this suggestion, because they hold the belief that only spontaneous sex can be enjoyable. However, as pointed out by McCarthy and McCarthy, people don't look any less forward to a concert if they buy tickets ahead of time. The task then becomes helping the couple figure out *how* they would like sex initiated when it is scheduled, and *what activities* they would like on the "menu."

Intensive therapy for low desire may be required when it is attributed to problems related to sexual abuse; has resulted from the aftermath of the discovery of an affair; if there has been a major life change, such as cancer diagnosis or entry into a new phase of life; or if the couple cannot resolve their problem with information and suggestions. In fact, low or mismatched desire is probably the most common candidate for long-term therapy because it represents an ingrained pattern in the couple's dynamic. Because even therapists can fall into a pattern of avoiding sex and getting onto other topics, when treating desire problems it is important to continually check with the client or couple to see if progress is being made and to make adjustments in treatment as required.

ACTIVITIES

1. Educate yourself about the importance and use of lubricants. You may wish to purchase a few different types of lubricant and "road test" them either through intercourse or simply on your fingers so that you

can make some comparisons on your own. Identify some places in your vicinity or online where clients can purchase these items; these days, I am told, even drugstores in remote Montana carry such products. Think about how you will talk to your clients about using lubrication.

2. Do the same with vibrators. If you have never used a vibrator or the vibrator in your possession is from the dawn of time, it is especially time to conduct some research. Become acquainted with the local toyshop. Employees are usually well trained and will happily explain each type of vibrator and allow you to handle it. Don't forget to look at options for partners, such as vibrating rings that go on the penis (aka "cock rings").

3. Journal about your experience of going to the toyshop. How will you present this option to clients who have an aversion or who have never been to a toyshop before? Of course, some toyshops are more pleasant than others, and if the one in your area is not up to snuff, then see if there is one in a nearby locale that you think mainstream clients will find acceptable.

4. Look online at various sites as well. Many sites try to have something for everyone, and some have a lot of educational information.

5. Consider the ethics of selling such items; see Chapter 19.

6. Identify gynecologists in your area who have an interest in sexual medicine and develop a cross-referral relationship. Be prepared to talk to the gynecologist about how you can help their patients who have sexual complaints.

RESOURCES

Cass, V. (2007). *The elusive orgasm: A woman's guide to why she can't and how she can orgasm*. Cambridge, MA: Da Capo Press.

Follie, S., Kope, S. A., & Sugrue, D. P. (2011). *Sex matters for women: A complete guide to taking care of your sexual self* (2nd ed.). New York, NY: Guilford Press.

Goldstein, A., & Brandon, M. (2009). *Reclaiming desire: 4 keys to finding your lost libido*. Emmaus, PA: Rodale Books.

Mintz, L. B. (2009). *A tired woman's guide to passionate sex: Reclaim your desire and reignite your relationship*. Avon, MA: Adams Media.

Ogden, G. (2008). *The return of desire: A guide to rediscovering your sexual passion*. Boston, MA: Trumpeter.

Solot, D., & Miller, M. (2007). *I love female orgasm*. Cambridge, MA: Da Capo Press.

SENSATE FOCUS ACTIVITIES

William Masters and Virginia E. Johnson were the originators of sex therapy and this is their classic activity for couples. This series of activities is designed to do a number of things:

1. Focus you on pleasure instead of performance; decrease anxiety.

2. Increase a sense of connection.

3. Establish or re-establish a good sex life.

Here is the basic exercise. Variations follow. Please note, intercourse is off limits until the later stages of the activity.

Sensate Focus I

- You will be taking turns sensually caressing, stroking, and feeling your partner's hands, arms, feet, and legs.

- Set aside 20 minutes, three times during the week.

- Select a setting where you will have uninterrupted privacy. You can make the scene romantic with music, candles, and so on.

- Agree to do this activity either clothed or lightly clothed, for example, shorts and tank top.

- You will split the 20 minute time into two 10 minute periods. One of you will be the receiver and one the giver of touch during each 10 minute period.

- You can use a coin to decide who will go first if you'd like. You can also decide ahead of time how you want to either plan or figure out who will initiate first.

- One of the reasons the word "focus" is in the title of this activity is that you are supposed to "focus" on your own sensations instead of your partner's responses (or what you *think* are your partner's responses). If what you are doing to your partner feels good to you, chances are very good it also feels good to your partner.

- Try to talk as little as possible during the exercise. You can give feedback later, perhaps the next morning or sometime before you repeat the activity. Refrain from giving feedback right after the activity when your partner's defenses may be down. They may feel too vulnerable then to take in your suggestions such as the fact that you need firmer touch.

Sensate Focus II

- Sensate Focus II includes exploration of the breasts and genitals.

- Follow the guidelines in Sensate Focus I regarding time, frequency, and tuning in to one's own sensations.

- Start the activity with general touching of the hands, arms, feet, and legs; don't move immediately to the breasts or genitals.

- You can do this activity nude or with light clothing, as you prefer.

- Try including a "hand riding" technique. When it is your turn to be the receiver, place your hand on your partner's hand to gently guide them into understanding how much pressure, how fast or slow, or what particular areas you like to have caressed. Don't take control; just add a little input to what the giver is doing.

Sensate Focus III

- Same idea as Sensate Focus I and II, but now the touching is mutual.

- Shift your attention to your enjoyment of your partner's body.

- If you become highly aroused, take a little break and resume touching. The point is to enjoy the journey, not just the destination.

Sensate Focus IV and V

- Continue as in previous activity sessions.

- At some point, move to the female-on-top position without attempting insertion of the penis into the vagina.

- In this position, the woman can rub her clitoris, vulva, and vaginal opening against her partner's penis regardless of whether or not there is an erection.

- Eventually, the woman can insert the tip of the penis into the vagina if there is an erection. Go back to nongenital pleasuring if either partner becomes anxious.

- After doing this type of play a few times, you will most likely feel ready for intercourse. Keep the focus on your sensations and on nondemand pleasuring.

From Buehler, S. (2011). *Sex, love, and mental illness: A couple's guide to staying connected.* Santa Barbara, CA: Praeger.

EXPERIENCING ORGASM

- Learning to self-pleasure through masturbation is the key to understanding what makes your body feel good so you can tell your partner during sex. If you have shame about your body or masturbation, talk to your therapist.

- In order to have an orgasm, you need to be aroused. You can become aroused by reading or looking at erotic material, having a sexual fantasy, or exploring your body.

- If it is difficult to get aroused, try relaxing first in the bathtub, listening to soothing music, or getting a massage.

- You will know if you are aroused if your genitals feel more sensitive. Usually, your vagina will also be lubricated. There may be other signs that are visible, like the clitoris growing larger. You can use a mirror to notice such changes and to help you understand your sexual anatomy.

- How much friction and pressure to apply to the clitoris is a personal preference. Sometimes women find that a very light touch is best. Others need a strong touch or even powerful vibration from a toy. Still others will rub the *mons pubis*—the fatty pad of tissue covering the pubic bone—while others rub or even gently tug the labia. There is no right way—so have fun experimenting!

- If you feel your excitement build, then you find yourself putting on the brakes, you may be afraid of letting go or getting out of control. Make sure your environment makes you feel comfortable—that the door is locked and you have privacy.

- To keep building excitement, try moaning, which sends a fresh signal to the brain that you are excited. Some women find it helps to move their pelvis around in small circles, or to rock it up and down. You can also massage your breasts, buttocks, or inside of your thighs to keep sexual energy turned up.

- Women experience orgasm in lots of different ways. You may feel warm tingles up and down your body. Your muscles may contract and let go. You may thrash around, or you may get very still. Some women simply have a feeling of bliss or peace. Enjoy discovering your own orgasm style.

- When you are ready, you can let your partner know what you like by describing it. Or you can show your partner by having your partner ride your hand. Of course, you can also learn to have orgasm with your partner's help, if that is better or more arousing for you.

- Don't get discouraged. Just enjoy pleasuring yourself whenever you feel like it, that is, when you feel aroused, have had a fantasy, or when you have private time to experiment.

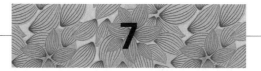

Men's Sexual Problems

A common cliché related to sexuality and gender is, "Women are so much more complex than men." Not so. Consider the example of a man who ejaculates more quickly than he'd like, who then develops a level of anxiety that impedes erections. This, in turn, may engender low desire and avoidance. In fact, men with sexual problems struggle just as much, if not more, than do women due to stereotypes like, "Men are always ready for sex," or "For men, sex has nothing to do with love."

According to the *DSM-5* (2013), male sexual disorders include

- Premature (Early) Ejaculation
- Delayed Ejaculation
- Erectile Dysfunction
- Male Hypoactive Sexual Desire Disorder

In men, the sexual response from desire to arousal to climax tends to be more linear and reflective of the Masters and Johnson model, as men experience a considerably more automatic response to sexual stimulation. Interestingly, until a few decades ago problems related to erectile function and ejaculation were thought to be primarily psychogenic; treatment consisted of psychoanalysis or marginally successful behavioral interventions. Currently, the field of sexual medicine believes male sexual dysfunction is mainly due to physical problems. But there is still a place for mental health professionals in treating male sexual dysfunction, since medical interventions are not always dependable or effective on their own, and there still exist cases that are more psychological than physical.

SOCIAL MYTHS AROUND MALE SEXUAL FUNCTION AND EXPRESSION

Despite major shifts in gender roles in American society, men are still raised with high performance standards. Boys are expected to demonstrate control over their inner life as well as physical capabilities to demonstrate their strength. Sports often dominate a boy's life, and this is an area where performance demands are often first internalized and carried into adolescence and adulthood; in adulthood there are demands to be successful on the job and provide for one's family.

Many men get no more sex education from their parents than a warning to prevent pregnancy and sexually transmitted diseases (STDs), contributing to a hands-off, "boys will be boys" approach to sexual development. Add to this a social atmosphere in which boys and teens learn about sex from their peers, who may brag or even exaggerate about sexual experiences.

Conversely, they may be influenced by religious messages that prohibit sex until marriage. Since 60% of male adolescents lose their virginity during high school (Halpern & Hardon, 2012), men who wait until adulthood are often behind the curve, which creates feelings of inadequacy and possibly disappointment for a partner due to their lack of technique. They may also be sexually inhibited and unable to identify or express sexual needs, which can lead to unfulfilling sexual encounters.

Men are bombarded with almost as many models of physical perfection as women are. A large upper torso and biceps and small hips create the "ideal" male figure at a time when male obesity is higher than ever, creating anxiety over appearance. Men are also getting more plastic surgery, with facelifts, chin implants, and even "pec" implants. In reality, not every man is a movie star or celebrity athlete. Men are not superheroes. They are just what they are: human beings, with feelings and thoughts about themselves. In the wake of all the messages about masculinity and power, devastating looks, and fabulous income, it is no wonder that many men doubt themselves in the bedroom.

WHEN ERECTION DISAPPOINTS

While the prevalence of ED varies according to study, about 20% of men over the age of 30 have had some experience with this disorder, defined as the inability to attain or maintain an erection as desired (Albersen, Orabi, & Lue, 2012; Dandona & Rosenberg, 2010). The older a man is, the more at risk for developing problems with erections. In order to be diagnosed, ED must be associated with personal distress.

ED is considered a harbinger of cardiovascular disease, particularly atherosclerosis (hardening of the arteries), affecting blood supply to the penis (Tan, Tong, & Ho, 2012). This symptom is commonly treated with medications such as Viagra™, Levitra™, and Cialis™, which are known as *PDE5 inhibitors* (Wylie & Kenney, 2010). These medications work by stopping or inhibiting the chemical action that causes blood to leak out of the penis, thereby allowing the penis to appropriately fill with blood for an erection.

The medications for ED have created a vital pharmaceutical industry around sexual medicine. It is impossible to watch evening television without a reminder that a man can perform "when the moment is right," if he takes his medication. In my clinical observation, physicians are quick to prescribe PDE5 inhibitors, even to young men simply wanting performance enhancement, and often without examination. Because men frequently receive such prescriptions without counseling, they may hold a belief that taking a pill will cause an instantaneous erection, that the man's partner will be excited about the use of medication, or that medication will override problems such as performance anxiety and inadequate arousal (Gambescia, 2009). Lastly, men often don't recognize that as they age they have more need for foreplay in order to have an erection, inadequate arousal being the leading cause for discontinuation of medication (Stimmel & Gutierrez, 2007).

There are several other types of medical approaches to treating ED, which are used when PDE5 inhibitors are ineffective, or when side effects (runny nose, headache, backache, flushing, and eye disturbances) are intolerable. Before oral PDE5 inhibitors were invented, the same type of medication was injected into the penis using a syringe and a tiny needle. This treatment, called *intracavernous injection*, is still available, but has obvious drawbacks in that administration can be painful and injections can cause scarring. There is also a medication called MUSE that is a pellet that is inserted into the urethra through the tip of the glans. Finally, there is a surgical option of a penile implant, a device that pumps up the chambers within the penis to create an erection. This option is used when all other options have failed because it is irreversible and has all the risks inherent with other types of surgery. It is generally considered when a man is in a relationship with a sexually healthy and willing partner.

Additional ailments that can cause ED include neurological conditions such as multiple sclerosis (MS), Parkinson's disease, brain tumor, stroke, and epilepsy; diabetes; prostatectomy; Peyronie's disease (curvature of the penis); psoriasis; chronic pain; psychiatric disorders; and any trauma to the pelvic area (Wylie & Kenney, 2010). Hormone imbalances, particularly low testosterone, can cause ED. Another problem of which many men are unaware is cycling, as the posture and seat on the bicycle can lead to compressed nerves (Sommer, Goldstein, & Korda, 2010). Medications can also be culprits, particularly psychotropic medications, cardiovascular medications, and medications that affect the endocrine system (Baldwin & Mayers, 2003).

Psychological issues, especially anxiety and depression, commonly contribute to ED (Baldwin, 2001). It can be fruitful to assess how a male client copes with any and all kinds of stress. Does he expect himself to be able to perform under any circumstance? Men who abuse alcohol (Atjamasoados, 2003; Fahrner, 1987), chronically use marijuana or other street drugs (Johnson et al., 2004), or who submit themselves to unrelenting work stress are also at risk for ED. Men affected by posttraumatic stress disorder (PTSD), whether due to past sexual abuse, service in the armed forces, or from disaster, may also struggle (Buehler, 2011).

STEP INTO MY OFFICE...

Mitchell, a medical student who had just turned 26, visited several physicians to figure out why he could no longer perform sexually with his girlfriend, of whom he was very fond. When no physical cause could be determined, he was referred to me for assessment. Mitchell denied any anxiety, and indeed, he appeared to be a self-controlled, confident man—which also made him fairly well defended. After three sessions I uncovered the fact that he had tried to have sex while recovering from bronchitis. When his body hadn't performed as expected, he became even more tired and felt "bad all over." It seems he had developed symptoms of depression that he did not recognize. Once we created a timeline of symptoms and sexual problems, things began to make sense. Mitchell came to session four to thank me; no additional treatment was needed.

Like Mitchell, many men don't recognize symptoms of depression in themselves. Because they are socialized to hold in their feelings, they do not experience sadness or report it to others. Thus, they may not connect grief, loss, ending of a relationship, or other stress with ED (Gambescia, 2009). ED may obscure a man's underlying relationship problems, such as high levels of conflict and lack of intimacy, feeling undesired, or a partner's lack of response to romantic or sexual overtures. ED may also be a response to a partner's sexual dysfunction (Metz & McCarthy, 2004). Issues concerning pregnancy and disagreements about starting or adding to a family can erode a man's desire for intercourse.

IMPROVING ERECTILE FUNCTION AND SEXUAL CONFIDENCE

Even if the cause of ED appears clearly psychogenic, refer male clients to an urologist specializing in sexual medicine (see *Resources*) for hormone testing and possible medication; men in their 20s or 30s who appear fit can have low testosterone. If low testosterone is the culprit, it may have done some psychological damage that you can help the client repair. Often, a PDE5 inhibitor is simultaneously prescribed to quickly provide sexual confidence; with older men, the medication may need to be used on a regular basis. You should also refer the client back to the prescribing physician if they are on antidepressant or other medication known to interfere with erections.

There is a lot of erroneous information on the Internet, so plan to spend time educating the client and his partner about mind/body connections and ED; that is, the same nerves that contribute to an erection also create the experience of thoughts and feelings. When thoughts and feelings conflict with pleasure signals in the brain, a man's erection can disappear. Clients can also benefit from lifestyle changes, including losing weight, exercising, and quitting tobacco (Metz & McCarthy, 2004). Deep breathing and head-to-toe relaxation on a regular basis help create a new baseline from which a man can better cope with stressful demands. They can also help the client to slow down and get in touch with the sensations of his body, which can aid in arousal. Tips for changing one's lifestyle and improving erectile function can be found on the Client Worksheet, "Tips for Better Erections," at the end of this chapter.

Counseling men regarding PDE5 inhibitors can be essential. These medications are among the most prescribed in the world, but in my experience their use is not well understood by men or their partners, and physicians who prescribe don't necessarily take time to counsel. Men need to know they need stimulation in order to get and stay aroused, otherwise the nerve signals to the penis and the tissues within it will not be able to do their job, with or without the medication. You will need to counsel men to identify what they like—and don't like—in the bedroom and to communicate it to their partner.

Intensive therapy is generally recommended if problems with erections are long-standing; there is excessive guilt and shame associated with sex; the client is an adult virgin or delayed first intercourse until late in life; there is a history of molestation; the couple is recovering from infidelity on the part of either partner; there is a comorbid psychiatric disorder; or the client is experiencing the loss of a marriage or partner, whether through divorce or death. Men who have little insight may also need more sessions to help them understand how their inner life is affecting their sexuality.

From a behavioral standpoint, Masters and Johnson originally developed sensate focus activities to help men and their partners eliminate performance anxiety (De Villers & Turgeon, 2005). As written, they seem pretty straightforward, but their application—in private, in the comfort of the couple's bedroom—can be revelatory. For example, a man may have difficulty receiving touch, perhaps because he feels he doesn't deserve it, that it isn't manly to need touch to stay erect, or because he doesn't think of himself as "touchy-feely." Sensate focus activities may be exactly what is needed for the couple to learn or relearn how to play and experience each other without pressure. A worksheet and information about the use of sensate focus activities can be found in Chapter 6.

Intensive cognitive therapy is sometimes necessary to correct sexual myths, cope with anxiety, and increase sexual self-esteem. The client is advised to log his thoughts about sexuality between sessions to discern themes and then create counter statements. You can also work directly with myths such as, "I should always be ready for sex when my partner wants it," "Intercourse is the only kind of sex worth having," "I need to be able to perform like the men in porno," and so forth.

THE PROBLEM OF EJACULATING QUICKLY

Early, or premature, ejaculation causes frustration and embarrassment in males (Althof, 2006; Jannini & Porst, 2011; Palmer & Stuckey, 2008; Rowland & Cooper, 2011). It can lead to performance anxiety and thus can be a contributing factor to ED or avoidance of sexual activity. Couples where the male ejaculates quickly may feel that they are missing out on the emotional closeness brought by intercourse. Unfortunately, partners are not always kind when a man cannot control his ejaculation. They may feel that their partner is being inconsiderate and has no interest in whether or not they achieve orgasm. In single men, early ejaculation can create low self-esteem and an unwillingness to enter into a new relationship, particularly if a past partner expressed disappointment. In all men, the shame of early ejaculation can lead to an avoidance of sex and low desire.

Early ejaculation (sometimes also referred to as "rapid ejaculation") is sometimes considered to be the most common male sexual problem. If, however, the International Society for Sexual Medicine's (ISSM) *Guidelines for the Diagnosis and Treatment of Early Ejaculation* (2010) is used, only about 1% to 3% of men have early ejaculation:

> *A male sexual dysfunction characterized by ejaculation which always or nearly always occurs* prior to or within about one minute *of vaginal penetration, and the inability to delay ejaculation on all or nearly all vaginal penetrations, and negative personal consequences, such as distress, bother, frustration, and/or the avoidance of sexual intimacy.*

Although the ISSM definition appears accurate, it has also been called problematic for a few reasons, one being that early ejaculation is defined within the context of heterosexual penis–vagina intercourse; what about oral sex or male with male sex? Also, it doesn't encompass the large number of men and their partners who suspect or perceive that they do not last as long as they would like from penetration to ejaculation, which averages about five minutes. Men may not meet the exact criteria for early ejaculation, but that doesn't mean that they couldn't benefit from or do not want to learn ways to increase ejaculatory control. All that being said, the majority of women do not have orgasm from thrusting during intercourse, so if a man desires to last longer it is good form to assess why that is and determine with the client if this is a worthwhile treatment goal. Additionally, a female partner may need to be educated that she needs clitoral stimulation before, during, or after intercourse if she wants to experience orgasm in the presence of her partner, rather than depending upon or demanding her male partner "give" her an orgasm.

STEP INTO MY OFFICE...

Jason called on a Tuesday morning, demanding to be seen quickly. It seems that his marriage had been on a precipice, and he had systematically gone about making repairs through several weeks of concentrated couples therapy. Now that his relationship was stable, Jason, a successful business man who traveled the world looking at investments, wanted to tackle a longstanding problem that he wanted to discuss in my office today!

What was this pressing issue, I wondered? His hurry should have clued me in: He complained of early ejaculation. After listening to him tick off all the things he had done to right his marriage—cut his travel, participated in family functions, took his wife out on weekends—satisfying his wife sexually was the last frontier.

What was happening? Hanging his head, Jason admitted that he usually lasted "only" about 10 minutes, a problem that had bothered him for years. It took almost 30 minutes to educate Jason that 10 minutes was more than respectable, that he shouldn't base his self-esteem on his ability to control ejaculation, and that sex didn't have to be a performance, and another 20 minutes for Jason to realize my point. In one session, a case of early ejaculation solved!

At one time, a man with early ejaculation was seen as neurotic and treated with psychoanalysis. Later, Masters and Johnson viewed early ejaculation as a conditioned response to be addressed through behavioral interventions, for example, the "squeeze" technique (the man stops intercourse and his partner squeezes the glans of the penis until the urge to ejaculate subsides) or the "stop-start" technique (the man stops intercourse altogether until he feels he has enough ejaculatory control to resume activity).

While most treatment still focuses on the development of ejaculatory control, early ejaculation is now viewed as the result of biological differences, psychological factors, or a combination of both. From a medical standpoint, rat studies have suggested that serotonin receptors in the brain may be at a lower set point in men with early ejaculation, creating more sensitivity in nerves leading to and from the penis. There have also been studies suggesting that early ejaculation may be hereditary. Early ejaculation may also be caused by thyroid imbalance, as well as *prostatitis* (inflammation of the prostate gland) or chronic pelvic pain.

DEVELOPING EJACULATORY CONTROL

Men who have early ejaculation often have a combination of low self-esteem and anticipatory anxiety, making it essential to build trust through good rapport; I personally find that I spend more time on the intake call than I do with individuals with any other type of disorder. Once rapport is created, the next step is to generate treatment expectations. Helping a man to have 3 minutes of control if he currently ejaculates prior to penetration may be realistic, whereas 10 minutes may not; another beneficial goal often is helping the client and his female partner improve the woman's capacity for orgasm.

Another aspect that needs to be brought up as treatment commences is the issue of using medication. Since men who take antidepressants sometimes complain of a side effect of delayed ejaculation (DE), pharmacists saw promise in paroxetine (Paxil™) as a medical treatment for early ejaculation (Ralph & Wylie, 2005), and it is in fact the treatment of choice for many men, who often have tried over-the-counter anesthetizing sprays, creams, and condoms without desired results. However, paroxetine can have unwanted side effects including nausea, sleepiness, and dry mouth. Like any antidepressant, it can also interfere with libido (Althof, 2006). Paroxetine also must be taken either about 4 hours before sexual activity to have the desired effect or daily in some patients. Nonetheless, it can be a viable option and needs to be discussed with the client as either a complete or adjunctive treatment. If the client chooses medication, then a referral can be made to an urologist.

In terms of education, keep explanations of early ejaculation simple to avoid "analysis paralysis" by an anxious male client. I like to use an analogy between nervousness and "noise." Any "noise" from anxiety makes the nerves to and from the penis and pelvic floor area overly sensitive to stimulation. Let the client know there are techniques to quiet the noise, including relaxation techniques such as deep breathing, progressive muscle relaxation variations, and the mindful awareness of one's body. Another way to increase control is through the strengthening of the pelvic floor muscles, which is thought to make them less sensitive to vibration (Metz & McCarthy, 2004).

Directed masturbation can also be recommended, and it is a particularly suitable activity for a single male client. Presented here is a variation on the various behavioral techniques such as "stop/start," where a man simply stops masturbating or having intercourse until his arousal subsides, or the "squeeze technique," where a man stops intercourse and has his partner reach down to squeeze the glans of the penis until arousal subsides. I would call it "mindful masturbation," because I emphasize to the client that he is to stay in the present moment and to pay passionate attention to what is happening in his body—to connect his physical feelings to levels of arousal.

The client begins by masturbating with a dry hand, stopping and starting as he would with a partner during sexual activity, and gradually increasing time to ejaculation and orgasm. He then masturbates with a well-lubricated hand to more closely approximate the human vagina. Finally, he can use a device called a "vaginal sleeve" such as a Fleshlight™, which replicates the sensation of intercourse. He can then generalize this to partner intercourse. Another technique is for a man to create a scale in which "10" represents the point of ejaculation when he masturbates. He then must pay attention to his body—his muscle tension and respiration and heart rate—to determine what a "9" feels like, then an "8," and so forth. He can then masturbate with the goal of staying at around 6 to 7 on the scale for increasing periods of time. The steps are described on the Client Worksheet, "Tips for Lasting Longer," at the end of this chapter.

Very little is made in the research literature of the connection between feelings and early ejaculation. Metz and McCarthy (2004) alone make mention of a man's need to identify his emotional feelings in order to get in touch with his physical feelings. What I have observed is that men with early ejaculation often rush through everything—they even *arrive early* to appointments. Feelings that go unexpressed are built up in the body and held in the musculature in ways that may not be well understood or realized by a man who is socialized to feel very little. When the opportunity to be sexual arrives, all the feelings that are stored up may break through in the rush of orgasm. I have learned it is often very helpful to have a man log his feelings throughout the day, at the same time practicing relaxation and mindfulness.

Just as important as feelings are the client's thoughts, which may be barriers to treatment. You most likely will need to help the client identify and counter negative thoughts such as "What if this happens again?" and "I'll never get this figured out." For example, the client can tell himself, "I am learning more control, which I may not always have, but I know I can improve" or "I'm developing improvement, not aiming for perfection." Cognitive therapy also can be used to increase self-confidence and dispel myths, such as a man's worth and identity are based upon how long he lasts or that he must be able to last a long time to help his partner have orgasm. The partner's myths can also be addressed, such as a belief that the couple's relationship depends upon length of intercourse or that the male is selfish or uncaring if he ejaculates too quickly.

Couples counseling may also be required. By the time couples reach out for help or the topic comes to light in the treatment room, they have experienced shame, sadness, anger, and blame over their seemingly lackluster sex life. Simply by normalizing to couples that this is a common problem that can be difficult to treat and removing blame by reassuring them that there was no reason for them to know how to treat this can help a couple feel relieved. Creating realistic goals such as having more fun and emotional connection whether or not intercourse lasts and a sense of being a team with both parties being responsible for their own sexual pleasure and self-esteem develop an optimistic outlook and bonds the couple.

WHEN EJACULATION DOESN'T OCCUR AS EXPECTED

Male orgasmic disorder, also known as delayed ejaculation (DE), is one of the least understood male sexual problems. DE is defined as a delay in, or absence of, orgasm in a male following normal sexual excitement and arousal during sexual activity. The *DSM-IV-TR* (2000) has been criticized for not including criterion that the man needs to feel distressed in order for DE to be diagnosed; the *DSM-5* now includes this criteria. In addition, there is no criterion for how long is too long in terms of delay; one man's frustration may be another man's triumph and vice versa.

DE can be lifelong, generalized to all types of sexual stimuli and/or partners, or situational. If it is situational, it may occur only during coitus, masturbation, oral sex, or other activity, or only while a man is with a partner but not when masturbating alone, and so forth. It is considered to be relatively rare; the Laumann study (1999) reported that it occurs in about 8% of the population, while another study suggests that lifelong DE is even rarer, about 1.5 cases in 1,000 (Waldinger & Schweitzer, 2005). In clinical sex therapy practice, however, I have found it to be a common complaint, perhaps because there are few places men can turn to when encountering this issue.

DE can occur because of low testosterone, traumatic or surgical spine injuries, or neurological disorders that decrease sensitivity in the genitals such as MS or neuropathy associated with diabetes (Richardson, Nalabanda, & Goldmeier, 2006). Pelvic surgery, for example, radical prostatectomy, can also cause DE. Some drugs, including SSRIs, tricyclic antidepressants, antipsychotics, or heavy consumption of alcohol, can contribute to delayed climax, as can the effects of aging, including sexual organ atrophy, lower testosterone levels, reduced erection quality (and therefore sensitivity), and decline in the intensity of orgasm. Beginning intercourse prior to an appropriate level of arousal may also be a factor (Rowland, Keeney, & Slob, 2004). Conversely, men sometimes develop a style of masturbation that makes it difficult to generalize the experience to other types of sexual stimulation, for example, vaginal intercourse.

Emotional and mental factors vary widely and include fear of pregnancy or contracting a STD, psychiatric illness such as depression or schizophrenia, environmental distractions, and chronic viewing of pornography. The latter activity can lead to the need for more stimulation than can be obtained in most ordinary sexual situations, as well as feelings of shame or guilt when the man is with his partner (Perelman & Rowland, 2006). Men also sometimes do not recognize their own need for sexual stimulation and arousal prior to performing intercourse; they assume that as long as they have an erection, they are ready for sex.

Myths exist that men who have DE have been viewed as being hostile to their partner or to have an excessive need for control. Female partners sometimes will blame themselves, fearing that their partner does not find them attractive. In reality, a man sometimes will work so hard at pleasing his partner that he forgets his own needs or loses awareness of his own arousal.

STEP INTO MY OFFICE...

The presentation of DE is varied, as is its treatment, as evidenced by the following two vignettes.

Travis

Travis is a 24-year-old newly married man who hasn't been able to ejaculate while having sexual activity with his wife. Travis and his wife were sexually active before marriage, except for intercourse, and Travis always assumed that once he was married and "everything was legal" he would have no problem ejaculating. Travis also had a history of panic attacks, so it was easy to assume that anxiety was the major contributing factor. However, upon thorough assessment, Travis admitted that from about the age of 15 he had been able to ejaculate while watching pornography with an interesting twist: he used a terry cloth hand towel to masturbate so that he could quickly hide any evidence of activity.

I gave Travis the suggestion of masturbating first with a dry hand, and next with lubrication, which Travis did without any problem. However, the DE showed no improvement. Now I recommended that Travis only ejaculate when he was with his wife. After 2 weeks, Travis reported that he had "almost" climaxed. I then met with the couple and we discussed that Travis might need more foreplay than his wife was used to if he was going to have orgasm with her. Two weeks later, Travis came into my office smiling, clearly pleased that he had resolved a problem he found most embarrassing.

Norman

At age 81, Norman was in seemingly good health but was bothered by his lack of erections and DE while his wife of some 40 years was still enjoying their sex life and regular orgasms. Norman visited an urologist, who administered an injection of alprostadil, which didn't help. Because of Norman's advanced age, the urologist could not recommend surgery for a pump, and referred Norman to me.

Norman was very open-minded about sex and we developed rapport quickly. I told him, though, that because of his advanced age we could probably assume that the small arteries going to the penis were hardened, causing his erection to be less firm and stimulation more difficult to perceive, which lead to DE.

Norman was surprised to learn that, in men, orgasm and ejaculation are two different events and that men are able to have orgasm without ejaculation. We discussed how different parts of the body—the so-called erogenous zones where skin is more enervated, the perineum, and the anus—might still have enough sensitivity to produce orgasm with adequate stimulation. Then I surprised Norman with two more suggestions: a vibrator and pelvic floor exercises. The vibrator would add more stimulation, and it and the pelvic floor exercises would bring blood flow and hopefully nerve growth to the penis. Norman left my office like a man on a mission to shop for sex toys.

LOSS OF SEXUAL DESIRE IN MEN

The *DSM-5* has made a significant distinction between low sexual desire in men and women. Male Hypoactive Sexual Desire Disorder (MHSDD) is now diagnosed when a man's desire is lower than would be expected for his age and stage of life. The existence of low desire must cause distress to the individual himself.

One of the most damaging aspects of HSDD in men is the myth that men *always* have more desire than women. However, sexual desire in men exists along a continuum from minimal to robust, and most sex therapists report they have as many calls for help from women as men with a complaint of low desire. Prevalence rates vary, ranging from 14% to 28%, with the largest increase in men over 55 largely attributable to *hypogonadism*, or decreasing levels testosterone (Dandona & Rosenberg, 2010). Hypogonadism has also been coined as *andropause*, which can be thought of as analogous to a woman's menopause. Symptoms of andropause include depression, fatigue, lack of energy, and poor concentration, as well as sexual symptoms like ED and low desire.

However, the concept of andropause is not well-researched, and its existence is still being debated, as these symptoms are also associated with normal aging (Pines, 2011). In all men, testosterone naturally decreases slowly over time, beginning at about age 35. By the time a man reaches his 40s or 50s, he may notice a decrease in sexual interest, which is considered normal. It is only when the decrease in an older man is more than might be expected—for example, decreasing from a desire to have sex 2 to 3 times a week to less than once a month—that unbalanced hormone levels and treatment with hormone supplementation needs to be considered.

That being said, low testosterone or other medical conditions can be a factor at any age. Medical problems affecting desire include cardiovascular disease and neurological problems from illnesses such as MS and Parkinson's disease (although the treatment for Parkinson's can sometimes cause an *increase* in sexual desire) (Dandona & Rosenberg, 2010). Medications can also cause decreased desire, such as selective serotonin reuptake inhibitors (SSRIs), antianxiety medications, mood stabilizers (e.g., lithium) (Baldwin & Mayers, 2003), drugs that treat cardiovascular disease like antihypertensives to control blood pressure (Neel, 2012), and recreational drugs including alcohol, nicotine, heroin, and marijuana (Buehler, 2011).

In cases where a man's testosterone levels are normal and he is otherwise fit, then problems such as comorbid mental illness or other sexual dysfunction such as ED or early ejaculation must be ruled out (DeRogatis et al., 2012). However, low desire can be lifelong, even in men who are healthy. Some men simply have less interest in sex than average. Clinically, they might report something like, "Sex is okay, but not as important as other guys think it is." They may also have a history of partners who have shared an observation that they don't seem very interested in sex.

Low desire in men, of course, can be situational. If a man masturbates when he is alone, even though his partner is available, he cannot be said to have low drive. He may turn to self-gratification because of difficulties with emotional intimacy and communication, relationship conflict, fear of rejection or partner's complaints about performance, and dissatisfaction with quality of sex. He may have become unhappy with physical changes in a partner over time, like weight gain, or even due to surgical changes as may occur with treatment for breast cancer. In terms of having a partner who is ill, men sometimes lose sexual interest because they do not want to intrude on their partner with their needs.

Additionally, men may develop negative beliefs about sex, particularly as they age and experience changes in their body, such as requiring more stimulation for an erection; they view themselves as sexually inadequate and lose interest. Beliefs about sexual inadequacy can also lead to diminishment of erotic thoughts; if you don't think of yourself as sexy, then you may not think about or initiate sex.

Clinically, depression is a common cause of low desire (Baldwin, 2001; Hickey et al., 2005). One of the symptoms of depression is *anhedonia*, or the loss of interest in something one used to enjoy, which includes sexual activity. Frequently seen in combination with *alexithymia*, or an inability to recognize or expressing emotions, a man may have difficulty understanding his body's signals that he has a need for affection or emotional connection. As a result, he may not receive the kind of stimulation needed to pique his sexual interest. Depression associated with bipolar disorder, generalized anxiety, schizophrenia, and personality disorders also can lead to low desire, as can past sexual abuse and associated shame and disgust regarding sex.

Additional problems linked to situational low desire include a man participating in atypical activities, such as cross-dressing, of which his partner may be unaware, or being involved in an extramarital affair. An increasingly common reason for situational low desire is over-reliance on pornography for sexual gratification. Unlike a relationship, pornography requires little forethought and no emotional demands, making it "Plan A" rather than "Plan B" and causing drive for one's partner to sink.

ADDRESSING LOW DESIRE IN MEN

Always ask the client if he has had a physical exam, and especially if he has had his testosterone checked. If not, make a referral. Men often want to try to solve problems on their own, but it is often a good idea to meet with the partner to assess the partner's level of support for the male client; how the couple communicates; the partner's level of frustration; and whether sadness, blame, or other negative affect threatens to undermine the relationship and needs to be repaired.

After ruling out medical and/or psychiatric illness, treatment of Male Hypoactive Sexual Desire Disorder will depend on subtype (Montgomery, 2008) and will generally require intensive therapy. If the male client has no medical problems underlying lifelong low interest, the goal is to help the client and his partner cope with the reality that their drives may always differ in strength. The focus can be on creating other attachment behaviors that help the couple express and experience love in other ways. For example, they may both enjoy massage, playing a game of tennis, or cooking a meal together. Part of the idea is to take the pressure off the male partner to "deliver the goods" and build confidence that he can please his partner in many other ways.

It is also critical to dispel the myth that "the man always has more desire." This damaging belief can lead to a man believing he is abnormal, and a woman feeling inadequate, that there must be something very wrong with her or the relationship if the male partner isn't "always" thinking about sex. Shifting perspective and educating the couple that, like other human characteristics, desire doesn't fall to gender stereotype.

If a man is unable to generate interest in a partner where interest would be expected—that is, the couple has a good relationship with a willing female partner—then individual psychotherapy is generally recommended, with strong emphasis on family of origin issues as well as cognitions about sex, love, and women. Strong rapport is needed if a man is going to reveal deeper connections between his psyche and his sexual behavior. This is when problems such as enmeshment with mother or the so-called "Madonna-whore" syndrome in which a man has difficulty directing his "dirty" sexual needs to his "innocent" and idealized partner are revealed. Long-standing but unrecognized problems with attachment, especially in men with an avoidant style, may also be identified, explored, and worked through.

As previously stated, sometimes men will express that they have "no" desire, but upon assessment you may learn that they masturbate daily. In addition to careful assessment, consider some individual sessions to allow the male to ventilate about what is bothering him and to sort out treatment goals, which may range from better communication about sexual wants or needs to admit that his marriage or relationship is so dissatisfying that divorce or termination may be indicated. If relationship issues are identified, then the work will become how to communicate these to the partner so that they are heard and to create a sense of team-building in order to rectify them, all in the name of building a better sex life. However, a better sex life may not occur automatically; you may need to further help the couple reconfigure their expectations and approach for the life they are leading now.

You will also want to assess for issues that seemingly have little to do with sex and more with self-esteem, such as feeling the effects of aging; job stress or possible pending layoff and financial strain; failure to meet life goals (including whether such goals were ever realistic); poor body image;

or conflict with family of origin members or in-laws. Generally, these issues are associated with subclinical depression; as they are addressed with cognitive therapy, mood improves and desire may return.

ACTIVITIES

1. Conduct a web search of the following terms and read some of the results. As a mental health provider, what biases do you notice? Are there any myths that are perpetuated—or dispelled—by the material you find online?
   - ED cures
   - Early ejaculation cures
   - DE cures
   - Penis size cures
2. Write your own ad, web copy, or blog entry on the topic of help for ED or early ejaculation. What is your perspective on these topics on how psychotherapy can help? Try to write a piece that will motivate a man with psychological problems to get help.

RESOURCES

Kerner, I. (2004). *She comes first: The thinking man's guide to pleasuring a woman*. New York, NY: William Morrow.

Metz, M. W., & McCarthy, B. W. (2004). *Coping with erectile dysfunction: How to regain confidence and enjoy great sex*. Oakland, CA: New Harbinger Publications.

Metz, M. W., & McCarthy, B. W. (2004). *Coping with early ejaculation: How to overcome early ejaculation, please your partner, and have great sex*. Oakland, CA: New Harbinger Publications.

TIPS FOR BETTER ERECTIONS

- Maintain a healthy weight and diet. Men who are overweight can produce too much estrogen in their cells, effectively feminizing the body. A Mediterranean diet of vegetables, fruits, lean protein, and unsaturated fats like olive oil can accomplish both.

- Exercise can keep cholesterol low, which means that the arteries that feed blood to the penis will function better. Exercise also helps manage stress.

- If you smoke, stop. Smoking damages arteries that send blood to the penis.

- Limit or learn to better manage stress so that when the opportunity arises to have sex, you are ready. Be protective of time set aside for relaxation. Try taking a different perspective, like being less serious about problems at work or home.

- Understand your body and sexual arousal. Tune in to your fantasies to figure out what is a turn-on for you. Explore your entire body, not only your genitals.

- Do pelvic floor muscle exercises, which help strengthen erections.

- Communicate with your partner about your sexual preferences.

- Realize that every man, at any age, occasionally has problems with erections. Don't let a temporary problem turn into a chronic one.

- Keep alcohol use to a minimum. A recommended limit on alcohol is two 1-ounce drinks of hard liquor or 4-ounce glasses of wine per day.

- See your doctor annually. Make sure your hormones are in balance. Also be sure to ask your doctor if any of your medications can interfere with sexual function.

- Get proper sleep. If you snore, get checked for sleep apnea, which can keep the body's tissues, including the penis, from getting oxygen.

TIPS FOR LASTING LONGER

Early ejaculation can be frustrating, but most men can improve ejaculatory control. Set a realistic goal for yourself and realize that, like any behavior, change will take time.

- Masturbate to learn more about your body. Take your time to enjoy your body first, then move to masturbation. Learn to tolerate higher levels of sexual stimulation.

- When you do masturbate, try creating a scale of excitement, with "0" being not at all aroused and "10" being the "point of no return." What does your body feel like at a level 6 of arousal? At a 7, 8, or 9? Try to stay at a level 7 for awhile, allowing yourself to slowly build to higher levels and ejaculation.

- In partnered sex, it can take pressure off if you help your partner have an orgasm first, then move to intercourse or other activities.

- During intercourse, move in circles or shallow thrusts to keep stimulation minimal.

- If you have a short refractory period (rest period between erections), go for a second round of intercourse. Men usually last longer during second intercourse.

- Exercise the pelvic floor muscles with Kegel exercises. These muscles help men have a stronger erection and develop ejaculatory control.

- Last but not least, do not let your self-esteem be affected by how you feel about early ejaculation. Feeling bad is more likely to make you anxious, which can lead to less control. Realize that you have many other ways to please your partner besides lasting longer during intercourse.

8

Common Problems in Couples Sex Therapy

It has been said that when a couple's sex life works, it accounts for 15% to 20% of their relationship satisfaction, but when it doesn't work, it accounts for 50% to 70% of their dissatisfaction (McCarthy & McCarthy, 2003). Couples committed to one another—whether gay or heterosexual—most often describe sex as providing a meaningful expression of love for one another. When a couple's sex life falters or stops altogether, they eventually feel emotionally disconnected. When sex goes, love withers.

Sometimes, a faltering sex life cannot be avoided. Couples can get derailed due to phase of life changes such as the birth of a child; chronic illness or cancer; or temporary unemployment. Most couples will work their way back to being physically intimate, though some may need a little nudging from a sex therapist. Other couples never get back on track—if they were ever there to begin with.

Sexual dissatisfaction in couples can be attributed to numerous issues, including being naive about sex; difficulty talking about sex; having unrealistic expectations; mismatched desire and lack of differentiation (Bowen, 1974; Schnarch, 1991); chronic unresolved conflict; mismatched sexual tastes; and overinvestment in domestic roles (Perel, 2007), while allowing passion to fade (Fisher, 2004a).

An ecosystemic assessment can help the therapist determine such factors and create an appropriate treatment plan (Buehler, 1999). For example, if one partner reports growing up in a sexually restrictive family environment, the treatment plan might be cognitive therapy to address irrational beliefs about sex that developed in the microsystem. When couples have disagreements about how frequently they should have sex or report differences in sexual tastes, then the therapist can address such issues in the macrosystem, using couples therapy techniques. Recognizing common problems can also help the therapist hone in on issues to assess and explore.

The last part of this chapter is devoted to a brief examination of couples who are interested or involved in polyamorous relationships—a topic that most therapists who study couples therapy do not get exposure to in graduate studies. A polyamorous relationship can take multiple forms, from couples that agree to be nonexclusive when dating, to married couples who choose to have an open relationship, permitting each other to have sexual and/or emotional liaisons with other adults. Whether a therapist is in the "live and let live" or "no way" camp, polyamory is increasing as a lifestyle choice and therapists must be prepared for the possibility of this topic arising in the treatment room (Zimmerman, 2012).

BEING NAIVE ABOUT SEX

Couples may display an astonishing lack of knowledge about sex. Generally, the more religious and conservative the couple's upbringing, the less they may know about basic sexual anatomy, arousal, and orgasm. The naive couple is also the most likely to contact the therapist with a complaint of vaginismus that has made consummation of their marriage difficult or impossible. Another common presentation occurs when one partner becomes more comfortable with his or her sexuality, while the other lags behind or resists.

Letting the couple know that they have come to the right place; that thousands of other couples have the same problem; and that they will not be judged for their lack of knowledge can help them relax and develop trust in the therapist as a mentor. The next task is to rule out past trauma, as this sometimes contributes to a partner's avoidance of knowledge with sexual content (Buehler, 2008; Maltz, 2012). If there is no trauma, or indication of any individual pathology, then the couple can be given psychoeducation about the human sexual response and sensate focus activities to facilitate pleasurable exploration. Depending on the couple's philosophy regarding visual material, there are also excellent DVDs in which actors demonstrate sexual technique. The Client Worksheet entitled "Talking to Each Other About Sex" (page 116) can also help couples learn about each other's sexuality. If the couple resists watching such material, there are, of course, many sex manuals that describe ways to attain sexual pleasure.

COMMUNICATING ABOUT SEX

Sometime couples—like therapists—have more difficulty communicating about sex than almost any other topic. (Other couples can't wait to start talking about sex, so much so that the therapist may need to slow them down in order to take a history.) Thankfully, helping such couples talk about sex is rewarding, as many couples express appreciation for the opportunity to reflect upon, open up, and discuss their sex life. Normalize for couples that the inability to talk about sex often occurs because most people learn to talk about sex as something forbidden. Another belief is that if one's partner is truly attuned, then there is no need for verbal communication; a loving partner *just knows* what to do. These beliefs mask vulnerable feelings, in that people frequently fear that their partner will reject their expressed sexual wants and needs. Soon, though, most couples learn that discussing sex represents an opportunity to become more intimate. Unfortunately for some couples, this new level of intimacy is threatening, requiring more intensive therapy to improve tolerance for emotional and physical closeness.

The therapist's task is to create a safe space to practice, facilitate, and model good communication so that the couple can negotiate a realistic bedroom contract, such as "We will have sex twice a week unless one of us is ill. Sam will initiate most of the time, and Jane will initiate when the couple is celebrating something in Sam's life," or "Kyle will give Meg oral sex to orgasm before intercourse, and Meg will give Kyle oral sex to ejaculation once or twice a month" (Metz & McCarthy, 2010). To facilitate such communication, couples can be assigned the task of completing an activity such the Client Handout "I Like / Don't Like" at the end of the chapter. This type of conversation starter can make it easier to break the ice when talking about sex as a new experience. Couples may or may not share their contract with the therapist; what is important is that they talk to one another freely.

CONTRACEPTION

Little has been written about the issue of contraception in the therapy office. In clinical experience, I have observed this to occasionally be a major contributing factor to a couple's sexual dysfunction. Couples occasionally may disagree over the type of contraception they will use. For example, the female partner may not want to take any type of oral contraceptive, while the male partner may dislike using condoms, leaving them to use the particularly unreliable withdrawal method. This, in turn, can lead to low desire or avoidance. A man who feels forced to use condoms, on the other hand, may develop erectile dysfunction or delayed ejaculation. Even a vasectomy can lead to psychological problems such as low desire or feeling less pleasurable orgasm. Thus, an assessment of a couple's past experiences with and methods of contraception can open up areas of conflict and power struggles that affect sexual expression. Obviously, a referral to the appropriate medical provider may be in order, but a worksheet on various types of contraception is provided at the end of this chapter to facilitate productive discussion of birth control options.

ADDRESSING UNREALISTIC EXPECTATIONS

Most sex therapists agree that the goal is not helping couples learn the latest and greatest technique for creating sublime orgasmic bliss, but to have a regular rhythm of activity that is alternately fun, passionate, serious, or playful as mood and need dictate. Individual partners and couples often come to therapy with unrealistic goals, including having the same level of desire; experiencing the same passion as when they met; showing a particular physical response as a demonstration of love, for example, a woman's body producing natural lubricant; or a partner attaining instantaneous skill as a lover. Couples may also have in mind that because the problem is "just sex," treatment will go quickly. They may be unaware of or simply not wish to address other relationship issues, with the hope that if their sex life is repaired, everything else will fall into place.

Setting a goal often requires educating the couple as to what is realistic *now*, given their current lifestyle with its demands and time constraints, their health status, and their age (Southern & Cade, 2011). Pointing out that at varying times in a couple's life, sex may need to be renegotiated (Metz & McCarthy, 2010). For example, sex may become more or less frequent or activities may need to be modified due to physical changes in the body, for example, muscles may not be so elastic or joints may ache. Finally, settling upon a goal that signals that therapy is both successful and coming to its natural end creates motivation during treatment.

CHRONIC NEGATIVE PATTERNS OF INTERACTION

Sexual problems can create conflict, and conflict can create sexual problems (Metz & Epstein, 2002). Naturally, nearly all couples experience conflict; it is the way in which couples manage conflict that makes the difference in the overall quality of the relationship (Gottman & Levenson, 1992). When partners face problems directly, speak assertively, and work cooperatively toward a solution, conflict is generally resolved. Partners that act aggressively, withdraw, make contemptuous statements, and engage in power struggles may have ongoing conflicts that undermine most attempts to engage in intimate behavior. Unresolved conflict can break down attachment bonds, affecting not only marital satisfaction, but the trust and safety needed if a couple is to comfortably explore their sexuality. It is nearly impossible to treat sexual problems until a couple learns how to manage conflict. If a couple's interactions are relatively calm, then it may be possible to treat how they manage conflict concurrent with sex therapy. Sometimes, problematic interactions and a couple's sex life are so entwined that they need to be treated separately, with other conflicts addressed first, such as problems with in-laws or finances. Finally, when a couple presents with severe conflict, sex therapy is contraindicated, and referral to someone who specializes in high conflict couples may be in order.

Occasionally, couples that report little conflict may use the bedroom as the place where they can focus all of their emotional distress. Perhaps this is because there is an association between the "dirtiness" of sex and the "dirtiness" of expressing negative feelings that creates the association and compartmentalization. In working with a seemingly cooperative couple's sexual problems, it is not unusual to reach an impasse as underlying tensions are revealed. Common conflicts include the ways in which partners use their leisure time, both individually and together; differing rhythms, such as sleeping and waking patterns; issues with one another's need or lack of need for order; and varying need for emotional closeness or distance. The couple needs to learn how to communicate more assertively about such issues, learning to bring them to one another's attention and talking them through until they are resolved, even if it means acknowledging they sometimes have very different opinions.

MAINTAINING PASSION IN THE FACE OF DOMESTICITY

As Perel has written, couples that "mate in captivity" lose the erotic charge of their early courtship (2007). It is almost farcical to expect couples to shed the mantle of domestic life at the end of the day and act out their sexual lust. The roles and tasks that create a stable home life make a couple more like "ma" and "pa" than lovers. On the other hand, the idea that couples are meant to stay romantically and sexually involved with one another throughout a long-term, committed relationship is relatively new, perhaps a reflection of media ideals and the fact that birth control allows for a more stress-free sex life. In most cultures, traditional couples focus their energy on creating financial and emotional stability for the family.

If we are to believe evolutionary anthropologists like Fisher (2004), then the true nature of the human pair bonding relationship is for serial monogamy. In conducting functional magnetic resonance imaging (fMRI) studies of people reporting to be at different stages in their relationship, Fisher has identified three stages of falling and staying in love and ultimately parting ways.

Stage 1: Being in Love

This stage is characterized by high energy, emotion, passion—and stress. People feel magnetically drawn together, but the question of whether or not this will be a favorable union hangs in the air, creating insecurity. Hormonal levels reflect this, with evidence of increased levels of norepinephrine, which acts as adrenaline; dopamine, which creates a feeling of reward; and serotonin, which creates the high of optimism. For most people, Stage 1 lasts approximately 6 months to 2 years. Many people mourn the passing of this stage, often by expressing a fantasy or wish to return to it.

Stage 2: "Passionate Love"

During this stage, passion still runs high and stress is minimal as the couple forms a more secure bond. Chemicals associated with happiness—oxytocin and vasopressin—are produced in the brain, and are thought to create the feeling of being bonded. Stage 2 can last for several years.

Stage 3: "Companionate Love"

Feelings of passion decrease, while commitment and safety increase. This stage is characterized by deep feelings of friendship, which is reflected in levels of oxytocin and vasopressin. Many relationships never make it to Stage 3, breaking up on average in their fourth year. Fisher points out that 4 years is about the time it takes for a couple to meet, mate, and produce offspring that grows to age two, at which time a woman might stop breast-feeding and be ready to mate with a new partner.

Of course, many couples manage to stay together long after the 4-year mark, and among those couples, a small number still express a feeling of passion for their partner. For those couples who complain they no longer feel passion, explaining these stages as having a biological and social basis can help answer the mystery of what happened to their love, removing blame and soothing disappointment. Once soothed, couples need to plan for times when they can fully embrace each other in the role of lovers. This may require discussion and the awareness or creation of opportunities for erotic trysts. Being able to put aside domestic tedium for orgasmic bliss is one key to keeping a long-term relationship sexually gratifying.

Aside from scheduling time for sex, there are other ways to recapture at least some of the excitement of passionate love. One is to engage in novel activities, both in and out of the bedroom. Doing so has the effect of raising oxytocin and dopamine levels, the former being associated with security, and the latter being associated with reward and excitement. Couples can be reminded that in the early stages, they tried all kinds of things together, including seeking out special restaurant experiences, taking romantic trips, and talking about what they'd like to do to one another when they got home to the bedroom. Looking forward to doing new things is also, in itself, rewarding. Couples in my practice have even benefitted from changing their bedroom environment, for example, ditching the parents' old bed set and choosing one that reflected their taste, then adding accessories that delighted them both.

Another is to brave the territory of frank eroticism, or the exploration of what is sexually exciting to oneself and one's partner (Kleinplatz, 1996). Eroticism is created when couples entice one another to enjoy sex through an exquisite arousal of the senses. Eroticism requires trust and the ability to make one vulnerable to one's partner as that partner attends to sexual needs, as well as a willingness to take a risk when reciprocating. Sharing erotic fantasies increases self-knowledge and provides "self-affirmation and validation." Intercourse is only one activity; whatever excites is erotic. When partners are attuned to one another's desires, able to tease one another to an appreciable level, sexual problems may dissipate.

Another unique way to attune partners to each other emotionally and spiritually during sex is to introduce the practice of Tantra. Tantra is actually a branch of yoga that has, in part, a focus on procedures and rituals designed to put the practitioner in touch with what is divine or sacred. Practitioners like Anand (1990) and Richardson (2003) have brought Tantra to the West with a focus on what is sometimes called "sacred spirituality" that employs techniques such as deep breathing and eye gazing, chanting, and erotic massage before and during intercourse. Although Tantra may be inappropriate for clients who have their own spiritual practice or, conversely, who have no interest in spirituality, some clients welcome Tantra as a way to access feelings of deep connection with their partner.

WHEN THE PROBLEM IS ATTACHMENT

The need for attachment is also primal, and most adults will search for someone who will fulfill relational and emotional needs when comfort is needed. However, not every adult is capable of healthy attachment, which occurs when partners demonstrate trust and are attuned to one another's needs. Instead, some adults are *anxiously attached*, causing them to fear that the partner will be unavailable during times of need and increasing cognitions and behaviors that they suppose will bring security. Others are *avoidantly attached*, meaning that they tend to be distrustful of others, causing them to operate more independently and to decrease intimacy-seeking behaviors.

Each partner's attachment style influences the couple's expression of intimacy (Resnick, 2012). Foreplay, with its inclusion of close proximity, caressing, and eye gazing, forms the basis for an adult bond. However, sometimes partners lack the education or experience to engage in foreplay, so that their sexual experience becomes replete with dissatisfaction. Fortunately, partners that are generally securely attached—who trust and are close in other ways—are the most likely to benefit from brief interventions in sex therapy. Such couples will read therapist-recommended books, experiment with sexual activities, and demonstrate more affection and openness as therapy progresses. They are, on many levels, the ideal clients for sex therapy.

When partners have attachment problems, they are often played out in affectional and sexual interactions. A common pattern occurs when an anxiously attached woman demands from her avoidantly attached husband more affection, causing him to withdraw because he doesn't understand his wife's desire for closeness, fears he cannot meet his wife's demands, and wants to avoid conflict. Or, an anxiously attached man may see his partner's lack of lubrication to mean she may be unhappy, increasing his fear of abandonment, as well as his demands of proof. In actuality, she may have a hormone imbalance, a yeast infection, or simply not be as aroused because she is distracted, but no matter to the anxious male partner. An avoidant woman, on the other hand, may refuse sexual contact not because she has no desire, but because she doesn't wish to risk becoming more intimate with her partner.

Identifying each partner's attachment style can help the couple better understand what unmet needs are causing distress. The therapist can reflect that what the wife wants is to know that her husband loves her, and what the husband wants is to know that his lovemaking is adequate for her. Couples respond to one another with empathy; trust is built; and repetitive, problematic interactions are circumvented.

The most recent neuroscience studies suggest that humans are socially, but not sexually, monogamous. That is, there are social expectations as well as social reasons for couples to form a monogamous pair bond, such as providing a more stable, two-partner family, minimizing exposure to sexually transmitted diseases (STDs), preventing unwanted pregnancy through consistent use of birth control, and creating an emotionally secure attachment.

DIFFERENCES IN DESIRE

Couples who have differences in sexual desire make up a large population. Couples assign various meanings to this experience. For example, men may feel insulted or rejected when their partner doesn't want sex as often as they do. Women often feel especially forlorn when a male partner has lower desire because of the widespread myth that men *always* want sex more often than women. Many people believe that if partners love one another equally, then they should equally want to have the same frequency of sex. Why this myth persists perhaps has to do with lack of differentiation—a desire to be merged with a partner, to feel secure by knowing one's partner is just as fully invested in the relationship (Schnarch, 2011).

Educating a couple that it is normal to have differences in desire, just as it is normal to have differences in any area of life, from taste in cuisine to how frequently one wants to spend time with relatives, is sometimes enough to stop a cycle of conflict. Some couples, however, use differences in desire as a struggle for power and control. The lower desire partner is naturally viewed as dictating when the couples will or won't have sex, while the higher desire partner is seen as being a demanding nag (Weeks, 1987). Generally, both partners feel misunderstood and annoyed with one another.

The therapeutic remedy is to generate compassion for each partner's position, for example, the lower desire partner may feel guilty for not meeting the higher desire partner's needs, or the higher desire partner may feel lonely or sad that the lower desire partner doesn't want to connect as often. Additionally, what needs to be ruled out is whether there is a genuine cause that is contributing to the discrepancy in desire, other than the natural differences that occur. Often couples that present with discrepant desire have poor problem-solving and conflict resolution skills that manifest in other areas of the relationship, so a thorough assessment of how the couple habitually handles conflict can help the therapist determine how to improve communication and differences of opinion or experience.

Interviewing partners separately can help parse out if the lower desire partner has past trauma; is dissatisfied with the quality or some other aspect of the couple's actual lovemaking; or has some medical issue that hasn't been attended to. It can also help the therapist learn if the higher desire partner is using sex as a way to manipulate the lower desire partner into doing their bidding; as a stress relief; or is, in fact, hypersexual in a manner that suggests a mood disorder such as Bipolar Disorder II.

DIFFERENCES IN SEXUAL TASTE AND STYLE

Couples often covertly manage conflict about sexual differences. A common scenario is a woman withdrawing sexually from her generally passive partner in the hope that he will become more aggressive. This strategy leaves him bewildered, but it also reveals a wish that the male partner could read the female partner's mind. Or, to indirectly exert control a man may quote one of several authorities, frequently church-based, who believe that women need to supply their partner's sexual needs. In a specific case concerning control, a man with OCD required his partner to be absolutely still so as not to disrupt his ritualistic method of attaining climax. While she acquiesced during sex to appear understanding, she found herself picking fights at other times.

A common overt conflict that couples have difficulty resolving is differences in sexual tastes, with the most frequently encountered problem possibly being that one partner is more sexually adventurous than the other. Imagining a sex therapist to be a *compadre* in adventurous sex, the more open partner brings identified patient (IP) into treatment with the hope that the therapist will persuade the IP to blossom—a recipe for therapeutic failure. Instead, the therapist can help the couple with problem solving. *Both* partners need to identify and communicate what they want, and why. Once they understand each other's needs, they can begin to identify behaviors that may be satisfactory to both, or negotiate a schedule or ratio of sorts, trading off whose sexual needs will be met.

Sometimes, solutions regarding sexual taste require that partners develop compassion or, minimally, tolerance, if they are to remain committed. For example, couples address the issue of a male partner's desire to cross-dress in various ways. In some cases, women actually assist their partner in his endeavors by buying clothing or polishing nails. In others, the solution is for the activity to remain completely private. Unfortunately, for some cross-dressers, engaging in the behavior results in dissolution of the partnership. Cross-dressing and other paraphilic behavior is covered in Chapter 18.

Differentiation and Sexuality

In Bowen's family systems theory (Bowen, 1974), couples in which partners are *differentiated* have the autonomy to feel, think, and act autonomously; couples in which partners are *fused* struggle with chronic anxiety, emotional problems, loss of identity, and relationship conflict. When a partner experiences fusion, he or she may feel lost or overwhelmed during sexual encounters and thus lack enjoyment or avoid them altogether. Fusion is perhaps most apparent in couples where there is a discrepancy in levels of desire, with the higher desire partner nagging the lower desire partner, blaming him or her for all types of relationship misery. The lower desire partner takes on blame and reacts by either creating conflict or withdrawing. Thus the couple remains stuck, unable to see the problem for what it is: two people who simply have different libidos, and who need to find an acceptable way to cope.

Fusion and associated relationship conflict plays out in other types of dysfunction, for example, when a woman cannot maintain appropriate feelings of self-worth if her partner has erectile dysfunction, perhaps seeking out an affair to compensate. Or I think of Vince, a man who came to my practice complaining of delayed ejaculation, who also could not commit to a relationship because he feared losing his individuality; he literally could not give himself over to a partner. To stop this pattern, couples can be educated about it and learn to label it when it occurs. They can develop empathy for one another's position, in that the higher desire partner needs to understand the guilt that the lower desire partner may experience, and the lower desire partner needs to understand the higher desire partner's frustration. Since this dynamic also becomes reflective of each partner's need to regulate emotional intimacy, it becomes important that they learn how to identify and verbally communicate their need for closeness or distance, rather than act it out.

POLYAMORY: A DIFFERENT VIEW OF ADULT RELATIONSHIPS

What is a monogamous marriage therapist, trained to treat monogamous couples, to do when faced with a person or persons who have multiple emotional and sexual relationships? When clients practice polyamory, defined most commonly as "maintain[ing] multiple love relationships and [being] open and honest within these" (Barker, 2005), it may present a challenge to a therapist raised in a culture and trained in theories that support the concept that adults normally develop wanting a relationship with one other adult (preferably heterosexual) whom they wish to marry and begin a life together. Polyamory (sometimes also called "non-monogamy" or "non-exclusivity") also challenges ideas of morality as well as conformity, as many adapters of polyamory view themselves pioneers, creating social structures based on choice rather than prescription. Among polyamorous heterosexuals, men may feel heartened that they no longer are constricted to having one sex partner, and there is some evidence that human males were not meant to be monogamous. Women may embrace being independent, rather than subsumed to the needs of one partner, and the rising number of women who engage in extramarital affairs confirms that the desire for more than one sexual partner isn't limited to men. For gay and lesbian couples, discussions of polyamory may be seen as validating alternate modes of relationship that they have created and practiced without benefit of social recognition.

A thorough discussion of the biological and social evolution of monogamy and the rationale for change in contemporary culture is beyond the scope of this chapter. What is important is for therapists who treat nonmonogamous couples is to recognize and set aside their biases in order to listen with compassion to what the client or clients might be saying about their feelings regarding social constriction or difficulties they may encounter in staying monogamous. Therapists must also be open to the idea that it is not for them to decide for clients what the best social structure may be. In some cases, such as when one partner identifies as heterosexual and one partner as bisexual, a polyamorous arrangement may be a viable option, or when partners are already engaged in extra-dyadic sex and want to continue the practice without deceit, shame, or guilt (Zimmerman, 2012). An individual who wants to practice solo polyamory may be seeking support for his or her decision in a monogamous world.

Zimmerman (2012) recommends that honesty and boundaries are the core issues that must be addressed when couples present or appear open to polyamory relationships. Being honest about one's sexual and emotional relationships, or the desire for them, allows couples to become intimate, while boundaries are the function that must be negotiated, particularly at the beginning stages. Zimmerman suggests that the therapist ask the partner about when and where sex with another or others can occur; how safe sex will be practiced; whether such relationships or events will be discussed; whether emotional attachment to others will be acceptable; how special occasions such as birthdays will be managed; and who will and who will not be informed about the open relationship. The question of what to tell children ranges from little or nothing, to sitting children down and giving them information directly, with assurance that the parents' relationship with them will remain unchanged in terms of love and security.

Open relationships, though touted as an evolutionary step up from those that are monogamous, are not without challenges. As Zimmerman points out, maintaining one or more additional relationships outside the primary relationship requires management of time and energy. There can be miscommunication about rules, leading to mistrust and jealousy. A lack of support from one's family or community for the open relationship may lead to a sense of isolation. Additionally, the power dynamics of the relationship may change, such as when the female partner in a heterosexual relationship initiates an open relationship: She appears to be more powerful than a female partner whose male partner initiates such an arrangement.

Perhaps tellingly, Zimmerman omits questions regarding what the clients might do if an unplanned pregnancy occurs; ostensibly, one of the "old school" reasons for monogamy is so that men knew they were the sires of their offspring. But even with the current availability of paternity tests, the emotional, physical, and spiritual consequences of an unplanned pregnancy cannot be overlooked as a topic for discussion. The point of doing so is not to create an atmosphere of judgment, but to engage clients in realistically assessing and addressing the risks involved in polyamorous arrangements.

STEP INTO MY OFFICE...

Eduardo came to the United States from Guatamala as an 18-year-old to join his family. He described that he had been sexually active from the age of 10 with a much older teen girl, a situation that he reported as (and insisted to be) consensual. Having had many sexual encounters since, he nonetheless married at age 22 to a highly religious woman about 10 years his senior who had been kind to him. He had great difficulty staying monogamous in the marriage and found himself wanting to have sexual and emotional intimacy with other men as well as women. We explored his sexual development, including his beliefs about monogamy. He determined that monogamy was not the path for him—at least not for the foreseeable future—and that as long as he was honest about his sexuality and desire for multiple partners, he could not see the harm in it. With much emotional wrangling, he decided to end his brief marriage so that he could pursue a solo polyamory lifestyle.

ACTIVITIES

1. Use your primary theoretical framework to consider how you might intervene to help couples struggling with sexual concerns. For example, in Bowen family system theory, the concept of *triangulation* is used to explain how some couples cope by bringing in a third individual to modulate anxiety or regulate intimacy. How might couples use young or dependent adult children to regulate sexual intimacy, for example, by having a child sleep in the couple's bed, or by being overly involved in an adult child's life?
2. What myths about sex in committed relationships do you and/or your clients hold? Write in your journal about how you might talk to clients about the natural loss of desire or sexual boredom. How might you motivate clients to stay together?
3. Would you recommend alternative lifestyles, for example, swinging or polyamory, to the couples that you see? Why or why not? Write about it.

THE LANGUAGE OF POLYAMORY

Partnered nonmonogamy: Committed couple that allows extradyadic sex.
Swinging: Nonmonogamy associated with a particular context called "the lifestyle."
Polyamory: Allows partners to have more than one relationship that is sexual, loving, and emotional.
Solo polyamory: Nonmonogamous individuals who do not want a primary partner.
Polyfidelity: Three or more people who have committed to be in relationship together.
Monogamous/nonmonogamous partnership: One partner is monogamous and the other is not.

RESOURCES

Anand, M. (1990). *The art of sexual ecstasy: The path of sacred sexuality for western lovers.* Santa Barbara, CA: Jeremy P. Tarcher.

Berman, L. (2011). *Loving sex: The book of joy and passion.* New York, NY: DK Press.

Gottman, J., & Silver, N. (2000). *The seven principles for making marriage work: A practical guide from the country's foremost relationship expert.* New York, NY: Three Rivers Press.

Nelson, T. (2008). *Getting the sex you want: Shed your inhibitions and reach new heights of passion together.* Beverly, MA: Quiver.

Schnarch, D. (2009). *Passionate marriage: Keeping love and intimacy alive in committed relationships.* New York, NY: W. W. Norton & Company.

TALKING TO EACH OTHER ABOUT SEX

Couples often talk about everything and anything—except sex. Take turns asking each other some or all of the following questions to learn about each other's sexuality.

1. Who taught you about sex?

2. What was the most ridiculous thing you ever learned about sex? How did you learn it wasn't true?

3. Before you had sex, what did you think about having premarital sex?

4. What did you notice about your parents' emotional and sexual relationship? How do you think it has affected you?

5. Did anything negative happen to you sexually? Is it something you would like to talk about?

6. What do you think about masturbation?

7. Do you have sexual fantasies? Are there any fantasies you would like to share?

8. Is there anything about having sex that you really don't like? Is there something about sex that we can change?

9. What causes you to lose your mood for sex?

10. What causes you to get in the mood for sex?

SEX, LOVE, AND CONTRACEPTION

Although it may seem unromantic to draw attention to the procreation side of sex, it is important for couples to discuss and agree upon a method of birth control that will work for *both* partners. Consider the level of birth control protection you need. If pregnancy is absolutely unwanted and you are certain you have completed your family, then a vasectomy is a better choice than natural family planning, which is associated with higher pregnancy rates. Ease of use, affordability, religious beliefs, acceptability to one's partner, and side effects are other factors that you may wish to consider with your prescribing physician.

The methods of birth control currently available include:

- *Barrier methods*: Male and female condoms, as well as the diaphragm, cervical cap, and contraceptive sponge.

- *Hormonal methods*: Examples include birth control pills, as well as the vaginal ring (NuvaRing), contraceptive implant (Implanon), contraceptive injection (Depo-Provera), and contraceptive patch (Ortho Evra).

- *Intrauterine devices (IUDs)*: Examples include the copper IUD (ParaGard) and the hormonal IUD (Mirena).

- *Sterilization*: Tubal ligation, Essure, or Adiana for women, and vasectomy for men.

- *Natural family planning*: Rhythm, basal body temperature, and cervical mucus methods.

- *Emergency contraception*: Morning-after pill, used to prevent pregnancy after unprotected sex.

A TRIP TO THE SEX TOY SHOP

A visit to the sex toy shop can be fun, educational, and even arousing. Choose a shop that is clean and tidy, with toys and other items on display that you can touch with your hands and examine with your eyes. Most good toy stores will have knowledgeable staff to answer your questions, which are perfectly acceptable to ask. Here are some guidelines for a fun and educational visit.

- Explore lubricants. There are water-based, silicone-based, oil-based, and natural lubricants. Some are flavored or have special properties like warming or cooling the skin. It is okay to ask for samples to try at home.

- Try your hand on a vibrator. There are small vibrators, medium vibrators, and jumbo vibrators, with motors that range from dainty to powerful. They are designed to stimulate different parts of the genitals or anus in various ways. Ask for a tour if you aren't sure what you are looking at.

- Some toys are designed for specific kinds of play. There are "nipple clamps" for nipple play, beads for anal play, and textured mitts for exploring different kinds of touch. Some will leave you with a question mark over your head, while others may excite you in a surprising way.

- A well-stocked store may also have all kinds of costumes, from innocent to dark in nature. It's okay to buy parts of a costume to make up your own ensemble.

- It is perfectly okay to laugh and have fun looking at merchandise. But be discreet, because one customer's joke is another customer's ideal.

- Don't make other shoppers uncomfortable by peering at what they are buying or making comments.

I LIKE / I DON'T LIKE...

Check off what you'd like to try with your partner. Trade lists; compare and contrast. Branch out, have fun.

- Have your partner explore your body with a fur mitt.
- Have sex blindfolded.
- Try sex outdoors.
- Try sex standing up in the shower.
- Engage in oral sex.
- Engage in anal sex.
- Play with syrup or whipped cream.
- Be lightly bound up with crepe paper.
- Lightly bind your partner with crepe paper.
- Use a feather to explore your partner's body.
- Pose for erotic photographs.
- Look at books of erotic photographs.
- Tell a sexual fantasy.
- Pretend to be strangers meeting for sex.
- Have fun grooming pubic hair.
- Engage in nipple play, for example, squeezing, tugging.
- Spend an hour in foreplay with no intercourse allowed.
- Try flavored lubricant.
- Do a strip tease or dance for your partner.
- Use a variety of sex toys in one session.

9

Parents' Questions About Sex

Couples, not just those with sexual and relationship issues, may ask therapists how to educate their children about a topic largely ignored in their own upbringing. While it may seem obvious that two fully mature adults who engage in intercourse already know enough to answer their children's questions, the fact that no one modeled how to talk about sex makes doing so fraught with peril. Parents learning about healthy sexuality also wonder how they can engender healthy attitudes in their children so that they don't suffer from the same misinformation.

As a therapist who is comfortable (or on their way to becoming comfortable) with sex, you are in a unique position to help the next generation avoid many of the sex and relationship problems you see in adults in your practice. You can give parents reassurance about normal childhood sexual behaviors, counsel them on how to teach their children in an appropriate way at each stage of life, and alert them of ways to protect their children from unwanted sexual touch.

Therapists, like their clients, often have grown up in a home atmosphere where sex wasn't discussed. Like their clients, therapists are also parents who may not have had the chance to talk to their own children. Those therapists who have not yet started families may also grapple when couples begin to ask questions about how to talk to their kids about sex.

Parents, of course, are the most appropriate people to talk to their children about sex for a number of practical reasons:

- They are the best judges of when to give their children age and developmentally appropriate information.
- They can teach their children about appropriate physical and emotional boundaries in relationships.
- They can convey their values about sexuality as they educate their children in making future choices.
- They can create an open atmosphere where children know they can safely come to their parents with any questions or worries about sex.

Krafchick and Biringen (2002) advocate for therapists helping parents with these important tasks that parents sometimes stumble on due to their own negative experiences with sex, lack of knowledge about sex, and lack of access to research-based information. Parents also need support in a culture of peers and media that holds values that may conflict with their own.

Much of what I have written in this chapter was acquired while working for a decade as an elementary school teacher, as well as being a parent. During the last part of my career, the Los Angeles Unified School District trained groups of teachers in recognizing and preventing child sexual abuse, and I was among the first selected for the training. As such, we were instructed in talking to staff, children, and parents about childhood sexual abuse, and the need for parents to talk to children about sex. Parents are the obvious choice, because they usually want and need to impart their own values about the role of sex in one's life.

Parents need to create a balance between being too open or closed about sex. Too much information can overwhelm or confuse a child; too little can lead to a belief that sex is something secretive or inappropriate. Children also can become upset by what they are told, for example, if the only time a mother talks to her daughter about sex is to confide that she was molested. They can also be confused, as when a father shows his son a collection of pornography and encourages him to enjoy sex "but wear a condom," making the teen feel pressured to become sexually active.

Generally, parents want to know:

- When to start talking to children about sex
- What to tell them about their bodies
- How to explain conception and pregnancy
- What to do if they discover a child masturbating
- How to prepare an older child for puberty
- How to talk about safe sex without condoning sexual activity
- How to convey values about sex without causing a child to become overly inhibited.

Use the Client Worksheet "Talking to Your Children About Sex" to guide a discussion in your therapy setting. An additional worksheet, "Talking About Sexual Values," may also be supplied to reinforce that talking about sex is an opportunity for parents to share their ideas.

WHEN TO START TALKING ABOUT SEX

The first year of life isn't too early to start talking about sex. When parents express shock at this, remind them that sex encompasses a wide range of behaviors and human experience. At age 1, parents can begin to identify parts of the body, such as *vulva* for the outer lips of a girl's genitals, or *penis* and *scrotum* for a boy's outward genitals. After all, a hand is called a hand, and a finger, a finger. By calling body parts something other than what they actually are, a parent does two things: (1) they convey their own discomfort about the body part and (2) the child learns that there is something about these body parts that needs to be hidden.

As children grow into toddlers, they often notice the bodies of other children and sometimes those of adults, perhaps while they are dressing. It is appropriate to answer a toddler's questions and give them reassurance that what they are seeing is normal. Toddlers do not need to know about the adult function of body parts. If a toddler views an adult woman's breasts, then it is fine to simply say what they are. If the toddler is curious and asks *why* a woman has breasts, it is best to explain in a context that they will understand, for example, an adult woman who has a baby can feed the baby with milk from her breasts.

Most toddlers learn indirectly about pregnancy if their parents become pregnant, or from watching or hearing other adults talk about pregnancy. Once again, a toddler doesn't need to know *how* a pregnancy occurred. A toddler can be told that a male and a female adult are needed to create life and that there is a baby developing within a mother's body, ready to be born at the right time.

A major part of one's sexuality is the ability to form a satisfying relationship and to express feelings. Toddlers can learn that, ideally, people who love one another form relationships before having a baby, so that the baby is loved, too. If parents hold expectations that people must be married before conception to ensure a good foundation for a family, or for moral reasons, then they can include their beliefs in a light-handed way. Toddlers can also be taught about expressing their feelings openly through parents' modeling. Feelings can be expressed verbally as well as physically. Hugs and kisses are one way of expressing love, but talking about one's feelings can make a person feel that their feelings matter and can make a difference in their lives.

As most children develop, their curiosity increases. Children as young as 5 or 6 may start asking *how* they were conceived, *how* a baby exits a mother's body, and *what role* the father plays. They also begin to learn about sex from the whispers of peers in the schoolyard and interact playfully with children of the opposite sex. They may be curious again about developing bodies, as girls as young as 9 today begin to show signs of puberty. Let parents know that it is best to react calmly if their child says something inappropriate about sex, instead of with shock and anger, which can create feelings of shame and guilt.

This is the time—not when a child is 10, or 12, or heaven forbid, 16—to talk more specifically about anatomy and basic reproductive function. Well before puberty begins, at around age 8 or 9—in part because puberty can begin younger now—it is time to talk about the normal changes they can expect in their own bodies, for example, pubic hair, underarm hair, and in the appearance of their genitals. They need to be told that these are signs that their body is being prepared for adult life—but that they are not yet adults.

Girls can be told they will have "breast buds" before they develop breasts. They need to know about the production of hormones that will regulate the menstrual period. It is time to show a daughter what feminine hygiene products are and to tell her that she shouldn't be embarrassed to come to her mother (or, if mother isn't around, her father) and let her know if she gets her period. I have even heard a nurse counsel girls that it is perfectly okay to use a wad of toilet tissue or paper towels in an emergency, because the nurse found that sometimes girls were so embarrassed to ask for napkins or tampons that they bled onto their pants.

Boys need to learn about the production of sperm and ejaculate fluid. A boy may find that he is having more frequent erections and needs assurance that this is nothing to be ashamed of. He may wake up from a pleasant dream and find that he has ejaculated. Instead of hiding this fact and feeling guilty, he can have a towel in his room so he can clean up, or change his sheets. He can be told (parents will love this) it is a sign that it is time to do his own laundry—no questions asked.

Masturbation needs to be a topic of conversation. Most boys begin masturbating around age 10 or 11, though sometimes as young as 7 or 8. At a younger age, they do not ejaculate, of course, but they can experience orgasm. Girls tend to be older when they begin exploring their own bodies—some not until well into their teens. It is helpful that boys and girls know that they may experience normal hormone surges that can create sensation in the genitals and subsequent tension in the body and that masturbation is an acceptable form of release. If a parent can't bring him- or herself to use the word "masturbation" (an ugly sounding word if ever there was one, certainly intentional), then "self-pleasure" is a good euphemism.

Discussion about "safe sex" can take place any time a child is curious about preventing pregnancy, or if they hear the term. If a prepubescent child hears about herpes papilloma virus (HPV) or another sexually transmitted disease (STD), then parents need to have a frank discussion that diseases exist that can be passed through sexual activity. Likewise, a prepubescent child may also know about unplanned pregnancy by watching television or, as frequently occurs, from an adolescent or young adult family member, creating another teaching opportunity for parents. Parents can let children know that sexual activity of all kinds is something that takes place between two mature, loving adults because it requires discussion and some planning; for example, they need to talk about preventing STDs and unplanned pregnancy. The best plan is for abstinence and to delay a sexual relationship until one is mature enough to have a conversation about the use of condoms and birth control. For some parents, "mature enough" means, "when you meet someone special and are in love"; for others, it means delaying intercourse until marriage.

Parents of children with special needs, including learning disabilities, autism, and attention deficits, may need additional assistance in communicating about sex. There are certified sex educators within the American Association for Sexuality Educators, Counselors, and Therapists (AASECT) who may be able to help with particular challenges, such as working with an autistic teen who begins to act out sexually with the opposite sex, or discussing the need for appropriate physical boundaries for a naive learning disabled student. Using visual imagery and storytelling, educators can help special needs individuals develop assertiveness and awareness that may prevent later heartache.

Either way, parents can be assured that, according to research, talking about sex openly and frankly *will not* cause their child to run off to buy condoms and have sex because they know they are "protected." The fact is about half of American teens begin having intercourse at age 15; by age 22, only about 10% of young adults have yet to experience intercourse (Mosher et al., 2005). Even American teens who are told in no uncertain terms that they must remain celibate for religious reasons may end up engaging in intercourse—or, more commonly, oral sex and other sexual play to avoid pregnancy. It seems that when teens have appropriate information, they grasp the serious side of entering into a sexual relationship and are more likely to at least delay having sex until they are older.

I handled this with my own daughter by reminding her that her task during her teenage years was to prepare herself for future goals—another important discussion that sometimes doesn't takes place—and that there would be time enough for a serious relationship later, when she was better prepared to handle one. At the time of this writing, she is a junior in college (sorry, darling, for sharing this, but I know you will ultimately approve) and has let me know that she has delayed intercourse by saying, "I haven't found the right boyfriend. I'm sure I could have sex if I wanted it—but why would I do that to myself? I would feel terrible if I did and then the boy didn't even talk to me! I've seen it happen! I feel sorry for girls who don't feel good enough about themselves to wait." Was I ever glad I talked to my daughter openly about sex! Talk about a proud parenting moment. Because I knew she had listened, I felt reassured she would, when the time was right, plan appropriately for safe and protected sex. Thus, a discussion of self-esteem, boundaries, and the ability to fend for one's self when it comes to sex can also be part of an open discussion.

In fact, youths are faced with a variety of sexual challenges, such as having comments (both welcome and unwelcome) made about their developing body, sexual advances made or rejected, hearing about the sexual escapades of their peers, and exposure to some element of pornography; about 42% of teens report having seen pornography, and 62% of those reported that the exposure was unwanted (Wolak, Mitchell, & Finkelhor, 2007). No parent can deny that it would be best to talk about these situations and welcome a teen's questions when and if these challenges occur. You cannot depend on a teen to have "common sense." The part of the brain that regulates planning and keeps impulses in check is still developing, which is why so many states have put more restrictions on teen driving. It is a parent's responsibility to let a teen know that they are aware of problems that can come up, not just with sex but with beginning efforts at romantic attachment, and can be a source of wisdom rather than shame.

ANSWERING PARENTS' COMMON QUESTIONS

In preparation for answering parents' questions, here are a few points of guidance:

- Normalize with parents that it is common to feel nervous talking about sex.
- Ask about whether sex was discussed in their homes and process any feelings about this.
- Normalize a child's questions or behaviors, unless they are cause for alarm, for example, their child is sexually overly aggressive with peers or has been caught doing something inappropriate such as texting nude photos.
- Role model what they might say to their child. Allow them to rehearse with you, or suggest they rehearse with each other.
- Offer age-appropriate resources that parents can read for themselves or give to a child to read.

My Child Touches Him- or Herself "Down There" All the Time! What Do I Do?

The parent needs to let the child know that while masturbation feels good, it is also a private activity to be done in the bedroom or shower. This is a matter of fact statement, not a scolding. If masturbation is truly constant, the child may be soothing him- or herself from anxiety, loneliness, boredom, or other uncomfortable feeling. Parents need to consider what might be causing the chronic behavior. It may be a wise idea to refer to a pediatrician, who can rule out any physical causes, for example, an infection.

Our Child Came Into Our Bedroom Last Night and Caught Us Having Sex. What Should I Tell Him or Her?

Depending on the age of the child—and what the child may have seen—the answer will vary. A young child who has expressed fear that "daddy was hurting mommy" may need reassurance that what was seen is the way adults sometimes play and show affection. An older child might be told that yes, his or her parents were having sex, like other adult couples who love one another. A teen can probably take a joke like, "Yes, your old parents still enjoy sex. Sorry to gross you out!" But then it would be wise to let the teen know that people really are sexual until they no longer have a partner or their health fails.

And then, get a lock on the door and tell children older than 4 or 5 not to bother mom or dad unless they are sick or there is an emergency, as everyone needs privacy sometimes. Parents can certainly keep the door unlocked at other times if they wish.

Our Male (or Female) Child Plays With Girl's (or Boy's) Toys. Does This Mean He or She Is Confused About Gender?

Possibly—but it is probably way too early to draw that conclusion. Instead of worrying about whether a toy or play thing is inherently male or female, it may be best to consider the *values* that the parent wants the child to learn through play (Freeman, 2007). In other words, if parents wish a boy to learn about nurturing, then they can permit play with baby dolls. If they want a daughter to learn about competitive sports, then they can allow rough play during a soccer game. When a child's interest in opposite sex behaviors consistently crosses gender, that may be an indicator of gender confusion, or perhaps an emerging transgender identity. In such cases, consultation with a psychotherapist who specializes in gender issues is recommended (see *Resources*) so that both child and parents can better understand the fluidity of gender (Malpas, 2011).

Another Child Touched My Child's Genitals.
Is This Sexual Abuse? What Should We Do?

If the children in question are about the same age, the child needs to be told it is normal for children of any age to be curious about each other's bodies and even to want to touch someone else, but that there are rules about touch, for example, the touch needs to be given with affection, it needs to be welcome, and it needs to occur in a place other than where one's bathing suit goes.

Of course, if there is real abuse, for example, an 11-year-old asking an 8-year-old to perform oral sex, then the parent or therapist may need to report the abuse, as a study by Shaw et al. (2000) suggests that the effects of child on child sexual abuse can be as damaging as adult on child abuse. Parents need to be alerted that the aggressor may need psychological help to understand appropriate boundaries. Both aggressor and victim will need to be assessed, the aggressor for possible past sexual abuse.

How Do I Explain Birth Control If I Want My Child to Wait
Until Marriage to Have Sex?

Telling a child *about* birth control is different from telling a child to *use* birth control. Birth control can be explained as *family planning*. This term makes it clear that birth control is used to prevent unwanted pregnancy for married or committed couples. Parents can explain that it is advantageous for adults to plan for pregnancy so that they can prepare for the responsibility of having a baby. This is another opportunity for parents to educate children about the serious side of sex. Planned Parenthood has good resources regarding family planning; see *Resources*.

My Brother (or Sister, or Fill in the Blank) Is Gay.
What Do I Tell My Children?

Assure parents that telling children about homosexuality will not make the child interested in becoming gay, as it appears that being gay begins biologically, before birth. A straightforward explanation is best, such as, "Sometimes two men (or two women) fall in love with each other." If the child is old enough to ask questions about the possibility of babies, he or she can be told that same-sex couples can have families in other ways, such as adopting babies who need parents.

If parents believe that homosexuality is "wrong" (or, if you yourself don't condone homosexuality, but your clients do) remember that, as a therapist, you are not to judge someone's beliefs, should they be different than your own. If it seems appropriate, you can explore why parents feel this way and, if there is good rapport, educate parents appropriately about LGBTQ people and any fears they have about children being exposed to a gay lifestyle.

Should I Tell My Child That His Father and I Were Sexually Active Before Marriage?

The question here is, why? If the parent wants to tell the child because he or she had regrets, it will suggest that they may have been coerced into having sex or had a weak will and gave in. If the parent wants to give the child permission to have sex before marriage, it probably isn't needed; let the individual figure it out at the right time to become sexually active. Unless the child asks directly—a situation that deserves a direct, but not detailed, answer—discussion of the parents' premarital activities, with each other or with other partners, is unnecessary.

My Teenager's Friend Showed Him/Her Pornography. Now What?

There are two issues here, the friend having pornography, and the child being exposed to material. In this case, the friend's parents need to be alerted that their child has access to pornography and to accept that it is time to educate one's own child about such material. Instead of creating a storm of worry and shame, begin by letting the teen know that people have almost always been interested in looking at other people doing sexual things because it can be exciting. Although there is nothing wrong with people having sex, watching pornography is like watching a cartoon, where people may not look or act like real adults having sex. Also, the parent can emphasize that in pornography there is no expression of feelings, which is what makes having sex with someone in a loving and safe relationship special. Finally, it is fair to let them know that, like gambling, sometimes people get so involved in looking at pornography that they forget to have fun and be with other people in real life. They may lose out on learning how to go about courting, dating, and, eventually, finding someone to love or marry and share a healthy sexual relationship.

Should I Let My Child Go to the Sex Education Class at School?

Explore why the parent is fearful about letting the child go to the class and educate the parent as necessary, for example, that the information is basically biological. Let them know this is a good time to share their values that the best sex takes place in a loving relationship or marriage.

My 5-Year-Old Found a Box of Tampons. What Do I Tell Him?

Tell him or her what a 5-year-old needs to know, that women release an egg every month and if it is not fertilized, there is some fluid that comes from a woman's body that is called a "period." When this happens, a tampon absorbs the fluid so a woman can stay nice and fresh and go about her day. If the child is older, mother can take out a book and show the path of the egg into the uterus and discuss the lining that is shed every month. She can also show how the tampon is inserted into the vaginal passage and let the child know that for most women, using a tampon is comfortable and that having a period is normal.

What About Sexual Abuse?

In the metropolitan area where I live and practice, barely a month goes by without a report in the newspaper of a teacher, coach, religious leader, or youth organization leader arrested for child sexual abuse. Such incidents make it imperative for parents to teach children how to protect themselves from unwanted sexual touch or activity. And, the fact is that the majority of children are molested by someone they know, such as a professional, a neighbor, or a relative. While no child can ever be held responsible if abuse occurs, children who know what it is and what to do about it are more likely to feel less shame and to tell an adult if something happens.

Children as young as 3 or 4 can learn that their body belongs to them and that it is okay to say no if someone wants to touch their body and the touch is unwelcome. They are especially to say no if someone wants to touch their genitals, or "where their bathing suit goes," unless it is a parent and only if there is a good reason, like if they have a rash or pain. Even a medical doctor should not touch them unless mother, father, or a nurse is in the room. Children can also be told the difference between "good" and "bad" touch, and to listen to their "inner voice" if something tells them that what someone older is doing to their body is wrong or gives them an "icky" feeling. They also should know the difference between "good" and "bad" secrets, with good secrets being those you can eventually tell, like a surprise party or a gift, and bad secrets being those you must keep forever.

Parents need to be alert to their child's whereabouts, and children need to know how to stay in contact with their parents, whether via telephone or by asking an adult to use their phone. When it comes to activities, parents need to drop children off and pick them up on time so that potential predators do not have access to their children. Parents should also screen people such as sitters or even people who perform services in the home. In California, there is a website where parents can look up a person's name to see if they have ever been arrested for any offense in connection with child abuse. I know that I once checked to see who, in my neighborhood, had been arrested as a pedophile and was shocked to find a former client listed. Lesson: You can never tell by looking at someone, so it is not being overly cautious to check someone's references.

Finally, children need to be told that if something happens that makes them uncomfortable, they should by all means alert the parent or, if the parent is not immediately available, another adult. When I was educating children about protecting themselves, we would tell children to "keep telling until you are believed." I even went so far as telling them that if it was a parent who was hurting them, they could come to a teacher; if it was a teacher, they could tell the principal; and so forth.

Educating parents how to talk to children about sex can be gratifying, once any discomfort is overcome. Such education often strengthens the treatment alliance with the couple, as healing takes place on multiple levels, both internally for the parents and within the family system.

ACTIVITIES

1. Select and read books from the *Resources* list so that you can make appropriate recommendations to clients. What type of client can you see yourself recommending which type of book?
2. Use your journal to reflect on how you will manage countertransference when parents' values differ from your own. For example, you may hold the belief that it is a good idea to have sex with someone before marriage to ensure sexual compatibility, while your clients believe that sex should be saved for after marriage. How will you speak to such clients about the reality that 90% of people age 18 to 27 in 2001 have had intercourse outside of marriage (Halpern & Haydon, 2012)?
3. Consider your own upbringing and how your parents did, or did not, speak to you about sex. What might they have done better? Was there anything that they did especially well? How can you use your own experience to guide therapeutic interventions in this area, while remaining respectful of clients' values and experiences?

RESOURCES

American Association for Sexuality Educators, Counselors, and Therapists certifies educators, some of whom specialize in working with children and teens with disabilities. Find a directory at www.aasect.org

Planned Parenthood has many resources regarding family planning and birth control at www.plannedparenthood.org

Haffner, D. W. (2008). *From Diapers to Dating: A Parent's Guide to Raising Sexually Health Children–From Infancy to Middle School.* New York, NY: William Morrow Paperbacks.

Harris, R. (2004). *It's so amazing!: A book about eggs, sperm, birth, babies, and families* (Ages 7 and up.). Somerville, MA: Candlewick Press.

Harris, R. (2006). *It's not the stork!: A book about girls, boys, babies, bodies, families, and friends* (Ages 4 and up.). Somerville, MA: Candlewick Press.

Madaras, L., & Madaras, A. (2000). *What's happening to my body? Book for boys: A growing up guide for parents and sons.* New York, NY: Newmarket Press.

Madaras, L., Madaras, A., & Sullivan, S. (2007). *What's happening to my body? Book for girls* (Revised). New York, NY: William Morrow Paperbacks.

Miron, C. D., & Miron, A. G. (2001). *How to talk to teens about love, relationships, and S-E-X: A guide for parents.* Minneapolis, MN: Free Spirit Publishing.

Roffman, D. (2001). *Sex and sensibility: The thinking parent's guide to talking sense about sex.* Cambridge, MA: De Capo Press.

TALKING TO YOUR CHILDREN ABOUT SEX

It is natural for children to express an interest in their bodies, the bodies of others, and the nature of sexual reproduction. Parents sometimes get anxious, however, about how to talk to their children about these topics in a way that is healthy but helps children to understand boundaries. What follows are some guidelines for talking about this topic.

Children can begin learning about sexuality as young as preschool. They can learn that boys and girls do have some different parts of the body, and they can be told the real terms for the penis, testicles, vulva, vagina, and clitoris. If you find your child touching his or her genitals, you can say something like, "Touching yourself feels good, but that is something people do in private," then lead your child to the bedroom.

Older children may begin to ask questions. In general, you do not want to overwhelm your child with information. Listen carefully to the question your child is answering. You can also ask some questions before answering, such as, "Where did you hear that?" or "What have you noticed?" Then you can answer the question in a straightforward way with exactly the information he or she is asking about.

Puberty is starting at earlier ages, so children as young as 9 or 10 may need to know about changes in their bodies that they can expect, or that they are observing in their peers' bodies. At this age, children need straightforward answers about the biology of reproduction, body hygiene, and maintaining appropriate physical boundaries with peers and adults.

As they reach preteen and teen years, they may experience sexual fantasies and urges. They need to know that these feelings are normal. They are at an age when they can understand that masturbation can be a healthy outlet and an alternative to acting out on sexual feelings. If this does not fit with your religious beliefs, then you should talk to the preteen about distraction techniques. They also should learn about the parents' philosophy on dating and premarital sex, if these discussions have not yet occurred.

TALKING ABOUT SEXUAL VALUES

Make copies for everyone in the home who is to be involved in a discussion of sexual values. (Adults partners may wish to have a separate initial discussion first.) Allow time for family members to mark where they stand, then have a discussion about the various topics.

1. Sex should never be a topic of polite conversation.

    Strongly disagree   Disagree   Neutral   Agree   Strongly agree

2. Most families are okay talking about sex.

    Strongly disagree   Disagree   Neutral   Agree   Strongly agree

3. Homosexuality is a choice.

    Strongly disagree   Disagree   Neutral   Agree   Strongly agree

4. Teenager girls should be able to get an abortion without parental permission.

    Strongly disagree   Disagree   Neutral   Agree   Strongly agree

5. There are types of sex that do not cause sexually transmitted diseases.

    Strongly disagree   Disagree   Neutral   Agree   Strongly agree

6. It is best to wait until marriage to have sex.

    Strongly disagree   Disagree   Neutral   Agree   Strongly agree

7. Birth control such as condoms should be made freely available at school.

    Strongly disagree   Disagree   Neutral   Agree   Strongly agree

8. Adoption is the best choice when a single teen becomes pregnant.

    Strongly disagree   Disagree   Neutral   Agree   Strongly agree

10

Therapy With Sexual Minorities

Several noteworthy events occurred just while drafting this book. An American president openly supported gay marriage; an American state, North Carolina, banned gay marriage; and a foreign country, Argentina, legislated that a person needed to merely complete a form to change gender rather than rely on medical and mental health professionals to make a decree. Notoriously, Robert Spitzer retracted his study suggesting that "highly motivated" gay and lesbian people could change their sexual orientation, and California made it illegal to run a therapeutic program to effect such change. Clearly, people around the globe are addressing the rights of sexual minorities, albeit in different ways, reflecting changes in social mores and beliefs about sexual orientation and gender. Although Americans who identify as lesbian, gay, bisexual, transgender, or queer (LGBTQ) (*queer* referring to those who refuse to choose or who question their orientation or gender) constitute 3.4% of the population (Gates & Newport, 2012), they are finding more acceptance and therefore more support for various causes, such as ending discrimination against gay volunteers in youth organizations or having equal employment protection under the law.

AVOIDING BIAS

In order to treat the sexual problems of LGBTQ individuals, it is critical to understand the role of homophobia. *Homophobia* literally translates to "fear of homosexuals," but is better understood as an aversion to LGBTQ people (Ahmad & Bhugra, 2010). Such antipathy is rooted in the belief that sexual practices of gay people are "unnatural" because they occur outside the sanctity of marriage and cannot result in conception. These acts were severely punished in early American colonies, though they were practiced by heterosexual couples. Many people today, both gay and heterosexual, view oral and anal sex as perverse. In recent decades, homophobia has been kept alive because of the appearance of HIV/AIDS, with gay sexual behaviors having been blamed for the spread of the disease, despite the fact that whether a man has been circumcised may play more of a role and the fact that the highest spread of disease may be seen among heterosexual American seniors (Nguyen & Holodniy, 2008).

The hatred of gays is so pervasive in American culture, and elsewhere around the globe, that many LGBTQ people develop what is called *internalized homophobia*, or self-hatred of one's sexual orientation, which can contribute to sexual dysfunction (Ahmad & Bhugra, 2010; Bhugra & Wright, 2007; Hinchliff, Gott, & Galena, 2005). For example, in one study of sexual dysfunction conducted in Hong Kong of Chinese men who have sex with men,* sexual problems such as painful sex, anxiety, and lack of sexual pleasure were all associated with higher rates of internalized homophobia and lack of social support (Lau, Kim, & Tsui, 2008). Internalized homophobia also causes anxiety and depression and can contribute to substance problems, all of which in turn affect sexuality.

Bisexual men and women and transgender people sometimes complain that they face even more discrimination than gay and lesbian individuals, because others (both gay and heterosexual) question whether or not the bisexual person's orientation is real, or a way to avoid declaring oneself as gay (Dean et al., 2000). Some of the confusion or doubt about a person's orientation may be due to the fact that orientation can be fluid (Nichols & Shernoff, 2007), particularly in women who may change the object of their attraction because of environmental and personal characteristics (Diamond, 2009). In any case, the combined effects of internalized and external biases against one's identity are painful to self-esteem, and therapists must examine their own homophobia if they are to be allies in healing this population.

Men who have sex with men (abbreviated MSM) is a term used by researchers to allow inclusion of men who engage in sexual behaviors with other men, but who may not identify as gay or bisexual.

EVOLVING ATTITUDES OF MENTAL HEALTH PROFESSIONALS

1952: Homosexuality was classified as a "sociopathic personality disturbance" in the first edition of the *Diagnostic and Statistical Manual* (*DSM-I*).

1963: Homosexuality classified as a sexual deviation in the *DSM-II*

1973: Task force of the American Psychiatric Association votes to remove the term "homosexual" from the *DSM*, replaced by the term "sexual orientation disturbance" (SOD)

1980s: SOD replaced with *ego-dystonic homosexuality* (EDH)

1987: EDH removed from *DSM-III*, eliminating homosexuality as a mental disorder diagnosis

2013: *Gender identity disorder* becomes *gender dysphoria* (GD) in the *DSM-5.*

THE TRANSGENDER EXPERIENCE

Transgender refers to the behavior, appearance, or identity of persons who cross, transcend, or do not conform to culturally defined norms for persons of their biological sex; *transsexual* refers to "anyone who lives socially as a member of the opposite sex, regardless of which, if any, medical interventions they have undergone or may desire in the future" (American Psychologist, 2012). No one knows how many individuals identify as transgender or transsexual, nor is anyone certain how a person develops a transgender identity. There is speculation that prenatal hormone levels, as well as a person's experience in childhood, adolescence, or adulthood, may contribute to the formation of a transgender (trans) identity.

Homophobia can make being gay challenging, but being a transgender individual is perhaps the most difficult test of being true to one's identity. Transgender people are probably the least well understood of the sexual minorities, in part because they tend to be deeply closeted, uncertain of the meaning of their own experiences and fearful of being judged negatively because not only their orientation but their gender is called into question.

In American culture, gender is taken for granted as a binary choice of either male or female. It is such a basic part of one's identity that most expectant parents are eager to know the sex of their offspring at the soonest possible moment so that they can begin planning for the boy or girl's life. The possibility of having a transgender child isn't even a consideration. Yet, transgender people have long been recognized as a part of the human population; for example, in Thailand, *kathoeys* are transgendered men who are as such because of their karma (Conroy, 2010). Recent media attention (movies such as *TransAmerica* and interviews with celebrity offspring) has provided some needed exposure and education. However, for most mental health professionals there is still a huge gap in knowledge, including the belief perpetuated by inclusion in the *DSM-5* that being transgender is a mental disorder.

People who are trans—or even suspected of being trans—are at risk for bullying, physical harm, and even murder. In one national survey of LGBTQ youth, 90% of students reported hearing the word *gay* used in a derogatory way (Kosciw, Graytak, & Diaz, 2008). The surveyed also noted that over 85% of youth reported that they were verbally harassed and 44% said they were physically harassed because of their sexual orientation.

Transgender individuals differ vastly on how they feel about their assigned and desired gender, from being open with family members and transitioning from one gender to another early in life, to completely suppressing their desire, often for years into adulthood (Brown & Rounsley, 2003). Those who are suppressed experience a great deal of inner turmoil, conflict, and depression. Transgender individuals have a high rate of suicide; if the transgender person is a member of a racial minority, they are at even greater risk for discrimination, with African American trans women experiencing lowest levels of self-esteem (Kuper, Nussbaum, & Mustanski, 2012).

Thus, transgender people are often in great need of psychological services. They need not only to address conflicted feelings and heal trauma related to possible bullying and rejection, but to be appropriately assessed before most medical doctors are willing to begin treatment with hormones and/or surgery. The World Professional Association for Transgender Health (WPATH) publishes in their *Standards of Care* (2012) that transgender individuals should receive a long course of psychotherapy and a thorough medical examination before a transgender person transitions from male-to-female (MTF) or female-to-male (FTM). Recently, however, transgender people are choosing to bypass the WPATH requirements by obtaining surgery in Thailand or somewhere else where procedures are less costly and can be obtained without a psychological evaluation (Mason, 2006).

When presented with a person who identifies as transgender or who is uncertain about gender, the diagnosis of Gender Dysphoria (*DSM-5*, 2013). A transgender person must be distinguished from a person who is struggling to identify sexual orientation, is suffering from trauma and abuse, or is severely depressed or psychotic. However, it is not uncommon for an individual with transgender issues to present in therapy as being depressed or anxious, which might be attributable to the frustration of feeling that they are trapped in the wrong physical body (Brown & Rounsley, 2003).

Thus, a paradigm shift may be needed, in which the therapist views the transgender person as suffering from social and family issues, not from being a transgender person per se. As Ross (2009) points out in his article on the ethics of gender identity disorder, being transgender is not a mental disorder akin to having a delusion. It is not repaired with psychotherapy or psychotropic medications. It is best to conceptualize the transgender person as having a medical problem that is corrected through surgery. Psychotropic medications would be used to treat comorbid depression or anxiety so that the person can benefit from improved mood and function.

Children and teens, especially, should not be diagnosed as being gender dysphoric if they are displaying nonconforming gender behaviors, for example, a boy who copies his older sister by painting his fingernails black may be somewhat unexpected, but not necessarily a symptom of GD (American Academy of Child & Adolescent Psychiatry [AACAP], 2012; Minter, 2012). Nor should a woman who adopts masculine dress and enters into a male-dominated career be considered confused about her gender identity or sexual orientation; this can be considered as *gender expression*, rather than orientation (American Psychologist, 2012). GD, however, can be diagnosed in people confused about their gender and distressed about it. The point is not to help people accept the outward markers of their gender, but to make choices about their gender that feel right to *them*—and not to society, family members, or peers. A discussion of managing the development of gender variant individuals is beyond the scope of this book; see the *Resources* section for an article discussing the AACAP practice parameters.

Transgender people make various decisions about how slowly or quickly they wish to transition, when to transition, and what to communicate to family, friends, and coworkers (Brown & Rounsley, 2003). One MTF woman made her transition between high school and college, so that when she arrived at her new school she would only be known as a person of female gender, while an executive with a prominent position needed to make the transition in a more public way, with support from her company's human resources department. A transgender person may decide to use hormone therapy to take on some of the characteristics of the desired gender, but not surgery because of its expense, doubt about its efficacy (research on FTM who have a surgically created penis suggest they are frequently disappointed with the result), and a desire to have a more fluid gender identity.

Transgender individuals may make any of the following decisions regarding the expression of their gender, and such expression may be fluid over time (WPATH *Standards of Care*, Version 7, 2012).

- Changes in gender expression and role (which may involve living part time or full time in another gender role, consistent with one's gender identity);
- Hormone therapy to feminize or masculinize the body;
- Surgery to change primary and/or secondary sex characteristics (e.g., breasts/chest, external and/or internal genitalia, facial features, body contouring);

- Psychotherapy (individual, couple, family, or group) for purposes such as exploring gender identity, role, and expression; addressing the negative impact of GD and stigma on mental health; alleviating internalized transphobia; enhancing social and peer support; improving body image; or promoting resilience.

STEP INTO MY OFFICE...

When the client came into my office, he was a severely depressed college student who identified himself to me as transgender female. Not only had she hidden her trans identity from her parents, she had been beaten by people in another country, making her feel more helpless and victimized. Determining that she needed her parent's financial support to complete a professional degree, she dressed in feminine attire on weekends, in private with her girlfriend. The goal of therapy was treating the client's depression so she could graduate and make an income that would allow her to transition on her own terms.

Any therapist who plans to work with the transgender population needs to take care that they are thoroughly familiar with the *Standards of Care* published by the WPATH. Because transgender clients can be high-risk clients, the therapist must be prepared to assess risk on a frequent basis and to refer the client for psychiatric or high levels of care. Episodes of suicidal ideation or attempts should not be criteria for ruling out the transgender individual's desire or plan for transition, but the therapist must do all that is possible to help the client reestablish mental health equilibrium. The importance of consultation with experts in treating transgender clients and additional education and training cannot be emphasized enough.

SEXUAL BEHAVIOR IN THE LGBTQ POPULATION

Most research on sexual behavior in the gay population is focused on risk-taking and the spread of HIV, which is associated with drug or alcohol intoxication; failure to use a condom; and having multiple sex partners. Much emphasis was also put on the fact that MSM do engage in anal sex, which increases risk because the tissues of the anus are friable or dry, making penetration more likely to create small fissures through which the virus may enter. In reality, gay men most often engage in other behaviors besides anal sex, including oral pleasure and mutual masturbation; they also frequently enjoy taking their time in pleasuring one another (Sandfort & de Keizer, 2001). Sometimes when gay men are in the process of coming out and experimenting sexually with same-sex partners, they express insecurity about engaging in anal sex—as do their heterosexual counterparts, as anal sex becomes a more common activity. The Client Worksheet on page 146 gives guidance on how to safely practice anal sex.

In fact some gay men do not engage in anal sex at all. Among men who do engage in anal sex, feelings may arise about being a "top" or "bottom" during activity. Feelings related to homophobia and anal sex may emerge in the course of sex therapy. A man in either position may associate it with being "more gay." One man who penetrates or "tops" another man may feel he is "less gay" because being the penetrator is viewed as more masculine, while another man who "tops" may feel he is "more gay" because he is more assertive about his sexual attraction. A man who is penetrated as a "bottom" may see himself as being "more gay" or more feminine. Being active or passive during oral sex may also trigger such internal conflict and confusion, which can lead to sexual problems that might be sorted out in therapy. Lesbian women engage in mutual masturbation, oral sex, caressing, and penetration with fingers or toys. One of the reasons lesbians may have a lower rate of sexual complaints is because more of their sexual behavior is what heterosexual women and men might consider to be foreplay. As lesbians continue in long-term monogamous relationships, their expression of love and caring may look different than what is expected in heterosexual and gay male relationships, with less emphasis on sex and more on affection (Nichols, 2005).

Transgender, or "trans," men and women may have varied sexual behavior depending upon orientation or attraction, which may be homosexual, bisexual, or asexual. For example, either an MTF trans woman or an FTM trans man may express a wish to engage in sexual behavior with a woman (Bockting, Benner, & Coleman, 2009). At one time, such orientation would call into question whether or not the person was "really" trans. However, the appearance and function of a trans person's genitals do not necessarily dictate the gender of the person with whom they will engage in sexual activity. An FTM man who has not yet had "bottom" surgery to create a penis and who has a vagina may engage in vaginal intercourse from his male partner, for example. This kind of behavior is sometimes given the label "gender bending," referring to the fact that sexual activity sometimes occurs outside of conforming ideas of male versus female roles and rules. If the therapist becomes confused, it's best to simply admit it. If the therapist becomes uncomfortable, then the therapist may need to seek supervision or make a referral.

Numbers describing the prevalence of sexual problems in the gay population are lacking, as large studies such as Laumann, Paik, and Rosen (1999) did not break down dysfunction by orientation. In one recent study of 200 gay men by Bhugra and Wright (2007), 97.5% reported sexual dysfunction over their lifetime, and 52.5% reported current dysfunction. The most commonly reported problems for gay men include erectile dysfunction and delayed ejaculation. Lesbians report a different experience from heterosexual women; in one study, while 48% of heterosexual women reported problems reaching orgasm, only 15% of lesbian women had this experience

(Meana et al., 2006). For lesbian women, anorgasmia is the most common sexual problem, followed by ability to become aroused or sustain arousal, and low sexual desire.

Sexual problems in the LGBTQ population are also associated with conditions such as depression, anxiety, and drug and alcohol abuse. People of sexual minorities seek psychotherapy at higher rates than the general population, not just for mental illness but for help with self-acceptance, negotiating romantic and sexual relationships, and dealing with problems between themselves and family members. The process of coming out, or disclosing one's sexual orientation, is also a substantive reason to seek services. When a gay couple differs in how "out" they are, it can affect expectations such as behavior in social settings and create tension that can affect emotional intimacy and sexual expression.

ETIOLOGY OF SEXUAL DYSFUNCTION IN LGBTQ POPULATION

As with heterosexual individuals, sexual problems in gay and transgender people can be physical, social, psychological, or interpersonal. Many of the physical and psychological issues have been covered in previous chapters, but the social and interpersonal challenges of gay people vary from those of heterosexual people. Low self-esteem can result from homophobic bullying and threats, as well as not fitting in with the mainstream and overt or covert disappointment or disgust expressed by family members.

STAGES OF GAY IDENTITY FORMATION

Cass (1979) first conceptualized the following stages of gay identity formation

  I. *Identity confusion*: Recognizes but does not necessarily accept gay thoughts and behaviors, even finds them unacceptable; seeks information on homosexuality.
  II. *Identity comparison*: Accepts possibility of being gay; may accept gay identity but not sexual behaviors, or accept sexual behaviors, but not gay identity.
  III. *Identity tolerance*: Accepts probability of being gay; seeks out meeting other gay people; feels part of community.
  IV. *Identity acceptance*: Accepts gay self-image and has increased contact with gay subculture; anger toward antigay society.
  V. *Identity pride*: Immersed in gay subculture, discloses identity to family members and coworkers; inclined toward confrontation with heterosexual establishment.
  VI. *Identity synthesis*: Gay/lesbian identity integrated with other aspects of the self.

Minority stress can also be a contributing factor, as a study of gay and bisexual men suggests that facing the double discrimination of racism and heterosexism may have a negative effect on sexual function (Zamboni & Crawford, 2007). In a survey of LGBTQ youth, rates of conduct disorder, depression, and posttraumatic stress disorder were similar to that found in representative samples of urban, racial/ethnic minority youths (Mustanski, Garofalo, & Emerson, 2010). Coming out can create ongoing strain, as it is a fluid process that may need to be addressed in different situations, such as job change or social events.

Lesbian women often bond very quickly, perhaps because women typically share emotions with one another more easily than do men (Nichols & Shernoff, 2007). This fact has led to speculation that one reason lesbian women sometimes complain of low desire and interest earlier in their relationships than do heterosexual women is that passion fades sooner. However, low desire in lesbian women can also be caused by similar issues that affect heterosexual women, including work stress, relationship conflict, depression, and anxiety. Lesbians may also experience internalized homophobia that adds strain and inhibits sexual expression. Finally, just like their heterosexual counterparts, lesbian women can experience hormonal changes as a result of changes in menstrual status, pregnancy, and postpartum state that can affect function.

Gay men may have nonmonogamous relationship and living arrangements that can cause strained relationships and sexual dysfunction (Shernoff, 2006). Because gay men generally do not have role models for same-sex relationships, they may need to create their own rules regarding fidelity. Gay couples enter into a variety of arrangements, including an open relationship, where each individual may have sexual experiences with others; limits may be put on those experiences, such as only allowing certain sexual behaviors. They may also have an open relationship, but one in which they only participate in sex with others when they are together as a couple. Such arrangements can be liberating, but it can also be stressful if a couple does not agree on boundaries, or if one partner experiences jealousy as the longevity of the partner's relationship with an outsider is extended.

STEP INTO MY OFFICE...

A gay male client came into my office complaining of erectile dysfunction. Previously he had been married, fathered two children, and been a respected member of a religious organization intolerant of gay people, which had made his coming out process quite complex. He had also been molested by an older friend, which contributed to early confusion about his identity. He had many things in his history that may have contributed to erectile dysfunction (ED), but then he told me that he was bicycling a lot of "centuries," or 100-mile rides. I suggested that his problem might be physical, and not psychological, because the pudendal nerve to the groin can be damaged by long periods of time spent on a bicycle seat. I armed him with information about cycling and early ejaculation, and he resolved to switch to another form of exercise. I received a call several weeks later from the client to let me know the problem had resolved. Lesson: Always do a thorough intake, even if you feel certain the client's mental status is the primary factor.

TREATING LGBTQ CLIENTS

The ethics of treating LGBTQ clients is specifically addressed in Chapter 19. LGBTQ clients require a neutral or affirming stance on the part of the therapist. LGBTQ clients may already have had bad experiences with psychotherapists or other health care providers who feel uncomfortable or are outright rejecting and may approach the current therapy with trepidation. It is also important not to assume that all problems the LGBTQ client brings into the office are attributable to orientation or gender, or that nonmonogamous relationship arrangements are indications of pathology. Acknowledgment and identification of one's homophobic thoughts and feelings must be processed outside of the therapy office, although they can be used to guide an empathic discussion of the client's own internalized homophobia.

For the most part, the treatment of sexual problems with LGBTQ clients parallels that of heterosexual clients, although the exact content may be different. For example, a gay male client's sexual aversion may express itself as being fine with receiving oral pleasure, while being disgusted by giving it. Homophobia may be a factor, but so might concerns about transmission of sexual disease or dislike of the taste or odor associated with oral sex practices. In transgender clients, there may be sexual problems related to body image and hatred of one's biological sexual characteristics. Normalizing such feelings and then supporting the client's wish to change such features will be more welcome than working on acceptance of the body in its current state. What is critical, in other words, is to stay with the experience of the client, avoid pathologizing the client's experience, and provide empathic information and therapy as required.

CREATING A LGBTQ-FRIENDLY OFFICE ENVIRONMENT

- Include statements on marketing materials as being "gay friendly" or affirming
- On forms, include "partnered" as a choice for relationship status
- In addition to a check off box for "male" and "female," include one for "both"
- In the waiting room and office, have magazines and reading material that appeals to all genders and orientations
- Do not assume a person's gender or orientation; ask
- If a person uses terms you do not understand, ask for explanation

ACTIVITIES

1. Make contact with the director or appropriate person at the nearest LGBTQ center. Learn about the services they offer and educate the contact person about your practice.
2. Reflect in your journal on your own internal homophobia. Can you create your own timeline of the creation and dissipation of internalized homophobia? Is there anything unusual about your journey?
3. If your religious beliefs create difficulty for you personally in working with sexual minorities, read the section "Homophobia and the Treatment of the LGBTQ Population," p. 257 in Chapter 19. Write about how you will handle your countertransference.
4. Read the American Psychological Association's "Transgender, Gender Identity, and Gender Expression Non-Discrimination" statement online at *http://www.apa.org/about/policy/transgender.aspx*

Discuss with colleagues or reflect in your journal.

RESOURCES

Brown, M. L., & Rounsley, C. A. (2003). *True selves: Understanding transexualism—for families, friends, co-workers, and helping professionals.* San Francisco, CA: Jossey-Bass.

Downs, A. (2006). *The velvet rage: Overcoming the pain of growing up gay in a straight man's world.* Cambridge, MA: Da Capo Press.

Green, J. (2004). *Becoming a visible man.* Nashville, TN: Vanderbilt University Press.

Herman, J. (2009). *Transgender explained for those who are not.* Bloomington, IN: AuthorHouse.

Kaufman, G., & Raphael, L. (1996). *Coming out of shame: Transforming gay and lesbian lives.* New York, NY: Main Street Books.

Kort, J. (2012). *10 smart things gay men can do to find real love.* New York, NY: Magnus Books.

McCoy, R. (2000). *Late bloomers: Awakening to lesbianism after forty.* iUniverse.

Stevens, T. (2006). *How to be a happy lesbian: A coming out guide.* Asheville, NC: Amazing Dreams Publishing.

PREPARING FOR ANAL SEX

- Always use a condom and water-based lubricant to ensure safe sex protection from HIV and other sexually transmitted infection.

- Only engage in anal sex if it is something you want to do; don't do it solely to make your partner happy.

- Practice the exercises that follow until you feel confident that you will be able to have anal intercourse.

  - Begin exercises in bed lying on a towel or lying on your back in a warm bath.

  - Raise your knees toward your chest.

  - Explore all around your anus with a lubricated finger. You can use petroleum jelly for this purpose, but only use water-based lubrication on a condom.

  - Create gentle pressure with a finger moving around the anus in a circle, which should cause the sphincter to relax enough to insert one digit.

  - Once the finger can be comfortably inserted, begin to stretch the sphincter by making circular motions inside the anus.

  - After doing the exercises several times, it should be possible to insert another finger and continue stretching.

  - Further relaxation can be accomplished by using an anal dilator or a toy called a "butt plug," which can also be left in the anus on a regular basis to keep the anus relaxed and stretched in preparation for intercourse.

11

Sexuality and Mental Health Problems

Numbers suggest a story about sex, love, and mental illness. According to the National Institute of Mental Health, approximately 26% of adults in the United States are affected by mental illness each year; meanwhile, 31% of men and 43% of women have sexual problems (Laumann et al., 1999). As of 2009, about 55% of adults are married or in a committed relationship; 15% of Americans had married more than once, including 12% who had married twice and 3% who had married three or more times (Kreider & Ellis, 2011). Clearly, there must exist overlap between the three domains, yet little research exists on the effects of each upon the others.

What is unknown is how many adults divorce a partner because of sexual dissatisfaction; how many divorce because of a mental illness; how much of mental illness is attributable to sexual problems and how much of sexual problems are attributable to mental illness. Also unknown is how frequently therapists inquire of couples in their practice whether a mental illness is present in one or both partners, and what the impact of that might be on their relationship and sex life, and vice versa.

My book *Sex, Love, and Mental Illness: A Couple's Guide to Staying Connected* is the sole volume available on this topic. It is a slim volume for a reason: very little research has been written about it. Whatever articles exist generally address severe mental illness such as bipolar disorder or schizophrenia.

In fact, almost every mental disorder can have an impact on sexuality, even those first diagnosed in childhood, such as learning disabilities and Asperger's syndrome.

Some of the text that follows comes from clinical observation, meant to guide clinical inquiry, as well as spur additional research. Much will depend on the demographics of the population being treated, the couples' understanding of mental illness, the resources available for treatment, the conditions under which the symptoms first appeared, the meaning of the symptoms in the context of sexuality and relationships, and so forth. As previously recommended, a systemic approach to assessment will serve best in these complex cases; treatment suggestions follow at the end of the chapter.

ASSESSING SEXUAL PROBLEMS CAUSED BY MENTAL ILLNESS

The assessment of a sexual problem can reveal an underlying or comorbid mental disorder, and vice versa. Investigation is required to see which is which. For example, if a client presents with depression, upon query, do they report that they have struggled with lifelong early ejaculation, which has contributed to low self-esteem and problems with mood? Conversely, when someone presents with a sexual problem, investigation is needed to assess whether there is another underlying issue. For example, early in my sex therapy practice, I had a client who complained of delayed ejaculation. Somehow, my treatment suggestions weren't working and I decided I needed to investigate my suspicion that he had obsessive-compulsive disorder (OCD). I learned that he once became so distracted during sex that he checked every single spring in his mattress to find the one squeaking! He also would fantasize during sex, but he would need to start it all over from point A if the fantasy were disrupted in order to ejaculate.

MOOD DISORDERS: DYSTHYMIA, MAJOR DEPRESSION, AND BIPOLAR DISORDER

Mood disorders are by far the most common mental disorders, and all can have a negative effect on sexual relationships. A hallmark of both dysthymia and depression is anhedonia, or lack of interest in what someone usually finds pleasurable. Pessimism and low self-esteem add to a bleak outlook on sex (Baldwin, 2001). A depressed mood can also make it difficult to become sexually aroused and to reach orgasm. The tendency for the depressed person to withdraw, isolate, or push others away can lead to relationship conflict and contribute to emotional disconnection and a decrease in sexual activity.

Sexual symptoms associated with bipolar disorder vary according to phase. In the depressed phase, a person who is bipolar may manifest the problems just described, but in a hypomanic or manic stage may become overly interested in sex (*DSM IV-TR*, 2000; McCandless & Sladen, 2003). This increased drive may lead to impulsive, risky sexual activity, not exclusive to one's partner. It isn't unusual for someone with an elevated mood to be involved in more than one extra-relationship affair or in soliciting sex illegally, with devastating effects on the primary relationship. Even when a partner is aware they are involved with someone who has bipolar disorder, they may be unable to separate disease process from issues of character. In fact, divorce rates among couples in which one partner has bipolar disorder are two to three times higher than the general population (Hirschfeld et al., 2002).

Medications that are used to treat mood disorders, including mood stabilizers and antidepressants, can cause sexual side effects such as low sex drive, problems with orgasm, and in men, erectile dysfunction or delayed ejaculation. Doctors are also beginning to recognize "post-selective serotonin reuptake inhibitor (SSRI) syndrome," in which sexual side effects persist long after medications are discontinued.

ANXIETY DISORDERS

Anxiety of any kind can interfere with sexual response (Elliott & O'Donohue, 1997; Fontanelle, Wanderson, de Menezes, & Menlowicz, 2007; Kendurkar & Brinder, 2008; Van Minnen & Kampman, 2000). The symptoms of anxiety are somewhat similar to those associated with sexual excitement, for example, sweating and rapid heartbeat, which can be confusing. Anticipating sexual activity can generate fears about sexual inadequacy, leading to inhibited performance, also known as *performance anxiety*.

There are differences in sexual symptoms that appear among the anxiety disorders. A person who has social phobia may have difficulty finding an appropriate sexual partner, becoming what is called an "adult virgin." Adults who delay first intercourse past the age of 25 or so often develop sexual dysfunction, such as inability to have an erection for males, or to have orgasm with a partner for females.

Although it happens rarely, sometimes a person with yet to be diagnosed OCD may come into the office with a sexual complaint, especially anorgasmia or delayed ejaculation. Any type of obsessive-compulsive activity may interfere (Abbey, Clopton, & Humphreys, 2007; Aksaray, Brkant, Kaptanoglue, Ofl, & Ozaltin, 2001; Stewart, Stack, & Wilhelm, 2008). For example, one man who eventually was diagnosed with OCD had delayed ejaculation because even the slightest sound would distract him from his sexual fantasy, causing him to start over again from the beginning, even during intercourse with his increasingly frustrated wife.

OCD with sexual content can be quite distressing (Gordon, 2002; Williams & Farris, 2011). It is thought to be more common than individuals are willing to admit due to shame or embarrassment, as well as the fact that it is a more covert than overt form of OCD. A common sexually related obsession is ruminating over whether one is or is not gay. (Apologies to gay, lesbian, bisexual, transgender, or queer [LGBTQ] readers who may be offended that an individual obsesses about what that individual finds to be unacceptable behavior.) The person with this type of OCD is terrified about the possibility of being gay. He (or less frequently, she) may question each interaction as proof that he is gay; may look at gay porn to check his response; or have peculiar thoughts running through his head constantly, such as the question, "Am I gay?" Someone may also obsess about having an affair with a person they would consider inappropriate; the obsessions differ from *limerence*, or romantic preoccupation, in that the person has no attraction; rather they *fear* that if they think about having an affair, they will act upon it, and so they ruminate over the possibility. OCD with sexual content requires the same specialized treatment as any other form of the disorder.

Those individuals recovering from posttraumatic stress disorder (PTSD) due to sexual abuse may, understandably, shy away from sexual activity (Buehler, 2008). They may dissociate during sex, leading to a lack of pleasure. Certain sensory experiences—a smell on a partner's breath or the lighting in a room—can trigger flashbacks of the sexual abuse, bringing activity to a halt. Even more complex can be the experience of sex as a performance demand, especially for male survivors who may have been expected to actively please an older, often female perpetrator.

While the effects of sexual symptoms in adults molested as children can have a most chilling effect on even the most stable relationship, PTSD from any horrific event can cause sexual dysfunction. Male soldiers with PTSD from battle action may not have much interest in sex, or may struggle to attain an erection (Buehler, 2011). PTSD can create nightmares, so that rather than associating evening time with sex and romance, it is associated with fears as well as insomnia. Understandably, sex may be the furthest thing from one's mind when recovering from a natural disaster, but when lack of sexual interest persists it can be a sign that the sexual symptom may need to be addressed more directly.

EATING DISORDERS

With a focus on the body and appetite, there can be overlap between eating disorders and sexual problems (Ackard, Kearney-Cooke, & Peterson, 2000; Conner et al., 2004; Lester, 1997; Wiederman, 1998). Experts sometimes point to the fact that anorexia nervosa often first appears in adolescent females as their bodies are taking on the proportions of an adult female. Ambivalence about becoming a woman balanced with a need to appear attractively slim as modeled in the media can lead to anorexia. People with anorexia characteristically don't wish to feel any type of hunger—not for food, but also not for sex. Anorexia also causes the cessation of menses, another indication that sexual activity is consciously or unconsciously unwanted. Emotions are often hidden, impeding the formation of an intimate relationship.

Those adults with bulimia may present with a different sexual history and drive than those with anorexia (Culbert & Klump, 2005; Quadflieg & Manfred, 2003; Wiederman & Pryor, 1997). Bulimia is associated with a lack of impulse control, which may generalize to sexual appetite as well. In fact, there is some speculation that females who are bulimic begin having sex at a younger age and have more sexual partners. They are also at risk for experiencing sexual assault, unwanted pregnancy, or contracting a sexually transmitted illness. Additionally, they can become so preoccupied with their need to binge and purge that their emotional and sexual needs become a low priority.

SUBSTANCE-RELATED DISORDERS

Sexual Side Effects of Alcohol and Recreational Substances

Various substances have sexual side effects (IsHak, Mikhail, Amiri, Berman, & Vasa, 2005; Smith, 2007), so it is important to assess for drug use when a client has sexual complaints. Aside from the fact that substances can negatively affect judgment, causing people to take unhealthy sexual risks and perhaps make ill-advised choices regarding partners (Hall, Fals-Stewart, & Finchman, 2008), they can have rather specific physical effects. For example, men who are chronic drinkers can experience problems with erections, low sex drive, and "feminization syndrome," which include shrinking of the testicles and development of male breast tissue (*gynecomastia*) (Fahrner, 1987). In women, alcohol may have the opposite effect, increasing testosterone slightly and causing more aggressive sexual behavior. Women sometimes become dependent on alcohol to help them express their sexual needs.

Smoking marijuana can enhance sexual experiences for some users, but in men *tetrahydrocannabinol* (THC), the active ingredient in marijuana, can lead to a decline in testosterone, causing erectile dysfunction (ED) and low desire. It can also impact a man's fertility. In women, THC may be stored in the tissues of the cervix and within the lubrication of the vagina, interfering with sperm's ability to reach the egg for fertilization.

Stimulants and barbituates also have their effects. Male cocaine users may initially enjoy delayed ejaculation because they believe they are pleasing their partner, but they may eventually become frustrated with the desensitization of their genitals. Conversely, males may also experience early ejaculation because of increased excitability. Crystal methamphetamine may also cause early ejaculation, but does not seem to be associated with other effects on sexual function (Smith, 2007). The street drug ecstasy is sometimes included in this class of drugs; ecstasy is said to create a feeling of bliss during sex, but can interfere with sexual performance (Smith, 2007). In practice, I have observed that ecstasy can create psychological dependence and disappointment with "normal" sex. Barbituates are sedatives that are occasionally used and even prescribed to decrease sexual performance anxiety, but they are also highly addictive, and an individual who uses them may be mentally and emotionally absent during sex.

Opioids include heroin, codeine, morphine, and the powerful prescription drug oxycodone. These powerful painkillers may have an initial euphoric effect, but over time men will experience a decrease of testosterone, leading to ED and loss of drive (Bang-Ping, 2007). Opioids can affect a woman's menstrual cycle and cause infertility. Hallucinogens such as LSD, mescaline, and psilocybin can heighten sexual pleasure, but they can also create nervousness and paranoia, which interfere with sex (Palha & Esteves, 2008). One very important recreational drug to know about and to warn clients about the effects of is alkyl nitrates, or "poppers." Poppers are used to increase sexual arousal by opening up blood flow to the genitals in a rush. If used while taking sildenafil (Viagra™), it can lead to severely low blood pressure.

Another name for alcohol is "liquid courage," and that pertains to an increase in sexual confidence and initiative (Fahrner, 1987; Johnson et al., 2004; La Pera et al., 2008; Sobczak, 2009; Turner & Dudek, 1982). Alcohol and other drugs disinhibit the frontal lobes and executive planning, allowing the expression of sexual impulses, for better or worse. While a small amount of alcohol can help a person relax and enjoy sex, a large amount can cause sexual problems, most especially ED in men. On the other hand, alcohol can help delay ejaculation, an effect that men who tend to have early ejaculation may use to their advantage. In fact, it is not unusual in my practice for a man who complains of early ejaculation to also report that previously he was a heavy drinker, but once he stopped the early ejaculation symptom recurred.

Women and men may find the effects of alcohol allow them to enjoy sex without guilt; they may become reluctant to engage in "sober sex." Unfortunately, sexual activity under the influence is likely to lead to poor judgment for both sexes, increasing the likelihood of an unwanted pregnancy or sexually transmitted disease (STD). And, relying on alcohol to enable one to be sexual indicates substance abuse, if not dependence.

STEP INTO MY OFFICE...

Paulette complained over the phone of her husband's lack of interest in sex. When Paulette and her husband, Al, arrived in my office, it was clear that Al wasn't in good health. His skin was chalky, his hair was dry and frizzy, and he seemed to be in a stupor. Al not only had a low drive, but he was unable to get reliable erections. A full assessment revealed that Al had been a chronic marijuana smoker for over 20 years. Al received education about the possible effects of smoking marijuana, such as a decrease in testosterone. However, Al had no interest in quitting his habit, choosing pot over his wife, who was left to decide if she wanted to remain married to a man who wanted to get high more than he wanted sex with his wife.

Other drugs, both prescription and non-prescription, have sexual effects. Painkillers such as OxyContin are the most commonly abused pills and are sedating, leading to low drive and difficulty with ejaculation (Palha & Esteves, 2008). Methamphetamines generally increase drive at the start, as well as lower inhibitions, which can contribute to higher risk for STDs and unwanted pregnancy. With long-term use, men can experience ED in a condition known as "crystal dick." Marijuana in some amount may lead to euphoria and sexual pleasure, but heavy use over time can cause sexual inertia, ED, and problems with ejaculation and orgasm.

Almost universally, substance problems lead to relationship problems. Sometimes, sexual dissatisfaction is the underlying cause of a partner's excessive use of alcohol and drugs, with the latter being a foil for the former. Even when one partner makes a decision to become sober, it can disrupt a couple's perhaps illusory social connection as well as the way in which they engage sexually.

SEXUALITY AND PROBLEMS GENERALLY DIAGNOSED IN CHILDHOOD

Attention deficit/hyperactivity disorder (AD/HD) (Betchen, 2003), Asperger's syndrome (Attwood, 2007), and learning disabilities can all have substantial effects on a person's ability to form an intimate relationship and enjoy sex. Each affects social development in different ways. They affect a person's self-concept and self-esteem, cause shifts in perception, and can make communication challenging. When these disorders are diagnosed in childhood, they are treated in various ways, including not at all. As people with these disorders mature, they may believe that they automatically shed their symptoms and sometimes partners enter into relationships without knowing of their existence.

Very little has been written about the sexual development of individuals with learning disabilities (LD), and the content here is based on my gleanings as an elementary school teacher, an intern in various agencies that served children, and my years as a sex therapist. There are many kinds of learning disabilities, some affecting the ability to read, some to write, and some with receptive and expressive verbal communication. Because the impact of LD is often apparent to peers when an individual is in school, children with LD are vulnerable to teasing and bullying, affecting self-esteem. Children with LD also tend to have trouble understanding social cues and can seem naive. Parents may become protective of offspring who have LD, which can contribute to emotional immaturity.

As the saying goes, a child with an LD becomes an adult with an LD. A common relationship dynamic is to have a person with LD dependent on an organized, well-functioning partner; however, this arrangement sometimes creates wear on the relationship. It also creates more of a parent–child dynamic that undermines sexual feelings between partners. Finally, people with LD sometimes have sensory processing problems. They may have difficulty discerning how firmly or softly to touch a partner. They may also be socially awkward when initiating sex, which can be a turnoff.

Children with AD/HD face many of the same problems of low self-esteem and missing out on social cues; they also may gravitate to a partner who comes to act as an organizing parent (Halverstadt, 1998). This disorder, however, creates a different set of problems in that adults with AD/HD sometimes become bored in the bedroom, which in my observation sometimes leads to behavior like masturbating to pornography. Women with AD/HD may have difficulty with arousal and orgasm, while men may complain of delayed ejaculation. Unlike antidepressants, medications used to treat AD/HD can actually be helpful during sex.

Asperger's syndrome (AS), which may or may not be a diagnosis in the next edition of the *Diagnostic and Statistical Manual* of the American Psychiatric Association, is a disorder on the autism spectrum that is characterized by severe difficulties in social situations. Children with AS struggle to make appropriate social connections; they are often thought of as being "little professors" as they lecture more than interact with others. They also may miss inflection in voice tone, and may speak in a formal way.

As adults, many people with AS learn ways of compensating, sometimes parroting the behavior of others. Because they tend to be highly intelligent, they are able to enter into stable careers, which can make them attractive to some as partners. But they can be frustrating to be with when it comes to sex and romance. Common complaints of partners of people with AS is that romance is "mechanical," that touch is "rough," and that they may need to initiate sex since the person with AS doesn't pick up signals that they are interested.

STEP INTO MY OFFICE...

When Rhonda first came to my office, she complained of low desire. As we explored her relationship with her husband, whom she had met as a teenager, she described an intelligent "computer geek" who was very inflexible, had poor hygiene, and regularly argued with nephews under the age of 10 about the rules of a video game. It sounded as if he might have AS, so I asked her to bring Anthony into the office on the next appointment. Anthony was dressed in nondescript clothing and looked unkempt. His affect was flat and he answered my questions in monosyllables, making it difficult to develop rapport. In a clear attempt to rescue Anthony from his obvious discomfort, Rhonda began to answer questions for him. It appeared that a parent–child dynamic, created by Anthony's inability to engage socially, was in force—not an especially sexually exciting one to Rhonda.

BODY-RELATED DISORDERS

Chronic pain, health anxiety (what was once called "hypochondriasis"), and body dysmorphic disorder have in common the misinterpretation of physical perception. Each has a different effect, though, on sexuality and relationships (Sanchez & Kiefer, 2007). Chronic pain, for example, can interfere because the sufferer may become preoccupied with their physical experience; they are also at risk for depressed mood and withdrawal from social interaction (Monga, Tan, Ostermann, Monga, & Grabois, 1998). Someone with chronic pain may also have trouble with foreplay or intercourse. One gentleman I worked with, for example, could not perform in missionary position because it created terrible discomfort in his knees. In another case, a man did not make the connection between his lack of erections and chronic neck pain for which he was about to undergo his third surgery.

Health anxiety can also cause a person to become preoccupied and withdrawn from a partner (Pearlman, 2010), but this disorder is especially disruptive when the phobia is focused on a sexually transmitted disease or problem with the genitals or reproductive system. In one case described to me, a man was so worried about illness that he not only wore a condom, but taped large squares of latex for several inches all around his penis.

The sexual effects of body dysmorphic disorder are readily discerned (Ackard et al., 2000; Conner et al., 2004). A person who is painfully self-conscious about any part of his or her body is unlikely to fully enjoy sex. One woman, for example, had so many surgeries to correct what she perceived as lopsided breasts that she lost all sensation in her nipples, causing such severe embarrassment that she vowed never to enter into a sexual relationship. Men sometimes become so concerned with penis length or girth that they undergo surgery; in one case, the man's penis became mangled to the point that he could no longer have erections.

PERSONALITY DISORDERS

Each cluster of personality disorders is associated with different effects on sexual and relationship function. Though many changes were proposed to the Personality Disorders in the *DSM-5*, they continue to be organized as belonging to Cluster A, Cluster B, or Cluster C. There is scant research on the sexual cognitions or behaviors that are associated with each personality type; here are discussed Antisocial, Avoidant, Borderline, Narcissistic, Obsessive Compulsive, and Schizotypal Personality Disorders. What follows is a description of the types of sexual problems associated with each type.

Antisocial Personality Disorder

Associated with sociopathy, a person with an antisocial personality disorder (ASPD) is a difficult one with whom to create an emotional tie. Generally, they exploit people who may genuinely care for them. People with ASPD may be promiscuous and engage in infidelity. Although someone may find the idea of healing a person with ASPD appealing through love and attention—and yes, sex—the fact is that people with ASPD rarely change (Millon, Millon, Meagher, Grossman, & Ramnath, 2004).

Avoidant Personality Disorder

Someone with avoidant personality disorder (APD) generally has experienced intense social anxiety, and so they tend to avoid social situations (Millon et al., 2004). Although they do not appear odd, they are very shy and may work in areas where little contact with others is required. Despite this, they do understand their own need for relationship and usually have a deep wish to develop a close connection. If they become involved, they may experience sexual problems such as inhibition or anorgasmia due to deep-rooted shame and inability to experience the required vulnerability (Buehler, 2011).

Borderline Personality Disorder

Borderline personality disorder (BPD) is characterized by an unstable sense of self and others as well as an inability to regulate emotions, making loving someone with this disorder a challenge (Bouchard, Sabourin, Lussier, & Villeneuve, 2009; Reise & Wright, 1996). They are generally certain that they will be abandoned, resulting in frantic and chaotic behaviors designed to prevent being left. It has been theorized that people with BPD may have been abused, which contributed to maladaptive defenses.

A lack of impulse control and need to avoid emptiness can lead people with BPD to have more sexual experiences than average. The BPD partner may sometimes belittle or criticize a non-BPD partner for lack of sexual experience, in part to keep the non-BPD partner off-balance. People with BPD can be variable in terms of their sexual wants and needs, leading to miscommunication and conflict. Although their defenses are maladaptive, people with BPD have great trouble giving them up, making them difficult also to work with in therapy.

Narcissistic Personality Disorder

Behind the mask of perfectionism, people with narcissistic personality disorder (NPD) are usually quite needy of approval, and will look for admiration, adulation, and subservience to maintain an inflated sense of self. A person with NPD may use sex to validate how attractive or special they are (Shafer, 2001; Sperry & Carlson, 2000). They may become hypersexual, needing multiple sexual partners to gratify their need for validation. The non-NPD partner often serves as a scapegoat for relationship problems, thus they are often blamed when sexual issues occur. For example, if a man with NPD develops ED, he may contact a therapist complaining that his partner is "boring," rather than looking for other causes.

Obsessive-Compulsive Personality Disorder

Obsessive-compulsive personality disorder (OCPD) is characterized by a preoccupation with rules and order. People with OCPD tend to be highly organized, demanding, and inflexible, and tend to be perfectionists. When others do not meet their standards, they become frustrated or angry. OCPD can interfere with many of life's pleasures, including sex. Males tend to suffer from performance anxiety and ED, as well as early ejaculation. For females, OCPD can interfere with the ability to have orgasm and, consequently, sexual desire.

Schizotypal Personality Disorder

People who are schizotypal are characterized by odd, eccentric behavior and peculiar beliefs. They also tend to be loners, and hence rarely enter couples therapy. When they come in solo, as they occasionally do in my practice, it is usually because they find sex confusing and do not understand what their partner wants from them. They rarely stay in sex therapy for more than a session or two.

SEXUAL SIDE EFFECTS OF ANTIDEPRESSANT AND ANTIPSYCHOTIC DRUGS

There are many neurotransmitters and brain activities associated with sexual function (Fisher, 2004a; Leiblum & Brezsnyak, 2006), including:

- Serotonin
- Acetylcholine
- Oxytocin
- Nitric oxide

- Dopamine
- Vasopressin
- Gonadotropin-releasing hormone

Serotonin and dopamine are neurotransmitters that are critical to sexual activity. Dopamine is an excitatory neurotransmitter implicated in sexual arousal and erections, as well as the reward associated with sex and orgasm; dopamine agonists that are found in antipsychotic medications can reduce sexual performance (Smith, 2007). Serotonin, on the other hand, inhibits sexual behavior; thus, SSRIs such as fluoxetene can interfere with sexual pleasure, drive, and performance. Only buspirone, an atypical antidepressant, can reduce the sexual side effects of SSRIs and is sometimes prescribed to enhance sex drive.

Increased use of antidepressants has multiplied complaints of sexual dysfunction. About 50% of men taking antidepressants will experience delayed ejaculation, and about 30% of men and women will experience delayed orgasm or anorgasmia (Stimmel & Gutierrez, 2007). SSRIs are associated with more sexual problems than are tricyclic antidepressants. Effects include loss of sex drive, erectile dysfunction, delayed ejaculation or failure, and anorgasmia. These effects remit in only about a third of clients who stop taking medication; according to Smith (2007) this is often because sexual effects are due to depression or other factors, and not to the medications themselves.

A large number of patients report sexual side effects from typical antipsychotics, which include thioridazine, trifluoperazine, and haloperidol. In addition to the agonist effects on dopamine, there may also be changes in the endocrine system, such as elevated levels of prolactin (Baldwin & Mayers, 2003). Men with high levels of prolactin may have trouble with erections, and women may complain of decreased overall sexual function. Delayed ejaculation as well as reduced volume of ejaculate—sometimes causing complaints of change in orgasm—can result from taking such antipsychotics.

Sexual effects with new or atypical antipsychotics may be less prevalent. For example, quetiapine is less frequently associated with hyperprolactin, while clozapine causes fewer problems with erection, orgasm, sexual enjoyment, and satisfaction than typical antipsychotics (Baldwin & Mayers, 2003). No antipsychotic medication is ideal, however, as clozapine, reperidone, and olanzapine have been reported to occasionally cause retrograde ejaculation and priapism.

MANAGEMENT STRATEGIES

There are several possible approaches to addressing sexual problems related to the use of antidepressants (Melton, 2012), the primary one being to ensure that the sexual complaints do, in fact, arise from the psychotropic medications. Ascertaining when the complaints began and if there is any prior history of such complaints can help rule out other factors. Some clients may require more than one strategy, and all strategies must be discussed with the prescribing physician.

1. See if the problem stops without any intervention as the client's body adapts to the medication.
2. Switch to another antidepressant that is known to have fewer sexual side effects.
3. Add buproprion to the regimen.
4. For men, add a phosphodiesterase type 5 (PDE5) inhibitor such as Viagra™ to improve erectile function. In women, a PDE5 inhibitor may improve vaginal lubrication and orgasmic response.
5. Be sure to rule out low testosterone as a contributing factor in male clients; if present, supplement with testosterone.
6. A "drug holiday," or short break such as over the weekend, may help those taking sertraline and paroxetine. A related strategy is to take the dose of antidepressant *after* sexual activity.

OTHER DRUGS THAT CAN CAUSE SEXUAL PROBLEMS

Many prescribed drugs can cause sexual side effects (Neel, 2012; Smith, 2007). Sometimes physicians don't realize that there may be sexual side effects, such as with finastaride, an antibaldness drug that many users complained lead to complete loss of erections and low drive, sometimes long after discontinuation of use (Irwig & Kolukula, 2011). A commonly used class of drugs, statins and fibrates used to treat high cholesterol, can interfere with the production of testosterone, estrogen, and other sex hormones, leading to ED and difficulty with orgasm. Blood pressure medication, also known as antihypertensives, are prescribed to reduce blood flow, which in men can reduce desire and lead to ED and delayed ejaculation. Women can experience vaginal dryness, low desire, and difficulty achieving orgasm. Diuretics, beta blockers, and alpha-blockers can decrease blood flow to the sex organs, but also interfere with the production of zinc, which is needed to produce testosterone.

Another class of drugs, H2 blockers, also known as H2-receptor antagonists, are used to treat gastrointestinal disorders such as gastroesophageal reflux disease (GERD) and gastric and peptic ulcers (Neel, 2007). H2 blockers such as Tagamet™ can cause ED as well as breast enlargement in men when taken over long periods of time. Finally, anticonvulsants, used to control seizures, are increasingly being used to treat other conditions such as chronic pain and migraines. Older anticonvulsants include carbamazepine (Tegretol™) and phenytoin (Dilantin™) can lower testosterone, which can cause ED for men and decreased lubrication in women (Neel, 2007). They can also cause difficulty with orgasm and low desire for both sexes. Newer anticonvulsants like gabapentin (Neurontin™) and topiramate (Topamax™) may have fewer side effects.

Sexual Side Effects of Psychotropic Medications

Drug Class	Drug Name	Sexual Effects
TCAs	Amitriptyline, desimpramine, doxepin, imipramine, nortriptyline	Women: breast enlargement and decreased orgasm Men: erectile dysfunction and decreased orgasm
SSRIs	Citalopram, escitalopram, fluoxetine, fluvoxamine, paroxetine, sertraline	Women: decreased drive and delay or cessation of orgasm Men: delayed ejaculation and erectile dysfunction
SNRIs	Duloxetine, venlafaxine	Women: delay or cessation of orgasm Men: ED and abnormal ejaculation
Norepinephrine and dopamine reuptake inhibitor	Buproprion	Rare; may improve desire and orgasm in women
Mixed-action agents	Trazadone, nefazodone, mirtazapine, vilazodone	Adverse effects rare; trazadone associated with priapism

TCAs, tricyclic antidepressants; SSRIs, selective serotonin reuptake inhibitors; SNRIs, serotonin-norepinephrine reuptake inhibitors.

Antidepressant Types and Symptoms of Sexual Dysfunction

Phenothiazines	Men: ED; delayed or retrograde ejaculation; reduced volume of ejaculate; priapism; reduced testosterone
Haloperidol	Men: painful orgasm, low drive, ED
Thioxanthenes	Decreased drive and anorgasmia Men: ED and ejaculatory problems
Olanzapine	Side effects rare, may produce priapism Women: improved menstrual function and reduced side effects from risperidone
Risperidone	Men: ejaculatory problems, priapism though rare; gynecomastia Women: amenorrhea and galactorrhea
Amisulpiride	Elevated prolactin, but lower rates of ED
Quetiapine	Decreased libido most frequently reported effect
Clozapine	Fewer sexual side effects compared to convention antipsychotics
Ziprasidone	Priapism possible
Aripiprazole	Decreased prolactin

ACTIVITIES

1. Reflect on how you might go about assessing sexual problems in the clients you see who come in for treatment for other concerns, especially those that are most commonly seen in your practice.
2. How might you address the sexual concerns of clients who are currently in your practice, but came in for other problems?
3. Explore the websites of organizations that advocate for people who have the types of illnesses you most often treat. Do they have information on sexuality to which you could refer clients? If not, might you be able to create such information for their site?

RESOURCES

Buehler, S. (2010). *Sex, love, and mental- illness: A couples' guide to staying connected.* Santa Barbara, CA: Praeger/ABC-Clio.

NAMI: National Alliance for the Mentally Ill. www.nami.org. The National Alliance for the Mentally Ill is an advocacy organization. NAMI has local chapters and many run workshops for individuals and their families to help cope with mental illness.

Woolis, R. (1992). *When someone you love has a mental illness.* New York, NY: Penguin.

WHEN A PARTNER IS MENTALLY ILL:
RELATIONSHIP TIPS

Being in a relationship when you or your partner has a mental illness—whether depression, an eating disorder, or recovery from substance abuse—can be very challenging. Different mental illnesses also can have different effects on a person's sexuality, which your therapist can explain. Here are some tips for coping when someone you love is mentally ill.

- Become educated about the problem. Read about the illness and its treatment. If there is a support group, attend some meetings, especially at the beginning of the diagnosis.

- Agree on communication about flare-ups of symptoms or signs that medication isn't working.

- Minimize stress and establish routines. A chaotic household or schedule can make mental illness worse.

- Accept changes brought about by the mental illness. For example, the partner may no longer want to participate in certain activities because they are triggers. Honor the needs of the mentally ill person.

- Realize you cannot fix your partner. No matter how much you may wish that your partner wasn't depressed or traumatized, you cannot take away the mental illness.

- The well partner may want to find activities to do when the mentally ill partner isn't feeling well in order to keep resentments from building.

- Anticipate setbacks. Even people with well-controlled mental illness can have problems with medications that once worked, or decide that they no longer need medications, creating a flare-up. Handle setbacks without judgment and by finding the best care.

- Attend couples counseling. Couples need to be able to communicate thoughts and feelings about mental illness if their relationship is going to withstand challenges.

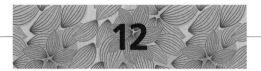

Sexual Recovery in Childhood Sexual Abuse Survivors

Perhaps the most difficult sexual symptoms to treat are those that arise in survivors of childhood sexual abuse (CSA). The sadness, shame, and embarrassment suffered by a survivor who cannot enjoy sex because of flashbacks or other symptoms of complex trauma is almost palpable. Yet, in my experience, as much as they clearly need help, they are sometimes the most difficult clients to keep in therapy. Going slowly and taking care not to retraumatize the client by being overly intrusive are two keys to early success in keeping the survivor in treatment. In addition, not every survivor of CSA will complain of sexual late effects. It is up to the therapist to ask, being certain to normalize that questions about sexual development are posed to almost every client.

POSTTRAUMATIC STRESS DISORDER VERSUS COMPLEX TRAUMA

Posttraumatic stress disorder (PTSD) is diagnosed when someone has specific symptoms in response to a single event, for example, an automobile accident, natural disaster, or sudden death of a loved one. Such symptoms include the "flight or fight" response; shock; extreme fear; helplessness; flashbacks; nightmares; and avoidance of any stimuli that reminds one of the precipitating event. In spite of such symptoms, the core self stays intact and there is generally minimal self-destructive behavior.

Complex trauma, on the other hand, is a response to repeated or chronic events (Courtois & Ford, 2009; Finkelhor & Browne, 1985), as might occur when a child experiences repeated molestation by one person, or is serially abused by multiple people, such as an uncle and a grandfather. The symptoms of complex trauma include those of PTSD, but go beyond them and become chronic. The likelihood of complex trauma occurring increases with incest (especially a female with a father or brother); repeated instances of abuse; penetrative sex (oral, vaginal, or anal, and with fingers, tongue, penis, or objects); and when threats were made to one's life or the life of family members (Browning & Laumann, 1997).

COMPLEX TRAUMA IN SURVIVORS OF CSA

Female survivors are more prevalent than male survivors. Current estimates are that one in four females and one in six males will experience CSA, but no one really knows the numbers because not all survivors come forward about their experiences. Females are also more likely to have experienced penetrative sex. Males, on the other hand, are less likely to admit abuse than females. They are more likely to have experienced a single incident of abuse or to have been abused by an older peer.

ASSESSMENT OF SURVIVORS

Biological Effects

CSA may cause neurological changes in the brain (Weiss, 2007; Wilson, 2010). Excitatory chemicals and stress hormones increase in such a way that the hypothalamus-pituitary-adrenal axis of the body, which regulates the body in preparation for stress (Friedman, Jalowiec, McHugo, Wang, & McDonagh, 2007), becomes disordered. Simultaneously, low cortisol levels disrupt the process of homeostasis in mind and body, making it difficult to modulate one's feelings and responses to stimuli, as well as potentially increasing the risk for inflammatory diseases in the future, for example, fibromyalgia or chronic fatigue syndrome (King, Mandinsky, King, Fletcher, & Brewer, 2001).

Physical changes in the brain may also account for the fact that some survivors act out sexually, while others develop a sexual aversion. Although the mechanism isn't well understood, researchers think that when abuse occurs at critical periods of sexual development, it can cause the emergence or suppression of sexual hormones. In either case, survivors may sense that they do not have complete control over their sexual behavior.

Somatization, or the development of physical symptoms in response to abuse, has been connected with the experience of chronic pain as well as "body memories" encoded as physical pain in the genitals or other body parts. Survivors make more trips to the emergency room than do adults who were never abused (Chartier, Walker, & Naimark, 2007; Newman, Clayton, & Zuellig, 2000). Women survivors sometimes develop fears regarding gynecological exams and labor and delivery (Leeners, Stiller, Block, Görres, Imthurn, & Rath, 2007).

Developmental Effects

When CSA disrupts attachment, a disorganized style is the one that most frequently emerges, exhibited by excessive help-seeking and dependency as well as social isolation and disengagement, impulsiveness, and inhibition, as well as submissiveness and aggression. *Traumatic sexualization* may also occur, in which inappropriate attitudes and feelings are formulated regarding sexual activity. All of this bodes poorly for future adult romantic and sexual relationships (Mullen, Martin, Anderson, Romans, & Herbison, 1994).

Sexual Late Effects

There are many sexual complaints associated with surviving CSA (Bartoi & Kinder, 1998; Cohn, 2010; Easton, Coohey, O'Leary, Zhang, & Hua, 2011; Maltz, 2012; Sarwer & Durlak, 1996), including low desire, difficulty with arousal, problems with orgasm, as well as sexual pain in males and females, while males may complain of erectile dysfunction and early ejaculation (Hall, 2009). However, not all survivors view sex negatively; sex is associated with attention, affection, privilege, and power, and some people also find that it is something that they are good at and truly enjoy.

In addition to having to overcome sometimes very powerful feelings of disgust, problems with self-regulation can make it difficult to attend to one's own thoughts, emotions, and physical responses during sex. Survivors often describe dissociating during sex, or engaging in "spectatoring," the sensation that one is removed from oneself, watching sexual activity as if from afar. They may freeze, numbing or turning off their sexual feelings as well as guilt and shame. Their partner may complain that they seem "absent" during sex; there may be sadness and tears after intercourse or even orgasm. Certainly, if someone isn't present for the experience of sex, they cannot experience sexual pleasure.

Aside from symptoms of PTSD—flashbacks, nightmares, and so forth—abuse survivors sometimes experience confusion about sexual orientation, or fear about becoming an abuser. It is not uncommon to express fears about the function of one's reproductive system and fertility.

Effects on Relationships

Survivors of CSA also run into challenges with almost every interpersonal relationship because of the trust and vulnerability required to be emotionally invested and available. Often there is strain in the survivor's family of origin, particularly if the family has split into factions of believers and disbelievers regarding whether or not the abuse took place. Interactions with family members who deny the abuse or who withhold emotional support of any kind put the survivor at risk of revictimization.

Couples in which one (or both) are survivors report higher rates of marital discord due to lack of trust, hostility, and poor communication, and higher rates of separation and divorce. Survivors more often report that they perceive their partner as uncaring and overly controlling, creating a rift when one might not otherwise exist.

TREATING SEXUAL PROBLEMS IN ADULT SURVIVORS OF ABUSE

Treatment can be challenging for therapists, not only because survivors require an especially gentle approach, but also because research suggests that many therapists have, themselves, been traumatized; in fact, a metaphor for a therapist that is often cited is that of the "wounded healer." Therapists who treat survivors, and who are survivors themselves, must take special care to maintain appropriate boundaries so as not to confuse their own issues with those of their client (Neumann & Gamble, 1995; Nutall & Jackson, 1994; Van Dernoot Lipsky & Burk, 2009). In fact, it could be said that no therapist is able to treat a survivor unless they, themselves, have been in treatment, lest the role of therapist does more harm than good to either party.

Therapists who treat survivors of abuse must be prepared for the client's resistance. Survivors are often reluctant to give up defenses that were adapted to keep abuse a secret due to shame. They may also misunderstand the therapist's motives for talking about sex; it is helpful to normalize that you are a therapist who speaks to all clients about their sexuality. Let the client know that they can express when they are having problems with trust or struggling with any aspect of treatment, which is generally long-term.

STAGES OF HEALING

Courtois and Ford (2009) suggests that there are three phases of healing, which are not necessarily linear and may need to be revisited at various times during the course of treatment:

- Stabilization: Developing rapport; creating safety; identifying and eliminating dangerous behaviors (e.g., drinking, engaging in promiscuous sex).
- Memory processing: Accessing and discussing memories at such as pace that the survivor doesn't feel overwhelmed, leading to avoidance and dissociation; addressing issues related to establishing healthy attachments.
- Personality integration and rehabilitation: Being able to function as expected for age and stage of life; developing greater capacity for physical, sexual, and interpersonal intimacy, as well as autonomy.

INITIAL SESSIONS

Helping the client identify sources of support they can turn to outside of therapy during treatment will buoy the client's emotional stability. Including the partner in initial sessions can be beneficial in assessing the strength of the relationship; to address any emotional fallout from the survivor's abuse that may have undermined the partner's support; and to establish boundaries, for example, putting intercourse and other sexual activities aside for the time being, if the survivor feels they need to take a break while trying to heal; a so-called healthy sex contract (Maltz, 2012) can be created later in which partners create an agreement about why they are having sex, what sex means to them, when sex may or may not occur, how they will communicate, and other related issues.

The beginning of therapy can also be devoted to educating the client about the biology of trauma, including over- or underreacting to sexual or other anxiety-provoking activity. (Fears about sex often generalize to other areas of a client's life.) Teaching the client how to self-soothe with techniques such as deep breathing, progressive muscle relaxation, and mindfulness—or some other self-identified practice—can be helpful both during and in-between sessions, and later in anticipation of sexual activity. Such activities, combined with ego strengthening to bolster low self-esteem, can generate self-efficacy and worth.

Cognitive therapy can be used to help the client recognize and redress negative thoughts and concepts about sex. Clients may give lip service to the idea that "sex is something that feels good and brings two people closer," but in truth feel not that way at all. It may take many weeks before the client can see that in their present life, sex can be an expression of positive feelings and an experience of pleasure, as well as an act one does for oneself, and not just to please one's partner or for the sake of the relationship.

In order to reinforce changes in thinking, behavioral changes must take place as well (Cohn, 2011; Maltz, 2012). The survivor may need to give him- or herself permission to say no to sex if they do not wish to engage, or to address any instances in which they feel coerced by their partner. They also must allow themselves the opportunity to do an internal check-in to ascertain what it is, exactly, that they do want from a partner, both in and out of the bedroom.

For survivors, flashbacks can be triggered during sex by almost any type of sensory stimulation, from the smell of a partner's breath, to the lighting in a room, to a certain touch on a certain part of the body (Cohn, 2011; Maltz, 2012). Sensations from within the body can also trigger flashbacks, such as a rapid heartbeat or hyperventilation. If the survivor can readily identify the triggers, they may be eliminated. Still, sometimes triggers cannot be eliminated altogether or a new trigger may appear. What can be helpful is for the survivor and partner to agree on a signal if the survivor is triggered; a common one is to say "yellow light" if the survivor fears being triggered, but wants to proceed regardless, and "red light" to stop altogether. When a "yellow light" situation occurs, the survivor can practice self-soothing techniques, but if it is a "red light" situation, the couple needs to stop. At this juncture, the survivor may try to self-soothe and regroup so that sexual activity can continue, or they may decide that they are too overwhelmed— but willing to resume another time. You can make a copy of the Client Worksheet "Understanding Sexual Triggers" as a handout for the client to take home.

An especially distressing triggering event occurs when a survivor has unwanted sexual fantasies, often cued during masturbation or other sexual activity (Wilson & Wilson, 2008). In a book regarding the nature of sexual fantasies (Maltz & Boss, 2012), the authors recommend:

- Analyzing the fantasy to explore its meaning, thereby diminishing its power.
- Creating a relatively stress-free environment for sexual activity, including having sex when one is more relaxed and practicing self-soothing techniques so that the survivor is less vulnerable to unwanted fantasies.
- Stopping sexual activity if the fantasy appears, resuming only when it dissipates.
- Changing the fantasy so that it becomes innocuous, for example, "bondage with ropes becomes bondage with spaghetti noodles."

A recent study (Wilson & Wilson, 2008) also suggests that the survivor can use aversion therapy, such as putting cayenne pepper on one's tongue when an unwanted fantasy manifests; however, many therapists may be hesitant to try such a procedure with a survivor of abuse.

RECOGNIZING AND DEALING WITH BURNOUT

Working with survivors of trauma seem to make therapists especially vulnerable to burnout or what is sometimes called "compassion fatigue." Signs of therapist burnout include the feelings that one's hard work is making little difference; physical fatigue; avoidance of work with clients, for example, being absent from one's practice or not returning phone calls; ruminating about clients' problems; insomnia; and symptoms associated with stress, depression, and anxiety.

Therapists are encouraged to engage in self-care activities, including:

- Scheduling time off from one's practice for refreshment
- Engaging in pleasurable activities with family and friends
- Getting exercise
- Developing an interest or hobby unrelated to one's profession
- Consulting with colleagues regarding difficult clients
- Seeking one's own therapy, especially if one experienced maltreatment similar to the client's
- Trying a centering practice such as meditation, writing in a journal, or prayer
- Avoiding depressing material, such as books or movies about traumatic events

ADDRESSING SPECIFIC SEXUAL DYSFUNCTIONS

In addition to general treatment suggestions, therapists may want to keep the following suggestions in mind.

Low Drive

- Normalize not wanting something that has been emotionally painful or confusing.
- Identify what thoughts or activities are more likely to lead to having sexual desire, for example, connecting emotionally with conversation or taking a scented bath.
- Teach Basson's "responsive" model of desire.
- Discuss with the couple that their sex life may not look like that of others; they are establishing what is normal for them in terms of frequency, type of activities, etc.

Anorgasmia

- Normalize the need for control.
- Use self-soothing, for example, deep breathing, mindfulness, or calming music and scents during heightened arousal prior to orgasm.

- Viagra has shown some potential in helping female survivors become aroused during sex (Berman et al., 2003).

Erectile Dysfunction and Early Ejaculation

- Both are relatively rare in male survivors.
- Encourage sensate focus activities and pleasure sessions.
- Consider use of PDE5 inhibitors (phosphodiesterase type 5 inhibitors, e.g., Viagra).

Hypersexuality

- Rule out concurrent bipolar disorder.
- Explore maladaptive reactions to feelings of sexual arousal and activity.

A FINAL WORD TO THERAPISTS ABOUT TREATING SURVIVORS

Therapists who treat PTSD are susceptible to "vicarious traumatization" when they engage empathically with survivors (Neumann & Gamble, 1995). Those who work with sexual problems of survivors of CSA may be especially susceptible because of their own discomfort with talking about sex, or because of the possibility that the therapist him- or herself has been molested. It is critical not to overly identify with the client and to remember the goal of healthy sexuality for the survivor; to build a network of supportive friends and family for oneself; and to find one's own self-soothing practice.

ACTIVITIES

1. Select two books from the *Resource* list and compare the authors' viewpoints on the following concepts:
   a. Victimhood
   b. Survivorship
   c. Sexuality
   d. Safety and vulnerability
   e. Partner considerations
   f. Explanation of trauma theory
   g. Recommendations regarding treatment
2. If you have not ever done so, write down some of your signs that you are overloaded or burned out by listening to sexual trauma. Then create a plan for addressing these signs, including limiting how many clients with trauma you will see; increasing self-care; getting more rest; talking to a supervisor or colleague; etc.

RESOURCES

Lew, M. (2004). *Victims no longer: The classic guide for men recovering from childhood sexual abuse.* New York, NY: Harper Perennial.

Maltz, W. (2012). *A sexual healing journey: A guide for survivors of sexual abuse* (3rd ed.). New York, NY: William Morrow Paperbacks.

Rothschild, B. (2010). *8 keys to safe trauma recovery: Take-charge strategies to empower your healing.* New York, NY: W. W. Norton & Company.

Van Dernoot Lipsky, L., & Burk, C. (2009). *Trauma stewardship: An every day guide to caring for self while caring for others.* San Francisco, CA: Berrett-Koehler.

MINDFULNESS AND SEXUALITY

Mindfulness, or staying aware of and living in the present moment, has many applications, including stress reduction and pain management. But it may also be useful in helping people with a variety of sexual problems, including low desire, difficulty with arousal, anorgasmia, erectile dysfunction, and early ejaculation. Mindfulness, which has its roots in Buddhist meditation, was brought to the West by Nobel Prize nominee Thich Nhat Hanh, while physician Jon Kabat-Zinn is credited with using mindfulness to help medical patients.

Living mindfully requires practice, but the payoff is inner serenity that can help you tune in to the sensations of your body. Mindfulness does this through both physical relaxation and nonjudgmental detachment from thoughts. As you are probably aware, the brain produces thousands of thoughts, most forming in nanoseconds. Some thoughts are important, but many are just noise. When people pay too much attention to the noise, they can start to make habitual, negative thoughts about one's self, one's actions, and one's body. Quieting the noise can help someone be more in touch with the present moment, bringing awareness and joy to sexual encounters.

The simplest mindfulness meditation is to pay attention to breathing and not much else, done without any real effort. Hanh suggests saying something easy to yourself as you notice: "Breathing in, this is my in-breath. Breathing out, this is my out-breath." If you add enjoyment to this act, you can make ordinary breathing into something pleasant as you realize that if you are breathing, you must be alive! Hanh calls this realization miraculous, but you can give it any positive meaning you wish: fundamental, real, good, wonderful, and so forth.

The next step is to add concentration, by aiding the mind to follow the body. If your in-breath lasts 3 to 4 seconds, then that can be how long you initially try to free your mind from thought. In this case, Hanh instructs that one says something like: "Breathing in, I follow my in-breath all the way through. Breathing out, I follow my out-breath all the way through." At first your mind may interrupt your concentration with thought, but eventually you will be able to breathe in and out with full concentration.

A third step is to link mind and body. This is where a connection can be made between mindfulness and sexual enjoyment. As you breathe in, you say, "Breathing in, I am aware of my body." As you breathe out, say, "Breathing out, I am aware of my body." When mind and body are unified, then you can pay attention to sensation as well as emotion. When you can calm mind and body during the initial stages of foreplay during sex, you can tune into what you are feeling and experiencing. This can increase arousal, emotional connection, and pleasure.

There are other ways to practice mindfulness, such as eating mindfully, doing walking meditation, practicing seated meditation, and so forth. Yoga can also be done mindfully. Yoga literally means "yoke," or linking together mind and body. It can also exercise pelvic floor muscles, make one more limber for sex, and can be done for either relaxation or invigoration, depending on the practice.

UNDERSTANDING SEXUAL TRIGGERS

People who have experienced sexual or other types of trauma sometimes experience flashbacks to different kinds of bad memories. These memories can occur because of "triggers," which can be a touch, a smell, a word, even a type of light that reminds or "triggers" a person's recollection of unwanted sex. Triggers can happen out of the blue, even with a loving partner during an enjoyable sexual encounter. That is because our bodies and minds store some memories in order to protect us. The body and mind cannot tell sometimes whether a memory is being appropriately triggered. This can make it very confusing when bad memories come up at the wrong time.

There are different ways to handle triggers. Here are some tips that may help.

1. Make sure you are relaxed both mentally and physically before you have sex. Massage, warm showers, or a long walk before sex can help.

2. Only have sex when you really want to. Remember, you always have the right to say no. That can prevent triggers caused by bad feelings.

3. Have a signal you can give your partner when you are being triggered. Agree that you will slow down or stop for a few minutes to see if you can relax and get back into the right state of mind to enjoy sex. If not, don't be angry with yourself. Just try again another day.

4. If you experience that you are starting to get triggered, try to ground yourself in the present moment. Remind yourself that you are in a safe place, with a safe person. Really look around the room and try to feel what is happening right now. Is your partner touching you? Are you touching your partner? Can you feel the bed or other surface?

5. Be sure to eliminate triggers. If you get triggered by the smell of beer on your partner's breath, ask your partner to brush his or her teeth before you have sex. If you get triggered by having your upper thighs or abdomen touched, let your partner know that, too.

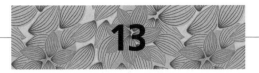

Sexual Pain Disorders

Sexual pain disorders plague millions of American women and men, though most mental health professionals would never know it as this topic is one of the most embarrassing for people to speak about (Donaldson & Meana, 2011; Jeng, 2004). In part that is because many physicians and psychotherapists mistakenly believe that painful sex is all in one's head (Slowinski, 2001), as reported to me by dozens of female patients.

It doesn't help that, as with other types of pain, there is often no visible injury at the site; also, physicians tend to be poorly trained in symptom recognition and the treatment of sexual pain disorders. What often happens is that when a woman makes a complaint of sexual pain to her gynecologist, the response might be a pat on her knee and a comment such as, "You just need to learn to relax," or, "Try a glass of wine first." Women often describe going from doctor to doctor in frustration, trying to relieve their physical distress, emotional desperation, and, quite possibly, their committed relationships (Connor, Robinson, & Wieling, 2008). Though in far less numbers, men also suffer from sexual pain disorders that are related to the prostate, as well as penile deformities about which they, too, feel embarrassment.

Fortunately, researchers, physicians, physical therapists (PTs), and psychotherapists have all taken recent interest in helping such women and men by expanding the understanding of why sex might be painful and how to treat it. Still, sexual pain disorders remain complex to assess and difficult to treat. Generally, it takes a team approach for successful treatment: a knowledgeable physician and a PT, both of whom are specialized in pelvic pain problems, and a psychotherapist who can help with processing the event of acquiring the disorder, recommending adjunctive treatments such as relaxation techniques, and counseling the individual who has the condition and his or her partner regarding intimacy and sexuality (van Lankveld et al., 2010; Slowinski, 2001).

UNDERSTANDING PAIN

Presented here is a simple explanation of the very complex problem of chronic pain. Begin with recognizing that there are two types of pain. *Acute pain* occurs when something happens, such as burning your finger on the stove. The brain receives the sensory input, and then signals for you to protect the area by pulling your finger away. The brain also signals for certain chemical reactions to occur, such as an immune response to aid in healing any wound. Acute pain disappears as the area heals.

Chronic pain is diagnosed when the area has healed, but the person still complains of pain, making treatment difficult. Chronic pain can be either nociceptive or neuropathic. Nociceptive pain occurs when nerve endings at the site of the pain, called nociceptors, keep sending signals to the brain that there is an injury. Such pain can be *somatic*, occurring externally as with provoked vestibulodynia, or *visceral*, occurring internally as with endometriosis. Someone with chronic painful sex also can have both somatic and visceral pain (van Lankveld et al., 2010).

The experience of pain is subjective—what makes one person writhe may be barely perceived by another—because of various factors, including individual differences in the brain, as well as the person's past experience with pain and other adverse health events, their psychological state, their ability to cope with discomfort, and even their relationships. The psychotherapist's role in treating any type of chronic pain is not to help the pain disappear, but to diminish its effects through better coping skills (Quartana, Campbell, & Edwards, 2009), including cognitive behavioral therapy (LoFrisco, 2011), relaxation techniques, and communication with one's partner (Connor, Robinson, & Wieling, 2008).

ASSESSMENT OF SEXUAL PAIN DISORDERS

Therapists cannot ethically or legally assess these problems on their own. A referral must be made to a physician who is knowledgeable in the medical treatment of provoked vestibulodynia (PVD), dyspareunia, and vaginismus. (Note that all of these sexual pain presentations have now been grouped together in the *DSM-5* [2013] as Genito-Pelvic Pain/Penetration Disorder. Other terms such as "vaginismus" are used here because they are prevalent in past research.) Therapists may, however, be the first stop when a woman has pain with intercourse, often because she and her partner are in psychological distress. In such cases, the therapist may serve the client by sharing their thoughts that this may, in fact, be a medical condition, and prepare the client for a doctor's visit.

Unfortunately, sometimes women have already been to several doctors without relief (Connor et al., 2008). It can be an important part of treatment to empathically listen to their story, and then normalize their experience, as it can be difficult to find a physician with the appropriate training. Making contact with physicians in your area—or as near to your area as possible—can help reassure a client that she will be directed to a medical doctor who can help; there are organizations listed in the *Resources* section of this chapter that can help you locate someone.

THE PSYCHOLOGICAL FALLOUT OF PAINFUL SEX

The inability to engage in sexual activity with one's partner can be distressing to the point that a woman may fear rejection and abandonment. Viewed through a feminist lens, this alone is problematic, as women can measure their worth beyond their ability to have intercourse (Farrell & Cacchioni, 2012). Nonetheless, this perception can lead to a behavior known as "pain catastrophizing," in which the painful condition is seen as the worst, most horrible event that could ever befall someone (Borg, Peters, Schultz, & de Jong, 2012). Other factors that lead to increased perception of pain include pain anxiety, fear of pain, and pain hypervigilance. Generalized anxiety and depression also contribute, as may negative emotions such as anger. When a woman feels helpless and hopeless about sexual pain, she may even express suicidal thoughts.

STEP INTO MY OFFICE...

With eyes cast down, Fiona told me the painful truth that she and her husband had been married for 8 years without having consummated their marriage. Although they tried to have intercourse, albeit with decreasing frequency over the years, penetration had been impossible. Fiona described that during first attempts at intercourse on their honeymoon, she had vomited from being so nervous. She occasionally still became nauseous when her husband attempted penetration.

Fiona had been molested by a neighbor, though at what age and how many times it had occurred she could not recall. She felt certain that it had included digital penetration. She had told a former therapist about the incidents, but never about the vaginismus. She had sought help from a physician who simply handed her a box of dilators and no other instruction. Now she wanted a baby. Could I help?

Fortunately, after 2 years of biweekly psychotherapy and a round of physical therapy specializing in pelvic floor dysfunction, Fiona and her husband became pregnant, fulfilling a long held dream to have a family together.

The state of a woman's relationship with her sexual partner, especially his response to her painful condition, can also generate an increase in the experience of pain. Ironically, *pain catastrophizing* can push away a potentially supportive partner, leading to miscommunication and emotional conflict (Quartana et al., 2009). Eventually, there can be avoidance of all sexual and physical contact, which can produce a further emotional rift in the couple's relationship. Couples affected by these conditions have complained of feeling emotionally numb or shutdown; restarting sexual activity can be awkward.

As with any individual who has a chronic pain or illness, there can be secondary gain that creates an obstacle to improvement (Rolland, 1994). For example, having chronic pain may be used to excuse one's self from participating in certain activities, staying home on disability from a job one dislikes, or receiving attention from health care professionals. And, in the case of sexual pain disorders, there can be secondary gain in terms of being able to control if, when, and how a couple's sex life will proceed. Thus, it is critical to have a complete sexual history in order to develop effective treatment goals, particularly to see if sexual dysfunction predated the development of sexual pain.

Although it cannot be said that sexual pain is directly caused by past sexual abuse, it appears that women who experienced molestation with penetration are at risk for increased pain when they develop conditions like dyspareunia (Leclerc, Bergeron, Binik, & Khalifé, 2009).

It is also important for the psychotherapist to understand that treating other symptoms of posttraumatic stress disorder (PTSD) will not automatically resolve such physical conditions, which must be treated as a separate issue. Additionally, women survivors of childhood sexual abuse (CSA) must be asked directly if sex is ever uncomfortable or painful, as they may be too embarrassed to report the symptoms unless asked. It is a simple matter to ask if sex has ever been more uncomfortable or penetration impossible, sparing a woman the perhaps difficult task of revealing that intercourse has been the source of disappointment and shame.

TYPES OF SEXUAL PAIN DISORDERS IN WOMEN

There are a variety of syndromes (defined as a collection of symptoms), infections, and diseases that underlie complaints of painful sex as described in a recent review article by van Lankveld et al. (2010). Sometimes these conditions overlap, which presents challenges in terms of treatment. Note, too, that as researchers and physicians work to understand painful sex, the terms are subject to change.

Provoked Vestibulodynia

Once called "vulvar vestibulitus," these conditions are characterized by pain in the vulvar area around the outside of the vagina. The most common reasons for provocation of pain are tight pelvic floor muscles, hormonal changes, and an increase in nerves in the vulvar area. Postmenopausal women are most likely to complain of PVD (Kao, Binik, Kapuscinski, & Khalifé, 2008).

Hypertonic Pelvic Floor Dysfunction

In this condition, the large pelvic floor muscles are too tight or hypertonic, making penetration of the vagina for intercourse, manual sex, or even tampon use extremely uncomfortable or impossible. Also frequently called "vaginismus," this is essentially a spasm of the muscles around the entrance to the vagina, bladder, and anus.

Vulvar and Vaginal Atrophy

Atrophy is diagnosed when the tissues of the vulva and vagina become dry, thin, and friable. It can happen as a result of menopause, but also hormonal changes due to use of oral contraceptives, removal of the ovaries, use of drugs to manage breast cancer, infertility treatment, and treatment of endometriosis. Women who have these conditions will complain that having intercourse "feels like being rubbed with sandpaper."

Vulvar and Vaginal Skin Disorders and Infections

Lichen sclerosis and *lichen planus* are skin disorders than can cause lesions and scarring on fragile vulvar and vaginal tissues. Both are sometimes mistaken as repeated yeast infection, which is unfortunate in the case of lichen sclerosis since untreated, it puts a woman at risk for vulvar cancer. All types of infections and sexually transmitted diseases also can cause painful sex, including chlamydia, herpes, gonorrhea, trichomoniasis, and yeast infections.

Pudendal Neuralgia

When the large nerve that transmits signals between the brain and the external genitals, the rectum, and the perineum (area between genitals and anus) becomes entrapped or damaged, it can cause excruciating pain that is difficult to treat. Women and men with pudendal neuralgia may also have pain with certain movements or even when seated, sometimes causing work disability.

Endometriosis

Endometriosis is diagnosed when uterine tissue associated with the menstrual cycle is found outside the uterus itself. Pain that occurs during the thrusting of intercourse or sex play, known as *dyspareunia*, is often caused by endometriosis.

Interstitial Cystitis and Irritable Bowel Syndrome

When the tissues of the bladder and urethra become inflamed, intercourse can become painful. IBS can also lead to *dyspareunia*, or pain with thrusting associated with intercourse.

TREATMENT OF FEMALE SEXUAL PAIN DISORDERS

The Role of Health Care

Treatment depends on the type of pain disorder that is diagnosed. With mild cases of provoked vestibulodynia where pain is more somatic than visceral, treatment might consist of practical suggestions, including the avoidance of any fragranced tampons or pads; using only warm water to wash the genitals; wearing cotton underpants during the day and none at night; a diet low in oxalates (a chemical found abundantly in some foods such as spinach and tomatoes); and taking time for relaxation (Coady & Fish, 2011).

When additional treatment is necessary to diminish pain, women may be prescribed topical estrogen to help heal dry vulvar and vaginal tissue (van Lankveld, et al., 2010). The painkiller lidocaine may also be applied in cream form to the introitus before intercourse. Antidepressants such as Zoloft™ or Cymbalta™ sometimes are prescribed to change the brain's response to pain. Antidepressants also come in cream form so that they can be applied directly to the pain site.

Treatment of visceral pain also varies with diagnosis. Pain associated with the pudendal nerve may be treated with nerve blocks or surgery. Endometriosis is often treated surgically. Pain from interstitial cystitis (IC) may be treated with nonsteroid antiinflammatory drugs, antihistamines, and tricyclic antidepressants. Pain associated with irritable bowel syndrome (IBS) may be treated with diet and medications to regulate bowel function, including antidepressants. Whatever the type of pain or whatever its cause, however, women may need to undergo a variety of treatments or combination thereof to obtain symptom relief.

THE ROLE OF PHYSICAL THERAPY IN THE TREATMENT OF SEXUAL PAIN

Treating women and men who have complaints of sexual pain often requires collaboration with a team of specialists, one of whom may be a PT who specializes in treating disorders of the pelvic floor. In an interview of PT and sex therapist Talli Rosenbaum (Al-Juraifani, 2012), she states, "The pelvic floor is a physical manifestation of an emotional state." Pelvic floor PTs who examine and touch women in order to treat them can be among the first to see manifestations of anxiety, aversion, and pain avoidance. Generally, pelvic floor PTs can help their patients not only by releasing tension in the interwoven muscles of the pelvic floor, but by teaching them techniques such as deep breathing and coping statements to help them tolerate discomfort. Pelvic floor PTs can also teach the patient about sexual anatomy, overcome shame about their bodies, understand how to make sex pleasurable, and how to talk to their partner about sex. A knowledgeable pelvic floor PT will generally be very open to collaborating with a patient's psychotherapist to provide good quality care.

Vaginismus is often treated with the use of vaginal dilators that are graduated in size (Kleinplatz, 1998). Dilation does several things, including desensitizing a woman to having something inserted into the vagina; helping pelvic floor muscles to relax; teaching a woman more about her anatomy; and increasing self-efficacy and control. Beginning with the smallest dilator, they are inserted daily for 10 to 15 minutes. When a woman can successfully insert one size without discomfort, she then tries insertion with the next size up. After using the dilators on her own, she can show her partner how to insert the dilator, allowing some shared control over her body, increasing trust, and preparing the couple for intercourse. Please note, it is important to ascertain with the couple whether or not they want to become pregnant immediately and to counsel them to obtain appropriate birth control if pregnancy isn't desired right away.

Physical therapy can be employed to relax hypertonic pelvic floor muscles through biofeedback, internal massage of soft tissue, external massage to muscles, and even corrections to a woman's posture (Rosenbaum, 2010). PT is used for all types of sexual pain disorders (van Lankveld et al., 2010); sometimes it is prescribed postsurgery as part of a program of healing. Physicians may also have their own treatment protocols, such as application of capsaicin (from a pepper that contains oils that burn) in a homeopathic attempt to halt nerve signals, or an injection of botox to immobilize the muscles.

THE ROLE OF MENTAL HEALTH

Woman who receive both medical treatment and cognitive behavioral therapy (CBT) have better results in the long-term than those who receive medical treatment alone (Ventolini, 2011). Such treatment can take place individually or in a group format. Women can be asked to keep a pain diary, noticing under what conditions pain is increased or decreased, which can bring insight regarding the contribution of stress, diet, type of activity, or pain hypervigilance. They can also record thoughts related to the perception of pain that they can learn to counter with standard cognitive techniques. Additionally, progressive muscle relaxation can help manage stress, thus decreasing pain signals, as can deep breathing, which can also help during sexual activity. Mindfulness has also been suggested as a way for a woman to connect with the present moment as a distraction from pain and a way to connect thoughts and feelings (Rosenbaum, 2013); see page 172 for a worksheet on mindfulness and sexuality.

Cognitive therapy can also help a woman who has been turned off by the whole idea of sex to put her sex life into a new perspective, particularly if the focus can be taken off mechanics and onto the need for touch and emotional intimacy (Lo Frisco, 2011). A woman can identify her own meaning of sexual activity so that it is more than simply pleasing a partner, which can lead a woman to feel duty bound to provide intercourse. Learning to assertively communicate needs and wants to her partner during sex is also beneficial. Assertive communication can generalize to interactions with medical providers. Copy and use the client worksheet on "Understanding Pain Management" as a place to begin work.

When a woman is in a committed relationship, the partner generally needs to be involved in treatment, and in fact in one study women expressed that they preferred couples over individual therapy (Connor et al., 2008). Couples' relationships sometimes suffer from emotional distress prior to diagnosis; they may blame each other or build up resentment. Thus, reparative measures need to be taken, such as normalizing their frustration and engendering a dialogue of forgiveness. Couples can benefit from supportive therapy as they narrate their experience; receive education about the disorder and its treatment; and learn to communicate openly about sexual and emotional needs and preferences. Most important, women who experience painful sex must learn to set boundaries—to say no to any sexual activity that they cannot tolerate or enjoy. It isn't unusual to find that clients with this presentation have a history of difficulty with setting boundaries in all kinds of relationships, from parents, to friends, to co-workers. Learning to identify one's own wants and needs, and to assertively communicate them, is a large part of treatment.

Couples often need counseling if they are to engage in sexual activities. In heterosexual couples, "sex" is often synonymous with "intercourse." Couples need to be reassured that all types of activity can be considered "sex," for example, manual sex, oral sex, or even frottage (rubbing one's genitals against the partner's body). Intercourse can also take place between a woman's thighs pressed together around a male partner's penis, or between her breasts or the cheeks of her buttocks. Some couples also will choose to engage in anal sex, which has gained more acceptance in the heterosexual community. They can also be encouraged to express their feelings in other ways, with affection, verbal expressions, little gifts and notes, and the like.

TYPES OF SEXUAL PAIN DISORDERS IN MEN

While women's sexual pain disorders have gotten some attention due in part to research spurred by organizations like the National Vulvodynia Association and the International Society for the Study of Women's Sexual Health, men's sexual pain disorders have gotten little, perhaps because they are more rare as well as more likely to have a physical cause. In their review article, Davis, Binik, & Carrier (2009) report that part of the problem has to do with the tendency of urologists to lump all types of men's pelvic pain disorders into one generic diagnosis of prostatitis. In fact, there are four types; two have bacterial causes, one has no known cause, and one has no symptoms. Most studies do not distinguish between types, however, so these three researchers coined the term chronic prostatitis/chronic pelvic pain syndrome (CP/CPPS).

Chronic Prostatitis/Chronic Pelvic Pain Syndrome

CP/CPPS pain can occur in the abdomen, lower back, upper thigh or groin, and in the testicles, the perineum, and penis (Anderson, Wise, Sawyer, & Chan, 2006). This pain makes many activities painful, including sitting, standing, and exercise, and is associated with urinary problems such as difficulty emptying the bladder. Clearly such symptoms may interfere with sex, but sufferers of CP/CPPS may also have direct sexual dysfunction such as pain with ejaculation, which in turn leads to ED, avoidance of sex, and low desire. All such symptoms can have an impact on relationship quality, and in a certain number of cases CP/CPPS has been blamed as a cause of divorce.

Peyronie's Disease

This disease, also known as PyD, is caused by fibrous tissue growth within the penis (Ralph et al., 2010). The growth can cause deformity of the penis, causing it to curve, dimple, shrink, take on an hourglass shape, or possibly become overly rigid. When the penis has too much curvature or rigidity, intercourse can become impossible. PyD can cause erectile dysfunction and penile pain. The condition can occur at any age. PyD reportedly occurs in about 5% of men, but PyD is thought to be underreported due to men's reluctance to admit to having this embarrassing condition.

Men with PyD may suffer profound psychological effects, including depression, low self-esteem, and relationship issues (Bella, Perelman, Brant, & Lue, 2007). In one survey of PyD males with a mean age of 54.5, 81% endorsed having emotional difficulties, while 54% reported relationship problems. Loss of penile length and inability to have intercourse increased the probability that a man would experience either type of problem (Smith, Walsh, Conti, Turek, & Lue, 2008). Married or single, a man with PyD may avoid initiating sex, fearing his partner's reaction to the appearance of his penis. The partner in turn may feel isolated and lonely within the relationship. Partners of men with PyD have been known to express disappointment, sadness, and even rage.

If PyD is not causing pain and/or interfering with a man's ability to have intercourse, then the treating physician may simply consult with the patient regularly to see if and when treatment might be warranted. There is no certain cure for PyD. It has been treated variously with oral agents, injectable medication, and surgery, each of which is associated with some type of side effect, including scarring with surgery.

Anodyspareunia

This is defined as painful receptive anal sex. While myths exist that *all* receptive anal sex is painful, researchers assert that such is not the case among men who have sex with men, with Damon and Rosser (2005) reporting just 14% of men in their sample identifying as experiencing anodyspareunia. They also report that "being psychologically unprepared, having a partner with a large penis, and inadequate foreplay" are common reasons for anal pain. There was no correlation, however, between internalized homophobia and the experience of anodyspareunia. Educating men about the need for foreplay, including play with fingers, dilators, and toys, prior to anal sex may help alleviate pain.

MENTAL HEALTH IN THE TREATMENT OF MEN'S SEXUAL PAIN DISORDERS

Since pain level is affected by mood and anxiety, then treating comorbid mental health disorders and teaching techniques associated with the management of pain, similar to those of stress management, can become initial treatment (Anderson, Wise, Sawyer, & Chan, 2006). In severe cases, referral to a pain clinic may be advisable (Luzzi & Law, 2006). Providing supportive therapy can be useful if the man is feeling embarrassed about medical treatment. Normalizing his embarrassment and helping him learn to be assertive with health care providers can be helpful.

Although there are no studies on the efficacy of any particular psychotherapy in the treatment of male sexual pain disorders, cognitive therapy may be used to address issues related to body image, loss of masculinity, and the meaning of being able to perform sexual intercourse as opposed to engaging in other types of sexual activity. Couples therapy may also be employed to address common problems, helping the couple to join in coalition against the pain and creating new ways to maintain physical and emotional intimacy despite challenges. Seeing that they can still have a satisfying and playful sex life by agreeing to other types of sexual activity, for example, showering together, massage, performing manual and oral sex, or using sex toys, can improve mood and outlook for both partners. The client worksheet on "Outercourse" can be used to spur sexual curiosity and activity.

ACTIVITIES

1. Research PTs in the area surrounding your practice to identify those who treat sexual pain disorders. Become acquainted with them and develop a cross-referral relationship.
2. Read 1 or 2 books from the *Resources* section to learn more about sexual pain disorders.
3. If you already treat clients who seek help for chronic pain, consider how you might use pain management or reduction techniques with clients who have sexual pain.

RESOURCES

Coady, D., & Fish, N. (2011). *Healing painful sex: A woman's guide to confronting, diagnosing, and healing sexual pain*. Berkeley, CA: Seal Press.

Goldstein, A., Pukall, C., & Goldstein, I. (2011). *When sex hurts: A woman's guide to banishing sexual pain*. Cambridge, MA: Da Capo Lifelong Books.

Wise, D., & Anderson, R. (2012). *A headache in the pelvis: A new understanding and treatment for chronic pelvic pain syndromes* (6th ed.). Occidental, CA: National Center for Pelvic Pain.

UNDERSTANDING PAIN MANAGEMENT

A referral to a psychotherapist for pain management can be upsetting to some people because they think it means that people think the pain is "all in their head." This is not true. Pain management helps you feel less stressed, anxious, or depressed so that your *perception* of pain changes. The pain may decrease and you may then be able to cope better.

There are two types of pain, acute and chronic. Acute pain is a signal that tells you something is wrong and you need to react, like touching a hot stove that can leave a burn. Chronic pain occurs when there is no longer a danger of injury but the signal stays turned on. Here are some tips for managing chronic pain:

1. Keep a pain log. Write down what time you notice the pain and rate it from 1 to 10. Also include what is happening, for example, you were driving on the freeway or talking to someone on the phone. This can help you and your therapist note patterns that you may want to change.

2. Practice relaxation. You can try mindfulness or another type of meditation. Deep breathing can also help. Breathe naturally, but from your diaphragm. Try to make your out breath longer than your in breath.

3. Use coping statements, which your therapist can help you develop. Examples include, "I don't like this pain, but if I relax I can learn to tolerate it better."

4. Take good care of yourself by getting enough sleep, eating a healthful diet, and exercising appropriately.

5. Find things that you can enjoy doing and that pain won't hold you back from. This can help take your mind off the pain and remind you that life can still be fun despite your physical discomfort.

OUTERCOURSE

While *intercourse* refers to penetrative sex of the vagina, anus, or mouth, *outercourse* refers to nonpenetrative sexual activity. Outercourse is a good alternative to intercourse when a couple wishes to avoid pregnancy; when birth control methods are unavailable or cannot be used for any reason; when couples want to avoid intercourse for religious or other reasons; when one or both partners feels too fatigued for intercourse; when intercourse is painful; or to learn more about one another's bodies.

Types of outercourse activities include:

- Kissing the lips and other parts of the body

- Masturbation, either each partner touching themselves or partners touching one another's genitals

- Frottage, or rubbing one's genitals against a partner's body

- Fantasy play, telling or sharing erotic stories

- Sex toys of all kinds can be used for stimulation

- Massage of the erogenous zones, for example, buttocks or breasts

Outercourse can help couples learn more about foreplay and the sexual response cycle and orgasm, especially in women. Caution must be used during outercourse, however, to ensure that preejaculate ("pre-cum") does not enter the vagina as this fluid can contain sperm and lead to pregnancy.

14

Sexuality and Reproduction

INFERTILITY

For many couples, having a child is what gives sex—and their relationship—its deepest meaning. Being able to conceive an infant, and being responsible enough to take care of him or her, can be a signal to parents and grandparents that one is now a fully mature adult. The imagined fun and pride of having children and building a family excites many couples into marriage. When pregnancy doesn't happen as expected, couples can become heartbroken, even causing them to question if they have married the right partner. Couples who are told they are infertile—which is defined as being unable to naturally conceive after one year of attempting pregnancy—may feel sad, stressed, depressed, anxious, and stigmatized as being "childless" or "barren." If they choose to undergo treatment, they may mourn a loss of privacy regarding their sex life, find their work life disrupted by doctor's appointments, and their finances drained by medical costs (Onat & Beji, 2012).

With many couples starting families later in life, plus the effects of health problems such as obesity on ability to conceive, infertility affects 7% to 17% of all couples (Smith et al., 2009). Male infertility occurs in 20% of all infertile couples, while couples with combined male and female infertility make up about 30% to 40% of couples. In about 10% to 15% of couples with infertility, there is no known medical cause. It is possible that many of these couples are dealing with a sexual dysfunction they are too embarrassed or unwilling for another reason to discuss it with their physician (Wischmann, 2010). Conversely, couples sometimes present with sexual problems in order to disguise fears about infertility.

CULTURAL CONSIDERATIONS

In the United States and most European countries, marriage is thought to be the culmination of romantic fulfillment, while in other parts of the world the purpose of marriage is to produce offspring. The wish for children reflects not only the couple's desire to create a family, but to please extended family members, who may wish to see the next generation carry forth name, wealth, and traditions (Greil, Slauson-Bevins, & McQuillan, 2010). In many countries, infertility carries a great deal of stigma and may be kept hidden from others. At the same time, for couples not as motivated by romance, sexual dysfunction may not have as large an impact on fertility, as the act of procreation is viewed through a different lens.

CAUSES AND TREATMENT OF INFERTILITY

In men, infertility is generally either due to a congenital problem, such as an undescended testicle that was never treated, or acquired through a disease like mumps or chemotherapy for cancer treatment (Smith et al., 2009). There are also several lifestyle variables that can affect sperm production, such as frequent cycling, soaking in hot water, wearing tight underwear, smoking, drinking alcohol, and exposure to environmental toxins. In a small percentage of men, hormone imbalances such as low testosterone, overproduction of prolactin, or hypothyroidism can create infertility. Besides low sperm production, there can be other problems with sperm such as motility or malformation. Finally, there can be mechanical problems such as blocked sperm ducts that prevent sperm from becoming part of a man's ejaculatory fluid.

In women, the most common reason for infertility is lack of ovulation due to hormonal imbalances; scarring of the ovaries, perhaps due to infection; early menopause; or failure of an egg to emerge from the follicle in the ovary. There can also be tubal diseases that prevent an egg from traveling down the fallopian tube to the uterus. Endometriosis, a disease that causes excessive growth of the *endometrium*, or lining of the uterus, causes infertility in women who have it. Lifestyle can also affect fertility, for example, smoking cigarettes or drinking alcohol, as can problems like anorexia, which can cause a woman's menstruation to cease.

Treatment of infertility depends on its cause (Greil et al., 2010), with some treatment being less invasive than others. For women with ovulation disorders, there are medications that can stimulate ovaries to release eggs. While such drugs can be effective, they need to be administered by injection and can cause unwanted side effects from bloating and weight gain to vomiting and migraines. Problems with the cervix, uterus, or fallopian tubes may be treated surgically, but are more often addressed with assisted reproductive technologies, or ART. ART includes in vitro fertilization (IVF) in which a woman's eggs are retrieved surgically, fertilized with the partner's or a donor's sperm, and then implanted in the woman's uterus 3 days later.

In men, sperm must be assessed prior to treatment, which requires that they produce a sample of sperm in the doctor's office through masturbation, a procedure which many conservative and non-Western clients have reported to be humiliating, if not impossible (Wischmann, 2010). As with women, there are drugs to correct hormonal imbalances and surgeries that may unblock the path of sperm. If surgery fails, or if a man is unable to ejaculate for any reason, then he may need to undergo a sperm retrieval procedure, which is an ejaculation produced mechanically by a physician.

When treatment fails, the couple can consider "third party conception," which includes using donor sperm, eggs, or embryo, surrogacy, or adoption. This may be a make or break moment, when couples must decide whether they are going to pursue such options, consider adoption, or accept that they are going to go on without children.

SEXUAL DYSFUNCTION AND INFERTILITY

Researchers report that sexuality and infertility can interact in a variety of ways (Greil et al., 2010; Kainz, 2001; Quattrini, Ciccarone, Tatoni, & Vittori, 2010; Wischmann, 2010). Sexual dysfunction can prevent a couple from having intercourse or cause them to avoid it, so that opportunities for conception pass by. Couples may also refrain from attempting conception once they find out about a diagnosis of infertility because of their feelings of sadness or anxiety. When couples affected by infertility do have sex to conceive, it can become more mechanical than romantic. Finally, the tests and procedures used in treatment of infertility can intrude on a couple's ability to express themselves sexually or to be spontaneous with their lovemaking.

Although there is sometimes a chicken-and-egg question regarding sexual dysfunction and infertility, one thing is clear: If a couple doesn't address their sexual problems, the likelihood of successful fertility treatment is diminished. The first issue is not a dysfunction, but rather a concern, in that many couples do not realize what is involved in becoming pregnant. Some have no idea how ovulation works. There is ignorance about timing of intercourse to conceive. While most doctors encourage frequent intercourse, couples sometimes refrain, saving up a man's sperm for the "right" moment at ovulation, which may already be too late. Infrequent intercourse may also occur because of sexual dysfunction such as low desire on the part of either or both partners.

In men, the most common sexual problem affecting fertility is early ejaculation, or being unable to control ejaculating before penetration occurs. Since couples often wait to conceive, making time of the essence, men in this circumstance will most likely be prescribed an antidepressant to slow ejaculation, but certainly they can use the recommendations outlined in Chapter 7. Conversely, delayed ejaculation (DE) creates an obvious problem in that the man may not be able to produce ejaculate at all. Erectile dysfunction (ED) is also reported, often because of pressure to produce sperm "on demand" when a woman is ovulating; female partners are sometimes overly demanding in this regard. The latter two problems may also occur when a man is required to produce a sperm sample for analysis. Sometimes, there are cultural and religious prohibitions against masturbation, while in other instances it is a matter of embarrassment or lack of privacy.

The most common sexual problem women face is either dyspareunia (painful intercourse) or hypertonic pelvic floor dysfunction (also called *vaginismus*, or inability to tolerate penetration for intercourse) (Furukawa, Patton, Amato, Li, & Leclair, 2012; Vercellini et al., 2012). If the problem is physical, as with hormonal imbalance, it will be treated medically; if viewed as psychological, often expressed as fear of pregnancy or labor and delivery, then a referral to a sex therapist is appropriate. In fact, many women with vaginismus don't schedule treatment until they are ready to conceive because they want to avoid confronting such fears. But other issues such as lack of orgasm or hypoactive sexual desire can affect fertility because a woman may lose interest in intercourse.

STEP INTO MY OFFICE...

Read these two vignettes below to understand different presentations of couples who experience infertility.

Tina

Tina, who grew up in a conservative Catholic country, had been molested as a child. When she married she learned she had vaginismus, but the couple decided intercourse wasn't important, as they could please one another in other ways. After several years, her husband decided they should begin a family and pushed Tina to do something about the vaginismus. During the assessment, she revealed that she was extremely afraid of the pain of labor, having watched her aunt experience a "traumatic" birth. In addition to the general treatment protocol, Tina also needed to find an obstetrician who would understand her needs. Although the vaginismus resolved and Tina was able to conceive, she requested a Cesarean section to avoid labor.

Ned

Ned married late in life to a woman several years younger. One of the reasons he had delayed marriage was because he did not want to have children. Now, however, he wanted to start a family. The problem was that he suffered from DE that became even more pronounced with more attempts at conception.

Although Ned didn't see much use for exploring his history, I prodded him to share his story. It seems Ned had traveled most of the world, staying in different countries for months at a time. As he talked, he remembered that his DE began when he met a woman who had tried to keep him in one place by becoming pregnant. Although he enjoyed the woman's company and especially her sexual companionship, he became increasingly angry when she tried to prevent him from withdrawing during intercourse, their way of birth control. Eventually, he stopped ejaculating with her altogether.

Once we connected the past pattern with Ned's current problem, he identified that he had some ambivalence about becoming a father. By working through his feelings and teaching him some relaxation techniques designed to help him let go, Ned was able to ejaculate with his wife and resume trying to conceive again.

EFFECT ON THE COUPLES' INTIMACY

For some couples, the process of treatment for fertility brings them closer, while for others it creates a painful divide (Jain, Radhakrishnan, & Agrawal, 2000; Onat & Beji, 2012; Smith et al., 2009). Partners can feel angry toward one another for many reasons, including the fact that one or both of them are infertile. They may find they have differing ideas about using ART. One partner may want to use every available type of treatment, while the other may have an attitude that if they are meant to have a child, they will become pregnant naturally. A partner may only object to a certain type of treatment, for example, the use of donor sperm. There may even be a large discrepancy between partners over whether or not becoming pregnant is a good idea, with one partner giving in to the other, sometimes with resentment. Whatever technology is used, each partner and the couple together must find ways to cope if treatment fails or the pregnancy results in a miscarriage.

Couples also find themselves scrutinized by others, who may ask when they are planning to have children. If people know they are having difficulties conceiving, the couple may be given unwanted advice including the unhelpful prescription to "Just relax!" One or both partners may feel anger toward others who are pregnant. They may complain that peer-aged family members who have been able to conceive with their partners get preferential treatment. They may also avoid socializing with other couples who have children and become isolated, which can have an unhealthy impact on relationship dynamics, causing the couple to become fused and organized around their problem.

Infertility can create a large emotional toll. A common pattern is for the female partner to express sadness or depression, which the male partner tries to fix. He cannot, so he becomes frustrated and withdraws, which only increases the woman's distress. Sex under such emotionally difficult circumstances may come to feel pointless or without meaning; couples may begin to question the viability of their relationship at all. If there were sexual or emotional problems predating the discovery of infertility, then the diagnosis may only exacerbate them.

ASSESSMENT AND TREATMENT OF INFERTILITY-RELATED SEXUAL PROBLEMS

In initial meetings, it may be preferable to meet with each partner individually so that they can speak freely about their feelings and relate details of the sexual issues. In addition to taking an individual history to rule out any mental health disorders, the therapist will need to:

- Ascertaining if the cause of infertility can be attributed to one or both partners, or is ideopathic
- What treatment is being used and its physical and psychological effects
- Whether or not there has been treatment failure
- How the couple feels about infertility and its treatment
- Whether the couple feels supported by one another and by extended family, if they know about the problem
- How the couple is faring emotionally under the strain of infertility
- What sexual problems the couple is specifically experiencing; whether the problem(s) predate the infertility diagnosis; and what the couple has tried to resolve them

Often one of the first goals of treatment is to normalize that sexual and relationship problems do occur in a number of couples in response to demands of diagnosis and treatment. Couples generally find it helpful to share their narrative of how they came to learn about the diagnosis and their journey in treatment. It is appropriate in initial stages to make referrals to sexual medicine specialists who may be able to prescribe treatment, such as phosphodiesterase type 5 (PDE5) inhibitor for early ejaculation and ED, or to a pelvic floor physical therapist who can help a woman resolve vaginismus. Specific treatment suggestions from Chapters 6 and 7 can and should be offered, as well as correcting any myths, such as the male needing to save up his sperm, thus refraining from frequent intercourse, or a woman only being fertile 2 weeks after her period has started. Bibliotherapy regarding sex and fertility can be recommended.

In regard to complaints that sex has become robotic or unromantic, there appears to be differing suggestions in the literature regarding how to make sex less of a chore during treatment. One school of thought is to encourage couples to make a commitment to have playful, creative sex no matter what. (As I recently told one client, most people would like to think that their parents had fun creating them!) If sex for procreation has become distasteful, couples may choose to take a temporary break from trying to conceive and focus on having pleasurable sex. A second school of thought is for the couple to accept that they will be having "target-oriented vs. pleasure-oriented" sex (Galst, 1986) in the hope that such clarity will make target-oriented sex easier.

Sometimes, the therapist has the task of preparing or supporting a male client who needs to provide a sperm sample. Cognitive therapy around any shame or guilt associated with masturbation will be helpful. However, sometimes men have difficulty because they feel embarrassed about looking at pornographic material in the doctor's office. Such men often report that they don't have sexual fantasies, either; they are usually from cultures that feature sexual oppression. Helping them to resolve any guilt about masturbation, as well as teaching them how to fantasize, can help them complete the task.

As always, good communication is key. Couples need to risk opening up to one another to share their thoughts and feelings about the diagnosis, the treatment, and any treatment failures. They can be encouraged to share disappointment or anger about their fate, or to mourn the loss of the opportunity to conceive "normally." At the same time, partners must recognize that since infertility is affecting them both, they may need to turn to outside sources of support. Trusted friends and family members may be depended on as confidantes, or they may be encouraged to attend a support group such as those offered by the organization RESOLVE.

SEXUALITY, PREGNANCY, AND THE POSTPARTUM PERIOD

Once a pregnancy is created and acknowledged, a couple's sex life can be affected in both positive and negative ways. Couples may be overjoyed about a pregnancy, or be completely surprised, needing to make major adjustments to their lives. The pregnancy can bring couples closer together as they share in the intimate changes brought about in a woman's body. Or, they can become anxious or preoccupied by the impending birth. The prospect of engaging in new roles and responsibilities can be overwhelming. Whether it comes as a surprise or not, the most precipitous time for a man to engage in an extramarital affair is during pregnancy.

At one time, research on sexuality and pregnancy was focused on whether or not intercourse during pregnancy could cause any harm to the developing fetus. In fact, coitus and orgasm can be detrimental at certain times, as when there have been several miscarriages; in cases where there is bleeding or signs of premature labor in the third trimester; or in term pregnancy (at 38 weeks or later) when membranes have been ruptured or the cervix is dilated, making it vulnerable to possible infection (Giannotten, 2008b). Otherwise, sexual activity is normal during pregnancy, does not harm the fetus, and will generally not induce labor until the very end of pregnancy, at which point orgasm can release the same hormones that obstetricians use to induce labor, namely oxytocin and prostaglandins.

Most recent studies show that while sexual activity declines significantly during pregnancy, the most frequent intercourse takes place in the first and second trimester, but wanes in the third trimester as she becomes fatigued and sexual activity potentially becomes awkward (Pauleta, Pereira, & Graca, 2010). But there is great variability during each trimester, with some women feeling sexually revved up and others having little desire. Much of this accords with the variability seen in sexuality prior to pregnancy and, in general, a couple's sexual pattern before pregnancy is reflected during pregnancy. That is, if a couple has an active and satisfying sex life before pregnancy, it usually continues as such (Giannotten, 2008a).

The experience of labor and delivery can also have an impact on a couple's sexuality (Polomeno, 2000). Some couples experience labor as an intimate experience, one that can even be erotic, as women are known to experience orgasm during birth. On the other hand, the birth process can sometimes be problematic, creating stress for both mother and father. While health care providers monitor mother and infant, the father may feel quite isolated with his fears. A few men who are present for the birth experience find themselves turned off by seeing the emergence of an infant from their wife's vagina. Fortunately, most couples recover adequately from labor, are happy with their new baby, and resume their romantic life at a later date, unless the labor was especially prolonged or complicated.

SEXUAL PROBLEMS DURING PREGNANCY

While some women and men have a positive sexual response to pregnancy, feeling closer than ever and aroused by a woman's growing curves, other couples are fearful of harming the baby during intercourse, and one or both partners may be turned off by a woman's "motherly" new body. Irrational fears about harming the growing fetus, causing miscarriage or blindness by having intercourse can affect partners of either sex. Thus, some couples refrain from intercourse during pregnancy, though they may engage in other sexual behaviors such as oral sex or anal intercourse.

The most frequent sexual complaints by women include low desire, dyspareunia, lack of lubrication, and anorgasmia. For men, the most common complaints are early ejaculation and ED, which is often related to fears about entering the vagina during intercourse and harming the fetus (Giannotten, 2008a).

SEXUALITY IN THE POSTPARTUM PERIOD

After delivering an infant, a woman's interest in sex is generally absent, particularly if she breastfeeds, which for some women can cause hormonal changes leading to vaginal dryness, dyspareunia, and overly sensitive nipples (Abdul, Thaker, & Sultan, 2009; Giannotten, 2008b). While couples are generally given the go-ahead to have intercourse six weeks after delivery, when the woman's body has healed from pregnancy, it may take much longer for a woman to catch up emotionally and sexually. A large majority of women experience sexual problems at 3 months postpartum; even at the 6-month mark, about 10% of women haven't engaged in intercourse due to lack of interest, discomfort related to scarring or breast engorgement, or confusion about resuming birth control methods (Pauleta et al., 2010).

Body image also plays a role in the recovering mother's sexual desire; while most women return to their pre-baby weight, some women are still heavier even 1 year after giving birth.

Even when couples engage in sex, a woman may find many changes in her body (Pauls, Occhino, & Dryfhout, 2008). The tone of pelvic floor muscles may be different, making it more difficult to achieve orgasm or causing intercourse to be less comfortable. Hormonal changes, especially when a woman is breastfeeding, can cause dryness and dyspareunia. Damage from episiotomy or trauma to the pudendal nerve can make intercourse extremely uncomfortable. Postpartum mood changes, whether exhibited as "baby blues" or frank depression, also impact sexuality. Women may complain of being "touched out" from handling the infant and find themselves not wanting to be held or cuddled by their partner.

Men can also have problems in the postpartum period. They, too, may suffer from exhaustion and related mood disturbance. Men sometimes feel jealous of the attention given to an infant or annoyed by the household chaos created by the infant's demands and care, though they may not express it, and sometimes respond by retreating into work or other activities. These issues need to be acknowledged and addressed in order to avoid marital problems.

TREATMENT OF SEXUAL PROBLEMS RELATED TO PREGNANCY AND CHILDBIRTH

Although it is rare for couples in the therapist's office to complain about sex during pregnancy, couples with sexual problems will often refer to pregnancy or the postpartum period as contributing to the demise of their sex life (Acele & Karaçam, 2012). Whether pregnant or a few months or even years postpartum, the couple can be asked about whether or not the pregnancy was planned; any difficulties regarding conception; ambivalence about parenthood; any history of miscarriage or abortion; complications during pregnancy or delivery; and questions about the use of contraception, either prior to or after the pregnancy. It is also important to assess whether the couple had any sexual concerns prior to conception.

For the most part, treatment consists of counseling couples that it is normal to experience a decline in intercourse, as well as to reassure them that unless told otherwise by their physician, intercourse is safe. Couples also need to be dispelled of myths such as sex causing harm to the fetus, or that the fetus "knows" that they are having sex. They can also be reminded that they can engage in other sexual behaviors, or, if they want intercourse, to try other positions and to use lubricant to increase comfort and pleasure. The client worksheet "Sex After Baby" can be used to facilitate the experience of restarting one's sex life.

After delivery, women who have given birth are often told that 6 weeks is the magical moment at which they can begin having sex. However, lucky is the couple whose infant is sleeping enough to give them respite. Women need to be reassured that they do not have to begin having sex until they feel their body has fully recovered. During that period, the couple may create intimate moments by exchanging massages, bathing in a tub or shower together, or snuggling on the sofa while they watch a movie. There is also nothing to prevent a woman from stroking or caressing her husband while he masturbates himself to orgasm.

ACTIVITIES

1. Make contact with the leader of your local RESOLVE chapter. If possible, attend a meeting. Ask the leader how she (or he) handles sexual problems of members when they arise. Perhaps you can offer to speak to the group, or to be a resource when the leader has questions.
2. Reflect in your journal about beliefs regarding sex during and after pregnancy. What might you explore when a pregnant woman wants sex, but her partner (male or female) does not? Or when the partner wants sex, but the pregnant woman does not? How might you counsel a couple that has not had intercourse during the entire pregnancy but wish to restart their sex life? What might you advise a woman who is afraid to have sex after pregnancy due to a physical or emotional trauma during birth?

RESOURCES

Jones, C. F. (2012). *Managing the stress of infertility: How to balance your emotions, get the support you need, and deal with painful social situations when you are trying to become pregnant.* Amazon Digital Services.

Kerner, I., & Raykell, H. (2009). *Love in the time of colic: The new parents' guide to getting it on again.* New York, NY: William Morrow Paperbacks.

Shapiro, C. H. (2010). *When you're not expecting: An infertility survival guide.* Hoboken, NJ: Wiley.

SEX AFTER BABY

The doctor said it: You can have sex 6 weeks after delivering a baby, and even sooner if you had a C-section. But just because your body is physically ready, you may not be mentally or emotionally ready for sex. Here are points of information and tips to help you ease back into sex.

- It is normal to have a vaginal discharge after childbirth called *lochia*. You should wait until the discharge stops to have sex to prevent infection.

- If you had an episiotomy during delivery, you probably also have stitches. Allow the body to take time to heal.

- While you are waiting to have vaginal intercourse, you and your partner can please each other manually or using toys—if you have the energy.

- Fatigue is the most common complaint after giving birth. Try to problem solve with your partner ways for both of you to get adequate rest so that you have some energy to be with each other at least romantically, if not sexually.

- Be open-minded about what you call "sex." Taking a warm shower together and toweling each other dry may count as "sex" during this time. It helps to have a sense of humor; maybe making toast can even be seen as an act of love.

- Sometimes women feel "touched out," or touched too much, from handling the baby or breastfeeding. Taking a break from infant care can help a woman recharge for giving and receiving touch from her partner.

- Breastfeeding can lead to some interesting situations, like milk letting down during orgasm. Accept these changes without embarrassment. Wear a nursing bra if you wish to prevent leakage or if your breasts are sore.

- Be kind to yourself about weight changes in your body. Do your best to exercise to perk up mood and improve body image.

- If you experience depression, don't hesitate to say so. Mild postpartum depression is common; just talking with a friend can help. If depression is moderate to severe, talk to your therapist and/or physician right away.

- Let your partner talk about his or her feelings without judgment. They may express jealousy or sadness that it is not just the two of you anymore. This is normal. Make sure your partner knows that, even though you feel too tired or overwhelmed with infant care for sex, you still love them and are looking forward to connecting again.

15

Sexuality and Medical Problems

Research and practical interest have grown over the past two decades about the impact of chronic illness on sexuality and relationships. In part, this is due to the fact that diseases that were once fatal, such as cancer, or extremely debilitating, such as multiple sclerosis (MS), are now better managed through medical treatment, making it possible for patients[*] to enjoy a better quality of life and to participate more fully in their relationships. Today, with the realization that with better quality of life individuals and couples may sustain some interest in sex, many national organizations that advocate for various chronic conditions now have website information, pamphlets, and books on the topic of sexuality, for example, the American Cancer Society.

However, simply providing a client with a brochure or website link may imply that the practitioner is uncomfortable actually discussing sex (Mercer, 2008; Taylor & Davis, 2006). Additionally, information may not be enough to resolve the sexual problems of some affected individuals. Despite the fact that researchers are encouraging physicians and nurses to discuss sex with patients, many are uncomfortable with the task or simply lack time to give individualized recommendations. Hence, there is a large population of patients for whom a referral for sex therapy is recommended or needed.

---

[*]"Patient" is used rather than "client" to denote that the person is receiving medical and/or psychological treatment.

When it comes to sex and illness, a multitude of problems can be created by the symptoms of the condition itself and/or its treatment, the psychological impact of such on the individual, and effect on the individual's partner. Each type of illness—viral, neurological, cardiovascular, hormonal, gastrointestinal, and so forth—affects sexual function and relationships in its own way. Sex may not be the same as it was before the illness was diagnosed, leading couples to understand and accept a "new normal" that may or may not include intercourse or some other sexual behaviors, but will hopefully include enough to make physical intimacy pleasurable and make up for losses in other areas.

Performing a literature review using the terms *sexuality* and *chronic illness* on PubMed produced 1,193 articles, many of which focus on sexual function and a singular topic, such as cancer, kidney disease, and arthritis. Medical and mental health providers who work with people with one particular illness may have some advantage in that their knowledge about sexual effects can be focused, but a therapist's practice may see patients with a broad array of medical problems, necessitating a systematic approach to collecting and understanding information in order to provide optimal treatment.

Rolland (1994) created a "typology of illness" across several dimensions:

- Acute versus gradual onset
  Illnesses with an acute onset will be unpredictable and may be more challenging that a gradual illness.
- Course of illness: progressive, constant, or relapsing
  Some people are always waiting for the other shoe to drop regarding their illness, which creates anxiety for both partners.
- Expected prognosis and quality of life
  Illnesses may affect a person globally, creating disability from work and other activities, or mildly, as in making it difficult to perform certain tasks.
- Degree of incapacitation of cognition, sensation, movement, energy, or appearance, for example, through surgery
  Obviously, the more the person is incapacitated by their illness, the more of an effect it will have on their relationship and their sexuality.

Using Rolland's typology, the therapist can make sense of the client's experience of illness, as well as formulate some hypotheses about the effects on the client's psychological status, self-esteem and body image, relationships, and sexuality.

EFFECTS OF ILLNESS ON RELATIONSHIPS AND SEXUALITY

Even a minor flu can create changes in relationship dynamics, perhaps when one partner—stereotypically the female—who is generally the nurturer becomes the patient who needs tending. Once the symptoms are resolved, however, the relationship reverts back to its usual pattern of interaction, including sexually. For some couples affected by chronic illness, however, the change in roles may vary depending on the course of the illness, or in some cases, become permanent. Couples who behaved independently from one another now may become interdependent, both because of physical care and the emotional demands of coping with an illness. The couple's quality of life may change due to physical changes imposed by the illness, but also because of financial and social changes to their lives.

All of these changes can have an effect on a couple's sexual relationship. Many people take their gender identity from particular roles. When a woman can no longer care for her family, when she is the recipient of care, and perhaps can no longer make grooming a priority, she may feel less feminine. When a man is no longer the primary breadwinner, depends on his partner (female or male) for medical care, and perhaps loses muscle tone because he can no longer work out, he may feel less masculine and disinclined to initiate activity. The couple may find they no longer have the same privacy they once did, and that their conversations between themselves and among family and friends are focused on the patient's medical condition.

The well partner may be marginally involved or critical in providing some degree of medical care, anything from sorting pills into containers to changing dressings or catheters. The home may become "medicalized," that is, the patient may be in a hospital bed in a room accessible by all family members, or there may be medical equipment or aids like a walker visible. Giving and receiving medical care from a partner is not only a reminder that all is not normal, it is also a boundary crossing, affecting how a patient may feel about his or her body, as well as how the partner relates to the body they are tending. There may also be scarring from surgery, rashes from medication, odors because bathing is difficulty, fatigue from the illness or its treatment, and guilt for not being able to meet a partner's needs that all interfere with sexual self-esteem. Such effects contribute to the mythical belief that people who are ill have little or no interest in sex, or that they become asexual. If the couples themselves carry this belief, then they may give up on having a sex life altogether, or the well partner may give up, not wanting to bother the ill partner with his or her needs. Finally, if the relationship was unstable or unsatisfactory prior to diagnosis, it may dissolve in divorce; in fact, the divorce rate for couples affected by chronic illness is higher than for well couples.

Some couples do draw closer because of an illness, especially if their relationship was a source of comfort and strength prior to the diagnosis. They may take the perspective that life is unpredictable or short, so they need to take care of each other even more now that one is sick. They may also have an extended family or other network of support, as well as financial resources to ease some of the strain of the effects of illness. However, even couples that cope as well as can be expected may have trouble reestablishing their sex life. They may not be prepared to discuss or have confusion about changes in drive, arousal, or ability to have orgasm. Couples who never imagined themselves in the therapist's office may feel quite embarrassed about their need for help. Fortunately, there is something to be done for these couples, as well as those who struggle more with changes.

What follows are examples of various types of illness and their sexual effects on the individual and partner. The client worksheets at the end of the chapter can be sent home with couples who feel ready to reengage in their intimate life.

CANCER

Treatment and quality of life for many types of cancer have improved exponentially over the past decades. Still, cancer can have sexual effects, ranging from low drive and difficulties with arousal and orgasm, to loss of erectile function and delayed ejaculation. Some effects are due to treatment, while others are attributable to psychological impact such as depression and anxiety. Changes in appearance due to procedures and medications can also impact the patient's sexual esteem and interest.

While almost every type of cancer can affect a person's sexuality, those affecting sexual characteristics have the greatest impact. Breast cancer and gynecological cancers (GCs) for women, and prostate and testicular cancers for men, make patients especially vulnerable. In U.S. culture, a beautiful body is a healthy one, and when one's sexual organs are affected by cancer, the patient often feels neither one.

Women's Cancers: Breast and Gynecological Cancer

In U.S. culture, the breast is the focus of much erotic attention, with many women seeking breast enhancement to feel sexy and more attractive. When cancer is found in the breast, there can be real feelings of depression and fear about remaining a sexual being, particularly if there is single or double mastectomy or, as occasionally happens, one or both breasts become misshapen due to biopsies and other procedures. Breast reconstruction cannot be performed in all cases, and even when reconstruction is undertaken, the results may be disappointing. In one case, a single woman who belonged to a large insurer was told she could have breast reconstruction, but without the addition of nipples because this would be too costly, leaving her needing to explain to each new partner how her breasts might be different from other women's breasts they had seen.

The treatment for breast cancer may include surgery, radiation, and/or chemotherapy in some combination. Treatment can lead to a number of changes in appearance, including loss of breast or breast tissue, decreased sensitivity in breast and nipple, scarring, hair loss, and weight loss or gain; many women with breast cancer experience poor body image (Katz, 2009). Tamoxifen is a medication that is used to keep the amount of estrogen in a woman's cells in check. Depriving a woman of estrogen can lead to all kinds of symptoms that can potentially interfere with sexual activity, including premature menopause and its accompanying joint pain, leg cramps, weight gain, and hot flashes, as well as vaginal dryness and dyspareunia (painful intercourse). Antidepressants are often used to manage hot flashes as well as mood changes; these medications can cause a further decrease in sex drive, arousal, and orgasm.

The treatment of GC may sometimes improve quality of life for a female patient, but it can also have a deleterious effect on sexual function (Krychman, 2007). GC can affect any part of a woman's reproductive system, including ovaries, uterus, vagina, vulva, and clitoris. Treatment is often a combination of radiation, chemotherapy, and surgery. Sexual risks of such treatments include vaginal shortening, decreased vaginal elasticity, vaginal bleeding, and fistulas, as well as changes in sexual arousal, lubrication, and orgasm (Gilbert, Ussher, & Perz, 2011). Women who must have a hysterectomy can experience sudden menopause and all of its symptoms, for example, mood swings, hot flashes, and insomnia. Hormonal imbalances and their treatment can create weight gain; chemotherapy can cause hair loss; and surgery can create scarring, all of which can diminish a woman's sense of femininity.

Changes resulting from surgery can have a dramatic impact on a couple's sex life. One woman I briefly treated was originally thought to suffer from repeated yeast infections, until it was discovered that she actually had lichen sclerosis, a skin disorder of the vulva, which unfortunately became cancerous. Treatment included radiation and surgery to remove her labia and clitoris. Her husband, who had tried to remain supportive through the ordeal, became depressed because although they could attempt intercourse, he had no interest in the cosmetic appearance of her genitals, and mourned the loss of the ability to give his wife pleasure through oral sex. The marriage ultimately did not survive.

Despite dramatic effects, medical providers sometimes provide little or no counseling to patients. One woman who had radiation to the pelvic area to treat a rare GC was given a box of dilators and told to use them, but was not told why, and so the box sat in a drawer until almost a year later, when her husband wondered if they were ever going to resume their sex life. Only when they tried but failed to have successful intercourse did she remember the dilators, which were prescribed to stretch the vagina after damage from radiation. After several therapy sessions and referral to a physical therapist for help, the couple was able to truly celebrate the woman's remission from cancer.

Men's Cancers: Testicular and Prostate Cancer

Testicular cancer is diagnosed most frequently in adolescent and young adult males, accounting for about 20% of cancers in that age group (Carpentier & Fortenberry, 2010). It is generally treated with surgical removal of one or both affected testicles, chemotherapy, and sometimes radiation. The psychological and sexual effects are more pronounced for teens and men without a partner. In one Danish study (Rossen, Pedersen, Zachariae, & von der Maase, 2012), 24% of survivors had reduced sexual interest, 45% reduced sexual activity, 14% reduced sexual enjoyment, 18% had erectile dysfunction (ED), and 7% had delayed ejaculation.

In the same study, 17% complained of problems with body image. Aside from changed appearance in cases where a prosthetic is not inserted, the inability to produce sperm in some cases can create a feeling of being de-masculinized. Teens and single young men sometimes aren't told to consider sperm preservation, or they decline preservation without giving the future due consideration. Those who have a partner may face fears about infertility, as well as the financial burden of treatment or its recurrence.

While testicular cancer affects young men, prostate cancer is mainly found among men over the age of 50 (Galbraith, Fink, & Wilkins, 2011). Like other cancers, prostate cancer is being discovered earlier, which means improved odds of preventing spread of cancer through the body and greater odds for longevity. Prostate removal surgery has also improved with the availability of so-called nerve-sparing procedures that protect the majority of men from experiencing incontinence or ED. Other treatment includes radiation, which has a small possibility of causing ED, and androgen deprivation therapy, which decreases testosterone and is associated with a variety of sexual problems including gynecomastia (male breasts), weight gain, genital shrinkage, ED, loss of desire, delayed orgasm, and infertility, in addition to diseases such as osteoporosis, diabetes, anemia, and obesity.

In addition to the sexual effects of treatment, many men experience sexual problems such as ED and delayed ejaculation *prior* to diagnosis and must cope with the psychological effects of dysfunction, for example, feelings of failure or performance anxiety. Partners can also experience distress, leading them to avoid discussing or initiating sexual activity. Men with prostate cancer may also have other illnesses that affect potency, including diabetes and cardiovascular disease. Also, older men who have had nerve-sparing surgery or other cancer treatment may find that their sexual function returns, but it isn't a return to their baseline level of function, with less rigid erections than expected, the possibility of "dry" orgasm, that is, orgasm without the release of ejaculate, or pain with orgasm.

Unfortunately, health care providers do not always address the psycho-sexual needs of patients, often because the patients themselves do not bring them up, fearing that they will be judged as "too old" to worry about such matters (O'Brien et al., 2011). Regaining sexual function can take months or as long as 2 years. Sometimes men understandably become impatient, and there are urologists who will agree to treat sooner with intracavernous injection therapy or a vacuum device. When these treatments are unsatisfactory, then a penile implant may be appropriate. Men who are older and have a long-term, committed relationship are more likely to engage in non-intercourse activities and less likely to pursue invasive treatment than are younger men who may not currently have a partner (Canada, Neese, Sui, & Schover, 2005).

CHRONIC FATIGUE SYNDROME AND FIBROMYALGIA

Chronic fatigue syndrome (CFS) and fibromyalgia are two different but related illnesses with unpredictable courses that can interfere with daily activities and relationship function. CFS is characterized by persistent or intermittent physical and mental fatigue that is not due to exertion, nor alleviated by rest. Minor symptoms include impaired memory, tender lymph nodes, muscle pain, and headaches. About 88% of women with CFS reported having one or more sexual problems, compared with 32% of women without CFS (Blazquez, Alegre, & Ruiz, 2009), with 81% having decreased sex drive, 32% difficulty reaching orgasm, and 31% experiencing "vaginal irritation."

Fibromyalgia is commonly comorbid with CFS. Fibromyalgia is characterized by joint pain, fatigue, and depressed mood. Antidepressants used to treat both CFS and fibromyalgia can contribute to low desire (Ryan, Hill, Thwaites, & Dawes, 2008). The experience of joint pain can cause the patient to avoid sexual activity. Sometimes, partners of people with these two illnesses suspect that the sufferer is using the condition as an excuse to avoid sexual intercourse. They may need to be educated that the complaints and symptoms are real, and that the couple must learn how to cope with the effect of symptoms on their relationship. In addition to common sex therapy recommendations, patients need to be counseled to increase self-care, pace their daily activities, schedule time for rest, and optimize sleep schedule and diet for improved energy.

DIABETES MELLITUS

Diabetes mellitus (DM) is a disease characterized by hyperglycemia, or high blood sugar. DM type 1 is caused when the pancreas produces little or no insulin and is usually diagnosed in childhood, adolescence, or early adulthood. DM type 2 is caused by decreased sensitivity of body cells to use the insulin that is produced. About 90% of DM2 is caused by lifestyle such as poor diet, lack of exercise, obesity, and genetics, and it is generally diagnosed in older adults (Giraldi & Kristensen, 2010). Even when properly managed,

both types of DM are associated with a variety of problems including neuropathy (nerve damage), poor cardiovascular circulation, and hormonal
imbalances, especially decreased testosterone in men.

Any and all of these problems can create sexual dysfunction. DM in men
is associated with ED, delayed ejaculation, and low desire (Jack, 2005); in
fact, sometimes ED is the symptom that leads a man to the doctor's office
and a diagnosis of DM. Men with DM may avail themselves of different
levels of treatment for ED, depending on the severity of their symptoms,
which may increase over time; they may start with oral agents and progress
through injection and implant if they are in adequate health to withstand
risks associated with surgery.

Women may report vaginal dryness and associated discomfort with intercourse; have increased risk of yeast and other vaginal infections that can lead
to sexual problems; and experience decreased blood flow to the genitals that
can make arousal and orgasm difficult. In addition to the remedies outlined
in Chapter 6, physicians will sometimes prescribe the Eros™ device, which
essentially works to bring blood flow to the clitoris and genitals, sensitizing
them for pleasure and orgasm. In addition to directly treating sexual dysfunction, people with DM are encouraged to improve their lifestyle, which
can reverse symptoms associated with high blood sugar as well as potentially lift depression associated with having and managing the disease.

NEUROLOGICAL DISORDERS

Any disorder affecting the central nervous system and brain, including
Parkinson's disease (PD), MS, spinal cord lesion (SCL), or stroke, has the
potential to interfere with sexual function. An examination of sexuality
and PD reveals, for example, potentially severe sexual effects (Bronner &
Vodusek, 2011). PD is a chronic neurodegenerative disorder, which progresses over time and causes physical disability. It is marked by tremor
at rest, muscle rigidity, dyskinesia, hypersalivation, sweating, and what is
referred to as a "masked" or expressionless face. Depression is an inherent psychological symptom, as is decreased self-esteem and negative body
image. In later stages, PD affects communication and mobility, making daily
activities challenging.

Sexual problems are common for people with PD, affecting quality of life
for the patient as well as the partner. In men, the most common SD is ED and
early ejaculation. Delayed ejaculation can also occur, which can lead to frustration and embarrassment. In women, vaginal atrophy, decreased lubrication, incontinence, and anxiety interfere, as does overall dissatisfaction with
their sexual experiences (Bronner & Vodusek, 2011). A patient's masked face,
sweating, and salivation, as well as being physically challenged, can prove
to be a turn off for both participants.

Treatment of PD can also be sexually problematic. Patients using a dopamine agonist such a levodopa may develop hypersexual desire, creating unwanted sexual demands on the partner, while antihypertensive and antidepressant medications can cause a decrease in desire. Both side effects need to be reported to the prescribing physician so that modification and changes can be made.

Men with ED are generally prescribed phosphodiesterase type 5 (PDE5) inhibitors, but may need to give oral medications more time to work due to slower digestion. When oral treatments don't work, then injections can be tried. The use of a vacuum pump can also be helpful, however, the patient needs to have manual dexterity to use the pump as well as place a band at the base of the penis once a rigid erection is obtained.

People who have experienced an SCL can be severely compromised (Parets & Schmerzler, 2008), though in what ways may depend, in part, on the stage of life in which the injury took place. For example, Ostrander (2009) writes that older women have a decreased sense of themselves as remaining a sexually viable person than do younger women. Mental and medical health professionals cannot assume that such injury will render a person disinterested in sex. If the injured person had a viable sexual relationship prior to SCL, then they are likely to want to continue a sexual relationship, though naturally it may take a revised script and expectations to incorporate new sexual behavior into a couple's repertoire.

Interestingly, many people with SCL experience heightened sensation in parts of their body that prior to the injury were not especially sensitive, such as ear lobes. They may also report that the area where sensation stops is highly sensitive and that stimulation to this area by self or partner can lead to orgasm. Men with SCL who wish to achieve and maintain an erection may be prescribed any variety of medical interventions, from PDE5 inhibitors to penile implant. Both men and women with SCL and their partners may need counseling to cope with changes in their sexual function.

SKIN DISORDERS

Skin problems, both those seen and unseen by others, can create stigma, low self-esteem, shame, and social isolation. It wasn't long ago that adolescents were told that masturbation could lead to acne. The skin is involved in the communication of feelings through touch; it is "part of the way we relate to our world; it registers and reflects our emotions" (Buckwalter, 1982). Psoriasis is a skin disorder that can create those negative effects in its patients. It begins with purple blotches almost anywhere on the skin, most often on the scalp, legs, and elbows, but also on the genitals and chest or breast area. The blotches develop into silvery patches, which then shed scales. Lesions on the genitals are especially difficult to treat because skin in this area is thinner and more sensitive.

Patients with skin conditions like psoriasis can experience self-disgust, to the extent that they ask themselves, "Who would want to touch me?" One study (Meeuwis et al., 2011) suggests that patients with psoriatic genital lesions have a worse quality of life than those with psoriasis elsewhere. They experience greater stigma and more desire to cover up lesions than patients affected by psoriasis in other areas of the body. More women than men report a decline in sexual activity associated with genital lesions, probably because women associate sexuality with physical attraction more so than do men. The treatment for psoriasis is also unappealing, usually with ointments containing corticosteroids. Severe cases are controlled with methotrexate, a type of chemotherapy that can cause ED.

ASSESSMENT

There are two types of couples affected by chronic illness who come into sex therapy for treatment, couples who generally enjoyed their sex life before the diagnosis and couples who always struggled. Couples and individuals who enjoyed their sex life will be most likely to quickly return to previous functioning with information and suggestions. In general, having regular sexual contact requires a measure of psychological flexibility, so these couples may also have an easier time adapting to challenges posed by an illness. However, couples who never experienced sexual struggles in the past may find changes in their sex life very stressful. And of course couples who struggled before the diagnosis of an illness may struggle most of all.

In the spirit of medical family therapy (Kleinman, 1989; Rolland, 1994), an "illness narrative" can be constructed in conjunction with the couple's experience of the disease's effect on their relationship and sexuality. A double timeline might also be constructed so that the couple can understand how they came to struggle. The therapist can also use this narrative or timeline to normalize the couple's experience. While the therapist is gathering information, the narrative can encourage the couple to begin talking about sexual symptoms, hopefully without blame.

Information needs to be gathered regarding not only physical symptoms and their treatment in the patient, but effects of illness on the couple's roles and boundaries. Feelings associated with confronting illness such as grief and loss, fear, and sadness can also be assessed and acknowledge. Inquire about how each partner coped with the demands of the illness; was it expected, according to usual character, or were they so overwhelmed that normally functional defenses failed? On the other hand, do not assume that couples fared poorly. In some cases, couples feel triumphant, for example, when prostate cancer is treated successfully. In the face of illness, couples may be more spiritually and emotionally bonded. It may truly be that sexual function is the only change that puzzles them.

Collaboration with the treating physician may or may not be necessary. In some cases, couples will express dismay that they weren't told about the sexual effects of the disease or its treatment; they may request referrals to other physicians who will be more empathic about sexual distress. Ideally, the patient or the couple may be empowered to communicate with their current physician about medications, including those for treatment of sexual symptoms; this approach has the advantage of the potential second order change in the patient-medical system relationship. Together, you can create a list of questions such as, Can I expect any part of my ongoing treatment to cause sexual problems? Which, if any, of my medications can cause sexual side effects? What options are available for sexual problems caused by my illness or its treatment?

TREATMENT

When couples are given a safe place to discuss their sexual concerns in the assessment, treatment is already underway. Normalizing problems with sex, as well as the difficulty in communicating with one another about sexual concerns, can hasten the process. Using the general recommendations for treating sexual problems in men and women covered in earlier chapters is a starting point for most treatment planning, but more work in other areas may need to take place before making specific suggestions. In addition, after assessing sexual problems, modifications may need to be made, as outlined below.

While normalization offers solace, the task of accepting a "new normal" may be a challenge for the couple. Only as you begin to discuss treatment goals may the couple realize their sex life, as they knew it, may be left behind them. Couples who believed they had put the initial shock of diagnosis and treatment behind them may be disheartened to learn that they have something else to grieve. Fortunately, most people will want to move forward quickly, realizing that being sexual in a new way is better than not being sexual at all.

Cognitive therapy can be used to address issues related to body image and self-esteem. Changes in one's body can be depressing or even shocking, but must be accepted. As with any distortion of body image, the patient and partner can be directed to focus on parts of the body that still work properly, or are still attractive. A woman's breasts may be irrevocably changed by cancer treatment, but she can play up her other features such as face or legs. Couples in early stages of treatment, perhaps those engaging in sensate focus activities, sometimes appreciate the suggestion that they keep on a bit of clothing, such as camisole or tank top and shorts.

Cognitive therapy also can be used to address myths and beliefs about "normal sex" (i.e., intercourse) and open people up to additional possibilities for intimacy, including hugging, caressing, massage, mutual masturbation, oral sex, and so forth. They can also be educated on the use of sexual aids, including medical aids like PDE5 inhibitors for men and topical estrogen to treat vaginal dryness for women. Other interventions include changing positions to take pressure off aching joints or to make penetration more comfortable. Couples can be educated to make use of furniture, such as sofa arms, pillows, and cushions to make sex more comfortable. Vibrators can be described and recommended to make orgasm easier to attain.

At the same time, couples can benefit from becoming less goal-oriented and more focused on increasing emotional intimacy. Spending time together doing things they both find enjoyable, sharing memories or looking at photos, and even discussing their strengths and weaknesses as individuals and as a couple can bring closeness when sex is difficult or impossible.

ACTIVITIES

1. Consider the following situations and reflect on them in your journal:
   - What recommendations might you make to a man whose wife has had a double mastectomy when he complains that he can no longer become aroused?
   - How would you discuss diabetes and ED with a man and his partner of three months?
   - What kind of referrals might you make for a woman who has eczema around her genitals? What recommendations might you make to her and her partner?
   - What recommendations would you make to a woman who is newly divorced and wishes to become sexually active?
2. Familiarize yourself with the prevention of sexually transmitted diseases (STDs) in one of the sites listed in the *Resources* section. Under what circumstances might it be important to provide education regarding prevention?

RESOURCES

American Cancer Society. The following web page has links to pdf copies of booklets on women or men, cancer, and sexuality. Retrieved from http://www.cancer.org/treatment/treatmentsandsideeffects/physicalsideeffects/index

Katz, A. (2009a). *Man cancer sex*. Pittsburgh, PA: Hygeia Media.

Katz, A. (2009b). *Woman cancer sex*. Pittsburgh, PA: Hygeia Media.

Kaufman, M., Silverberg, C., & Odette, F. (2007). *The ultimate guide to sex and disability: For all of us who live with disabilities, chronic pain, and illness.* San Francisco, CA: Cleis Press.

Krychman, M., Kellogg, S., & Firestone, S. (2010). *100 questions and answers about life after breast cancer: Sensuality, sexuality, intimacy.* Sudbury, MA: Jones & Bartlett Publishers.

National Multiple Sclerosis Society. *Sexuality and intimacy.* Retrieved from http://nationalmssociety.org/about-multiple-sclerosis/what-we-know-about-ms/symptoms/sexual-dysfunction/index.aspx

Roszler, J., & Rice, D. (2007). *Sex and diabetes: For him and for her.* Alexandria, VA: American Diabetes Association.

PREPARING TO ENGAGE IN SEXUAL ACTIVITY

Adapted from N. Parets and A. J. Schmerzler (2008). Neurologic disability and its effect on sexual functioning. *Medical Management of Adults with Neurologic Disabilities, 353–362*:

1. Select a time for sexual activity when you are both relaxed and have time and privacy.

2. If you are on a bowel or bladder routine, attend to it prior to sexual activity. Keep towels and cleansing cloths nearby in case of accidents.

3. Avoid drinking alcohol to prevent interfering with effects of PDE5 medications.

4. Use pillows or put pieces of furniture into use (e.g., arm of a sofa) to try different positions to make intercourse possible and/or more comfortable.

5. A vibrator can assist with achieving orgasm and/or ejaculation.

6. For women with neurological disorders, a water-based lubricant can make sex more comfortable.

TIPS FOR COPING WITH CHRONIC ILLNESS
OR CANCER TOGETHER

There are many movies and books about the triumph of overcoming incredibly challenging illness situations, some fictionalized and some true. Such stories are inspiring but may make it even more difficult to cope if you aren't really feeling triumphant. Here are some tips for surviving as a couple when one (or both) of you has an illness.

- Seek appropriate support. If you are the one with the illness, join a support group. If you are the well partner, find someone with whom you can share your feelings about the illness and its effect on your partner and your life.

- Don't allow illness to dominate every interaction and conversation. It will kill your romantic feelings for one another. Agree to put the illness or cancer on vacation, maybe sending it to the basement or little used room in the house for the afternoon or evening.

- Allow each other to spend time alone, to recharge or to collect thoughts. Being overly dependent on one another can also be a romance killer. Remembering that you are two people, leading two lives, can make your relationship more vital.

- Do what you are able to do romantically and sexually, and let go of the rest. Your sex life may look very different from what it was, but it is nobody else's concern. If you can only enjoy sex in one limited way, then enjoy it fully without shame.

- Be open about how you define "sex." "Sex" can be holding hands, gently rubbing each other's cheeks, trading foot or hand massage, making a favorite snack or beverage, or other loving gesture.

- If an illness should become terminal, know that some people can and do remain sexually connected until the end of life. Others are unable to do so. Do what feels right to the two of you. If you need medical intervention, such as topical estrogen for women or PDE5 inhibitor for men, let your physician know.

16

Sexuality and Aging

INTRODUCTION

The growth of the aging population in the United States is expanding, but our knowledge of sexuality among older adults is not keeping pace, allowing the ongoing perpetuation of myths about sexuality and aging. The perception that adults become asexual as they age is reflected in a comment made in my office by a man in his 30s. Distressed by his lack of sex with his wife (she had vaginismus), he blurted, "We need to get this resolved now, because we'll be in our forties and that will be the end of our sex life!"

Nothing could be further from the truth. The fact is that many adults in their 50s, 60s, 70s, and beyond maintain an interest in sexual activity, if the definition of "sexual activity" is broadened to include nonpenetrative behaviors such as manual and oral sex, cuddling, kissing, and frottage (rubbing genitals against someone to produce orgasm). Longevity, improved health through lifestyle and advances in medicine, and prescription and over-the-counter (OTC) sexual aids make it possible for aging individuals and couples to maintain sexual activity. Older adults are also exposed to articles and television segments devoted to the notion of "successful aging." However, when sexual activity comes to a halt because of dysfunction, aging couples must be cautioned that they are not seeking to restore the sexual health of their teens, 20s, or 30s, but rather determine realistic, attainable goals that may include a variety of changes in routine.

Despite the growing population of older adults, sexual activity among them is not well understood, except to the extent that pharmaceutical companies have underwritten research to determine efficacy of medical approaches such as phosphodiesterase type 5 (PDE5) inhibitors to treat erectile dysfunction (ED). What studies do exist are sometimes contradictory; for example, it has been commonly accepted that chronic illness impeded sexual function in older adults, but it may be that an individual's or couple's *perception* of the impact of chronic illness may be a more important factor. Additionally, the focus on sexuality in older adults is generally on those who are married, White, and middle class. Not much is known about the sexual behaviors of older adults who are actively dating.

The implication for treatment is clear, that therapists cannot simply accept that people may have reached the end of their sexual journey because of aging. Instead, therapists must be willing to explore various aspects of sexuality in the "third age" in order to compassionately and effectively treat sexual dysfunction in this population. The purpose for so doing is that older persons and couples who remain sexually active enjoy better physical and mental health than peers who do not. They also rate their relationships as more emotionally satisfying and report fewer problems with depression, anxiety, and stress.

MYTHS ABOUT SEXUALITY IN OLDER ADULTS

In another memorable anecdote, a student in a human sexuality course I was teaching related in an oral presentation that she had found evidence that her grandmother was still sexually active, bringing forth a rousing chorus of "Ew!" from classmates and reflecting, perhaps, some general disgust with the idea of older people making love—and enjoying it. Such stigma may prevent the elderly from initiating sexual behavior for fear of being seen as unseemly or gross, and in fact age-related decline in interest is more psychological than biological, as positive attitudes toward sex, body image, and the process of aging correlate with higher sexual satisfaction.

Media images about sexuality and aging add to confusing and contradictory beliefs. Aging rock stars may be portrayed as exuding a sexual aura, while an every day Joe in his 60s is portrayed as a pervert if he looks at a healthy young woman, and pathetic if he looks at a healthy young man. But if Donald Trump shows up at an event with "eye candy" on his arm, he not only exemplifies an older White stud, but sends a message that he can eschew women in his own age bracket who presumably are less attractive and, by deduction, less interested in sex.

Women fare no better, either in the media or the real world. Somebody, somewhere deemed that a face devoid of expression lines and character, artificially created by injections and surgery, was more beautiful than one displaying its path through life. Without such wizardry, women complain that they become largely invisible to the opposite sex. Doors are no longer held open and the figure no longer receives an appreciative glance—unless one decides to go on record as a "cougar," an older woman with the money and guts to fix herself up and go after younger men.

Further contributing to myths about aging, commercials for PDE5 inhibitors grace network television networks, suggesting that the only sex worth having is intercourse with a firm and ready erection ("when the moment is right," croons one ad). Men are encouraged to ask their doctors for prescriptions, which are readily handed out but often without any counseling. They may become disenchanted with the medication when they realize that they still need sexual stimulation to become aroused, or that having more sex doesn't make their life any better (James, 2011). Thus, James writes, Viagra is one of the most commonly prescribed medications worldwide, but has only a 50% refill rate. Few men and even fewer women realize that additional sexual stimulation, as well as other changes, may need to take place if the medication is to be efficacious.

The fact is that if someone thought of sex as important in youth, then it continues to be important in later life. Though average frequency of intercourse may decline to 2 to 3 times per month, it is still enjoyable for many couples, both straight and gay. Even people living in nursing homes may express sexual desire and engage in activity despite the embarrassment of caregivers. There has even been a recent movement to allow nursing home residents to engage in sex and to give them the privacy to do so (Caplan, 2012). Educating family members, who may be shocked or disgusted by their elderly relatives' normal sexual needs, is sometimes also required so that consenting elders can continue to enjoy sex.

What appears to stop older adults from participating is lack of partner. In his review article of sexuality and aging literature, DeLamater (2012) reports that men are more likely to stay sexually active later in life than are women, whose male partner is more likely to be in ill health or to die at a younger age. That does not mean, however, that all sexual activity stops; 46% of men and 33% of women age 70 and over engaged in solo masturbation. Interestingly, men in this group were more likely to masturbate if they did not have access to a partner, but women masturbated whether or not a partner was available.

However, there are differences among different cohorts of the aging population. Those adults in their 70s and 80s were born in the 1930s and 1940s, before the so-called sexual revolution prompted by the easier availability of birth control and the loosening of social mores such as premarital sex. They are more likely to have remained married to the same partner; that partner may, in fact, be their only partner. Roles may be more traditional, with the male partner expected to take the lead even in the face of flagging sexual and physical health. If they remarry after losing a partner due to divorce or a fight with illness, they may expect that being with a new partner will replicate early days with their original partner. They may have a more difficult time talking about sex with each other, let alone a therapist.

Those adults born in the 1950s and 1960s—the "baby boomers"—grew up largely with more permissive attitudes toward sex and thus have higher expectations of maintaining sexual interest and activity as they age. These adults may have had several partners and perhaps a couple of marriages or live-in relationships. If they are in a committed relationship, they usually enter therapy to find out how to stay sexually active despite challenges like prostate or breast cancer. Perhaps the biggest challenge with this population is acceptance that mind, body, and spirit may age at different rates.

There are also cultural differences in attitudes toward sexuality and aging. In one study of aging Chinese men and women, traditional views of sexuality prevailed, with sex being viewed strictly as intercourse and as an activity that a woman provides to her male partner (Yan, Wu, Ho, & Pearson, 2011). In Moore's study (2010) of 20 aging Japanese couples, 25% of men—and none of the women—reported engaging in extramarital relationships, in part because of the belief that wives were no longer interested in sex. In Africa, elderly people are rarely supplied with information about the transmission of HIV because of the belief that sex among older adults is impossible because of lack of energy.

UNDERSTANDING OBSTACLES TO SEXUAL ACTIVITY AS WE AGE

Using an ecosystemic perspective is ideally useful in determining the physiological, psychological, and relational factors that may deter a couple from remaining sexually active. For women, menopause is regarded as the biological harbinger of many changes, not only in sexual function, but also in psychological well-being. In men, changes in sexual status may occur more often due to illness such as cardiovascular disease, rather than to so-called *andropause*, or the gradual decrease in testosterone. For both sexes, treatment of sexual problems is often collaborative with physicians and possibly physical therapists. The role of the psychotherapist may be to coordinate treatment and to counsel the couple regarding any interventions recommended by health care providers.

BIOLOGICAL CHANGES AND AGING

It is considered common knowledge that older adults continue to be sexually active if they have a partner and are in good health. However, recent studies suggest that a person's *perception* of their health may be as or more important than their actual health status (Lindau & Gavrilova, 2010). Thus, a man with diabetes may feel fit enough for sex, even though his body is showing signs of damage to the penis and flagging erections. The reality of changes caused by illness, as well as medications used to treat varying problems, must be considered, as well as normal changes due to aging, when assessing older men and women.

Menopause

Menopause may occur at almost any age, and can be due to premature ovarian failure, hysterectomy with oophorectomy (removal of ovaries), medications such as tamoxifen used to treat breast cancer, or natural decline in sex steroid hormones such as estradiol and progesterone. The earlier menopause occurs, the more detrimental its effect because it can interfere with a woman's expected life course of pregnancy and childrearing. While the focus of this chapter is natural menopause and aging in women, many of the remarks are applicable to younger women who face early menopause.

Menopause is said to have occurred when a woman has ceased to have menstrual periods for 12 months. The transitional period leading to menopause is known as *perimenopause*, and the median age for beginning this period is 47.5 years of age, though some women experience symptoms in their 30s. Once a female enters menarche (the beginning of menstruation) her body adjusts to certain levels of hormones (Cobia & Harper, 2005; Davis & Jane, 2011). As these levels decline, the body exhibits symptoms that may come and go depending on changes in hormone levels. Such symptoms include irregular menstrual periods, hot flashes, sleep disturbances, and mood swings. Pregnancy, though rare, is possible until a woman is truly in menopause, so contraception needs to be continued.

Depression is also common, with about one-third of perimenopausal women experiencing its symptoms (Davis & Jane, 2011). Sad mood may be attributed to low estrogen, but it may also be related to insomnia. Psychologically, for some women menopause is a signal that one is aging and no longer sexually attractive. Women may also adopt an attitude that sex is pointless if there is no possibility of impregnation, and may mourn loss of fertility. In any case, depression can also contribute to decreased sexual interest and pleasure. The SSRIs used to treat depression may create further negative sexual side effects including problems with desire, arousal, and orgasm.

Sexually, the most common symptoms are low drive and changes in the vagina and vulva. Blood flow to the genitals is decreased, causing less lubrication, thinning of the vaginal walls, and loss of elasticity in the vagina, which may lead to discomfort and pain with intercourse. Like men, however, women often do not realize that higher levels of stimulation may be needed to experience the same level of arousal attained during premenopause status. They also may not be assertive in letting their partner know that they need additional help from an applied lubricant, leading to a cycle of painful sex, decreased arousal and desire, and more painful sex. Finally, it must be stated that the majority of women in menopause experience problems with pain or lubrication, so inquiries should be made.

STEP INTO MY OFFICE...

Mia is a 60-year-old woman complaining of painful intercourse. Unaware of the physical changes that come with menopause, Mia had consented to have intercourse with her husband without communicating that it created searing pain. Only when she could no longer tolerate the discomfort did she seek treatment from a physician, who prescribed topical estrogen. He also referred her to me because he learned that Mia and her husband never engaged in foreplay, which would help prepare her body for intercourse. In addition to education about menopause and the need to increase sexual arousal to make intercourse comfortable, I recommended that the couple engage in sensate focus techniques to help them reinforce to Mia that sex could be pleasant for both parties.

Male Decline in Sexual Function

Unlike women, men do not have a clear biological marker that age-related physical and psychological changes are underway (Feldman, Goldstein, Harzichristou, Krane, & McKinlay, 1994; Pines, 2011). Instead, testosterone levels in men gradually decrease over time, beginning as young as age 35. The treatment of this normal decrease of testosterone, sometimes referred to as *andropause,* or male menopause, is controversial and most recent information suggests that it be avoided except in men who demonstrate classic symptoms of hypogonadism, such as low energy and fatigue, loss of muscle mass, weight gain, depressed mood, and impotence.

What is known is that men are more at risk for ED as they age. In the European Male Aging Study, 30% of men ages 40 to 79 had ED, with a mean age of 60 (O'Connor et al., 2008). In one approximation, 322 million men will suffer with ED by 2025. The neurobiological factors affecting erectile function as men age is highly complex. Very simply stated, changes in blood supply to the penis and changes in the structure within the penis can make it difficult to attain or maintain an erection firm enough for satisfactory intercourse.

Aging men are also more likely to experience ejaculatory problems, with more cases of delayed ejaculation occurring due to changes in arousal. In one survey, delayed ejaculation was shown to increase with age, from 16% in men aged 57 to 64 to 33% in men 75 to 85 (DeLamater, 2012). The refractory period after ejaculation is prolonged; recovery may take anywhere from a few hours to a few days.

STEP INTO MY OFFICE...

Both Rick and Susan had been married before. Now in their early 60s, though, they both felt they were in love for the first time. Rick described having been married to his high school sweetheart. After their children had been born, his wife had lost all interest in sex and they were rarely intimate; in fact, it was one of the factors that led to their divorce. Susan reported she also married young to a man she now believed had Asperger's syndrome.

Susan, however, had dated several men since her divorce and had acquired quite a bit of sexual experience, while Rick had not. Rick admitted that he had trouble with erections and that led to avoidance of dating. The problems with ED were upsetting to Susan, who feared Rick may have found her too old to be attractive, which Rick denied. He did not know exactly when his erections had begun to falter, so I recommended a referral to a physician for testing. In the meantime, I gave the couple sensate focus activities so that they could begin enjoying physical touch and intimacy. Rick did have low testosterone, and was given a supplement plus a PDE5 inhibitor to use. Within weeks, Susan and Rick were on their way to having the rich sex life together that they had wanted all their lives.

Many times older men will report looking at pornography, seeking massages with "happy endings," or entering into extramarital affairs because they have difficulty becoming aroused with their wife or long-term partner. If they are able to have erections in these circumstances, then they may be diagnosed with problems with arousal or even relationship dysfunction, rather than ED. Men need to be counseled to take responsibility for communicating their need for increased stimulation, not only to increase arousal but also to enhance the effects of any oral PDE5 inhibitors that may be prescribed.

Despite what pharmaceutical companies and physicians may lead men and their partners to believe, PDE5 inhibitors do not cure ED. Such medications may improve erections, making them more reliable; however, the firm erection of youth may not be attained. Also, as men age PDE5 inhibitors have a lower response rate, so they are encouraged to take them frequently. Currently tadalafil (Cialis™) is recommended for daily dosing to make erections more dependable and sex more spontaneous, as the medication stays in the bloodstream longer. Testosterone is sometimes prescribed concurrently to improve the health of erectile tissue and nerve supply to the penis.

Contraindications for PDE5 inhibitors are multiple and include:

- Angina
- Recent myocardial infarction
- Heart arrhythmias
- Poorly controlled hypertension
- Use of nitrates, including amyl nitrate ("poppers") used recreationally
- Some eye diseases

Because of these contraindications, as well as the possibility of getting an imposter medication, men need to be referred to a physician for a physical examination and must not order such medications online.

When first-line oral vasodilators are ineffective—even after appropriate counseling—then there are other interventions to try. In ascending order from least to most intrusive, these include vacuum devices; medicated urethral system for erections (MUSE); intracavernous injection of vasodilators; and penile implant. With all types of interventions (outlined in detail in Chapter 7), it is advisable to include the spouse in the consultation as she needs to understand how the proposed treatment works and ways to incorporate it into the couple's sexual script.

THE RISING RISK OF HIV INFECTION IN OLDER ADULTS

According to the Centers for Disease Control, 12% to 22% of all new AIDS diagnoses are occurring among men and women over the age of 65 (2010). The majority of older adults with HIV experience both ageism and stigma from having the infection (Emlet, 2006), which has implications for sharing health status with a new partner or a medical provider. Younger carriers of HIV, of course, grow up into older adults who are carriers and who may spread the infection, while many older adults lack education about preventing HIV and other sexually transmitted infections (STIs). Older adults, therefore, may neglect to practice safe sex, for example, limiting sexual partners, requesting that their partner be tested before participating in sex, and using condoms for intimate encounters.

SOCIAL EXPERIENCES AND OBSTACLES OF SEXUALLY ACTIVE AGING ADULTS

Not every person ages in the same way, in part because of differing financial abilities to access appropriate medical care. Older adults who are members of a minority culture (or what was once a minority culture, e.g., in the case of Latino Americans) may be especially at risk for difficulties associated with aging, as they were less likely to have attained high job or social status (Burgess, 2004). Financial challenges may impede not only good overall health, but sexual health as well, as insurance may not cover or inadequately cover certain medications or procedures. For example, one patient described that his health maintenance organization only paid for a single PDE5 oral pill each week. As a man in a new relationship, he wanted more medication, but could barely afford it after paying for insurance and copays on other medications.

Laumann et al. (2006) conducted a global study of sexual satisfaction that suggested differences in cultures. In general, women and men from China, Japan, and Thailand reported lower levels of sexual satisfaction than Westerners, with the Asian women reporting the lowest levels of all. Older Asian men and women also engage in intercourse less frequently. In part this may be attributed to Asian cultural and religious beliefs that sex is for procreation, not recreation (Hillman, 2011). For example, in Taoism, men are encouraged to refrain from ejaculating in order to preserve *chi* or energy, which may be experienced as being in short supply as one ages.

There is very little information on the effects of aging on gay men and lesbian women. Because a large number of gays and lesbians in the aging population may not have embraced their orientation in younger years due to fears regarding homophobia (both in the general population and perhaps within themselves), they seem to be invisible from research. Feelings about aging, however, may not be so much related to orientation as to other factors, including how one feels about aging, including material and social resources, relationship history, and assigned meaning (Heaphy, 2007). On the other hand, ageism is reflected in the belief that it may be more difficult to find a partner if one is left alone, especially among gay men (Schope, 2005).

Invisibility is not just a dilemma of older LGBTQ individuals. Women in general often complain of becoming invisible in a society focused on youth and beauty. While men are seen as possibly becoming more dignified or distinguished as they age, women are judged more harshly. Nearly every actress in her 30s will report upon interview that she fears her days are numbered as her age increases, and that she will be relegated to throwaway roles rather than put center stage. As single women age, they find it more difficult to attract a suitable partner, as their male cohorts search for someone younger as a demonstration that they are still virile. Social rejection is an issue that may need to be explored as a source of depression in single women who are perimenopausal or in menopause.

PSYCHOLOGICAL CHANGES

As people age, they may experience a normal decline in cognition and memory. They also may face or be in retirement, a role change that some may find stressful if financially unprepared or depressing if they now feel themselves to be a nonproductive member of society. Loneliness can also be a problem if work relationships have ended and adult children have moved away; friends and relatives may also be dying, leaving holes in one's social network. A negative outlook toward aging and anxiety about fears of loss or one's own imminent death can add to a sad mood. The belief that older adults are asexual may also cause depression and avoidance of sexual contact—the very contact that might improve their mood.

RELATIONSHIP CHANGES

Couples who enjoyed an active sex life in younger years generally expect to continue as they age. However, sometimes couples have differing ideas about sexuality and aging, such as disagreeing on its importance, or one partner having a negative sexual self-image that creates avoidance (Bitzer, Platano, Tschudin, & Alder, 2008). In addition, aging accompanies other normative changes such as empty nest and retirement, creating new dynamics that are difficult to navigate. For example, a woman used to being on her own schedule may find it chafing to have her male or female retired partner at home more. Couples may find that they have little in common now that children are no longer dependent upon them. Conversely, adult children are more frequently remaining at home or returning to the nest after college, limiting privacy and opportunities for intimacy.

In fact, people in their 50s and 60s are more frequently than ever deciding to end marriages rather than continue a dissatisfying union (Kreider & Ellis, 2011). Sociologists Lin and Brown (2012) attribute this dramatic rise in part to the Boomer generation's emphasis on self-fulfillment. Additionally, once adult children leave home, some couples find they have little in common and, with perhaps many years of life ahead of them, they decide to head for greener pastures. More women have been in the work force, meaning that they have the financial means to take care of themselves, unlike women of previous generations who may have stayed in a marriage for financial reasons. Finally, boomers are more accepting of divorce than adults in previous generations.

But sexual expectations also may play a role in some unknown number of cases. Disappointment, depression, and hopelessness about the future of a relationship can lead to a break down in the couple's sex life. Differences in sexual interest can ultimately lead to tension, deterioration in relationship quality, and entanglement in extramarital affairs (Bitzer et al., 2008). Essentially, when one partner opts out of sex—perhaps due to low drive, perhaps to erroneous beliefs about sex and aging—it leaves the other feeling hurt and abandoned. Sexual dissatisfaction is likely one reason the divorce rate in older couples is increasing.

On the other hand, some couples find menopause, the empty nest, and retirement liberating. Such couples find that once the source of dysfunction is treated, they can have an even richer sex life than they did while engaged in childrearing or careers. One couple that I treated had been generally very conservative until he obtained a penile implant; the last thing I heard, they were off on a field trip to a sex toy store.

ASSESSMENT AND TREATMENT OF SEXUAL PROBLEMS RELATED TO AGING

In addition to a sex and relationship history (p. 60), the therapist needs to ask the couple the following questions:

1. What are the client's or couple's expectations regarding treatment?
2. Is sex still important to each partner? Why or why not?

3. If there is one identified patient, assess whether the other partner also has a sexual dysfunction.
4. What changes in either their relationship or sexual script does each partner wish to make?
5. How much inconvenience is the couple willing to cope with in order to have intercourse?
6. How has the couple coped with changes in roles, health status, and so on?
7. Has the couple been able to discuss sex with one another?
8. Is the couple in agreement over the use of sexual aids, for example, PDE5 inhibitors, lubricants, or vibrators?

Additionally, the therapist must attend to the entirety of each individual's experience of aging, as some of these psychological issues may manifest as sexual complaints. Using sex to relieve anxiety and depression isn't unusual, but in late age, when loneliness, grief, and regrets may be increasing, sexual complaints may indicate that an individual is having a tough time coping.

Setting goals may be an important part of treating a couple. They may need to be educated—and sometimes, to accept—that ideas about what sex is "supposed" to be need to be modified. If one partner has decided to cease sexual activity, then exploration must ensue. Is the reason based on the belief that sex at a certain age is unseemly? A physical challenge? Relationship distress? If the couple is anxious because of sexual dysfunction in one or both partners, then they can be reassured that they can continue a sexual relationship, though their sexual script may need to change either due to changes in activity or the incorporation of sexual aids and/or toys such as vibrators.

Couples often need counseling regarding the need for such sexual aids and toys. Prescriptions for Viagra™ and the like sometimes do not get refilled because people misunderstand how the medications work. They also may not realize that if oral medications prove to be non efficacious, then there are other treatments available. Women sometimes need to be counseled regarding the role of hormones in vaginal dryness and she and the couple educated about the various choices in lubricants. Many aging couples have never availed themselves of the thousands of toys available in specialty stores and online. One gentleman in his 70s was so happy to learn about a vibrating ring for his penis that might please his wife, too, that he left his session before it was scheduled to end to go purchase one at the nearest sex shop. In another case, a woman whose spouse was frustrated because he could not find the spot on her genitals to stimulate her to orgasm was encouraged to buy a pebble- or saucer-shaped vibrator that would stimulate the surrounding tissue as well as the exact spot.

Because finding one's sexual capacities changed or diminished can be difficult to cope with, it can help to focus one or both partners on finding a number of things in which they can still fully participate as they age. A discussion of successful aging might include recommendations such as increasing social contacts, developing new interests and hobbies, finding ways to be productive such as volunteering, and attending better to one's physical and mental health through diet and exercise. All of these suggestions can improve mood and outlook, which may ease acceptance of the aging process and make clients appreciate what they *can* do, instead of mourning what they cannot.

In terms of communication, normalize the difficulty of talking about sex. The belief that somehow sex is not as sexy if it is discussed may also need to be dispelled. Couples can share what they have enjoyed about their relationship together, such as feeling emotionally close. Use that closeness as a springboard to building trust and willingness to be vulnerable as the couple ventures into sharing what they need now to enjoy sex. Even couples who have been together and enjoyed their sex life for a number of years may need assistance in talking about the changes that have come with age, both sexual and nonsexual.

ACTIVITIES

1. Review images of couples over 50 on television, the Internet, and in print. What do you notice about how their sexuality is portrayed?
2. Watch a movie about love and sex in later stages in life and reflect on your thoughts and feelings in your journal. Some suggested titles are *Hope Springs, Something's Gotta Give, Harold and Maude, and Away From Her.*
3. If you have a relationship with an older adult with whom you can comfortably raise the topic of sex and love, initiate a dialogue about the topic. Ask their opinions about changes in perception of sexuality; the use of medications to extend the longevity of one's active sex life; and how they feel about adults staying sexually active into their 60s, 70s, and beyond.

RESOURCES

Lynn, D., & Spitzer, C. (2010). *Sex for grown-ups: Dr. Dorree reveals the truth, lies, and must-tries for great sex after 50.* Deerfield Beach, FL: HCI.
Price, J. (2005). *Better than I ever expected: Straight talk about sex after sixty.* Berkeley, CA: Seal Press.

ENJOYING SEX AS A MATURE ADULT

People are living longer and staying more vital than ever. Often, this means that there is still interest in romance and sex. There is no reason to let old stereotypes about sex being only for the young hold anyone back from staying sexually active. Sex may be different than it was in younger years, but that doesn't make it any less fun or interesting.

- Accept that your body isn't the same now as it was 10 years ago . . . 5 years ago . . . or even 6 months ago! Our bodies are always changing as we age, from the moment we are born. So go with the flow and enjoy life without regard for the number of candles on your cake.

- Sex requires energy. Get enough rest. Try to schedule sex when you know you are the most alert, maybe in the morning or early evening, rather than waiting for bedtime.

- Sex also requires stamina, so exercise is important for good heart health and good sex.

- Communicate honestly with your partner. You may find that you need more time to get turned on, or that you need more direct stimulation to your genitals to experience arousal.

- Don't be threatened or embarrassed by the use of sexual aids, including medicines like Viagra™, sex toys like G-spot vibrators, or the use of lubricant. These things are manufactured with pleasure in mind and they can make up for what nature no longer supplies.

- Talk to your doctor if you notice that you have no interest in sex or cannot get aroused. It may mean that you have a medical problem that needs attention or that your hormones are out of balance.

- Broaden your ideas about what constitutes "sex" so that if you are tired or not in the mood for sex, you can still connect with your partner. Cuddle up and watch a movie together while you munch a favorite snack, give each other a neck rub, or spend a few minutes kissing. Promise you'll rest up for sex another time.

17

Problematic Pornography Viewing Behavior

Internet pornography use has grown exponentially since so-called adult sites were first launched. Searches for Internet pornography are ranked number one, and visits to pornography sites are said to account for half of all Internet traffic. A joke recently circulated that a researcher wanted to conduct a study on men who had never viewed pornography, but he could not find a single subject, reflecting a belief that *all* men look at pornography. In my practice only men who grew up in conservative countries without early Internet access seem to have circumvented looking at explicit sexual material.

Whenever I speak to groups of mental health professionals regarding almost any topic related to sexuality, someone inevitably asks how to treat couples that complain about one partner viewing pornography. Although it may sound facetious, my answer is, "I treat using psychotherapy!" Therapists forget that they already have most of the tools to help these couples; instead they collude with the alarmist reactions of the injured partner and may carry their own similar disgust toward Internet porn. They are also under- standably confused, because even experts in the field cannot seem to agree on the definition of problematic use of Internet pornography. On one end of the spectrum are sexologists who argue that pornography is a healthy outlet when a partner is unavailable; when one has sexual interests that are difficult to satisfy, for example, certain types of fetish behavior; or as a way to learn about sexually satisfying behaviors. On the other end are addiction specialists who believe that pornography has no place in a person's life and that complete abstinence from all but partnered sex is required as a cure. Such disparate views are fascinating to ponder, but leave the therapist wondering what tack to take when a couple comes into the office on the verge of dissolving their relationship, or a single individual becomes aware that he (or less frequently, she) has grown to prefer Internet pornography to real sex with real partners.

To dispel confusion, I have decided to use the term "problematic pornography viewing behavior" (PVB) rather than "addiction" for a few reasons. One is that the word "addiction" carries with it moralistic connotations, similar to what was thought about alcoholism prior to the scientific understanding of the physiological nature of substance dependence. The word is also sometimes used as an insult to shame the pornography viewer, so it has a questionable place in the therapy office. The meaning of "addiction" also has become diluted as people claim that they are "addicted to chocolate" or "addicted to popping bubble wrap."

That is not to say that viewing Internet pornography has no relationship to addictive behavior. In a review article, Wetterneck, Burgess, Short, Smith, and Cervantes (2012) discuss the nature of PVB in terms of impulsivity, compulsivity, and addiction, making a case that impulsive use of pornography describes behavior that occurs without much forethought and generally for pleasure, while compulsive use concerns the repetitive urge to engage in such behavior, even when the behavior may have become uncomfortable. Addiction is associated with the mood-altering quality of viewing Internet pornography, which is similar to what happens when someone uses a chemical to alter mood or consciousness.

In fact, brain studies using fMRI suggest that the anticipation of using pornography sets in motion a cascade of reward chemicals, much like occurs in gamblers, shoppers, heavy exercisers, and video game users. Although there is no substance, and therefore no symptoms of physical tolerance or withdrawal, process addiction is similar to alcohol and drug addiction in that the process is often used to avoid, cope with, or change a negative mood state. By example, Wetterneck and his team (2012) identified that the more hours a person engages in PVB, the higher the likelihood they are trying to avoid negative affective states. Apparently, engaging in PVB potentially interferes with the brain's prefrontal cortex and its ability to evaluate the consequences of behavior or inhibit compulsive behavior (Karim & Chaudhri, 2012).

PVB can also be understood as a symptom of detached attachment style. Zitzman and Butler (2005) state that such behaviors created a "[p]rofound disconnection of the sexual experience from relationship context and meaning." In younger clients, PVB generally becomes an escape from potentially painful social and romantic interactions. They may flounder with creating an emotionally intimate relationship when the opportunity presents itself. In older clients, PVB may reflect the user's inability to get sexual needs met as sex with a familiar partner may not be as stimulating as pornography; the PVB individual, and possibly the partner, may not realize that emotional connection and secure attachment may compensate for lower levels of arousal.

Family therapists view PVB as a problem of boundary violations, inappropriate coalitions, secrecy, and poor communication (Ford, Durtschi, & Franklin, 2012). The individual with PVB may engage in the behavior because of relationship dissatisfaction, creating a coalition against the partner. The pornography use is likened to a relationship betrayal, similar to what happens with infidelity. In this regard, the couple must join against the problematic material and rebuild their relationship through increased communication. What separates PVB from infidelity, however, is that it is much simpler and usually more discrete to access pornography than it is a flesh-and-blood partner, making the attachment theory perhaps more applicable.

What perhaps can truthfully be said about PVB is that it may not be diagnosable in the traditional sense. PVB is perhaps best viewed as a socially and relationally constructed phenomenon, one that may violate some people's moral values, and which clients complain about and want curtailed or stopped. But how does one treat a problem that seems to be a matter of perception? As with other issues that come to light in the therapy room, the therapist needs to take a nonjudgmental stance, putting aside preconceptions about what PVB is or isn't to listen to the client's or couple's experience.

An ecosystemic framework may serve as a way to clarify understanding what the complaint means and how it might be resolved. For whom is this behavior problematic? What function is the behavior serving the individual and the system? How will solving the problem make things different? What is the goal of treatment? Is it to abstain altogether, to come to some agreement about when pornography is or isn't to be viewed, or is the couple going to find a way to make pornography part of their sex life together?

ASSESSMENT OF PVB

For some individuals, PVB began as a habit, as individuals who engage in problematic sexual behavior (PSB) often were exposed to such material at a young age, sometimes predating the Internet. One gentleman I worked with discovered, at age 8, two large drums of pornographic magazines and videos in an abandoned house. Somehow the client managed to keep his huge stash of material secreted away from his parents. Another client reported that he was an "early adopter" of the Internet in his preteens. His parents were naive and never realized that he was spending hours in his room masturbating to all kinds of sexual materials. For these men, using pornography became a way to avoid relationship conflict and deal with painful emotions, much as someone might use food or shopping.

PVB can be associated with major depression, the manic phase of bipolar disorder, anxiety, and attention deficit/hyperactivity disorder (AD/HD). In clinical practice, men who complain of PSB often have low self-esteem and tend to isolate themselves or become avoidant when they experience stress. During times of social withdrawal, they turn to pornography to relieve duress. Single men who compulsively use pornography may lack social skills; often they are lonely or bored. Men who are self-employed or who travel as part of their work seem to be, in my experience, more at risk for turning to the Internet for diversion and comfort.

Another variable that must be considered but is rarely addressed is whether or not there is a paraphilia involved in the PVB. In a presentation of 30 brief case studies, Levine (2010) suggests that men seek out cybersex for personal gratification; to practice a paraphilic behavior in private; and as an assertion of male privilege. Partners are sometimes shocked to learn that their mate is viewing material about bondage, wearing items of clothing, or involving scatological practices. Some partners may see this as positive, because it means that their partner is satisfying a sexual need without requiring their participation, while others find it gross or threatening enough that the viability of the relationship is threatened. In other cases, someone may receive a peculiar sexual request from a partner, such as a woman who asked me if it was "normal" for her husband to ask her to have sex with the family dog. The woman was very naive and it hadn't occurred to her that her husband may have gotten this idea from watching pornography.

STEP INTO MY OFFICE...

William, a young bisexual man dressed in a t-shirt and wearing flip flops, squirmed and laughed when he admitted to me he got sexually aroused by looking at men dressed in business suits and tuxedos. He had been able to hide both his interest and his sexual orientation until one day, feeling a little bored and sad, he decided to look at images on the Internet. Not only did he find images designed specifically to satisfy his interest, but also forums and chat rooms of other men who enjoyed dressing up. He made a decision to disclose his wish to his wife Kate that he wanted to make love to her while he was wearing a tuxedo. Although he protested that he had no interest in having sex with men, Kate still felt threatened and disgusted. Treatment consisted of finding ways to talk about William's bisexuality, his fidelity to his wife, and his seemingly odd fetish. Once Kate felt she could trust William not to stray into having sex with anyone else, she was able to concede that William could look at images as long as they maintained a healthy sex life together.

How do partners react when they discover PVB? In a strict addiction model (Carnes, 2001), the concept of *co-dependence* is used to describe the partner who becomes conflicted over stopping the behavior for fear that setting a firm boundary may lead to abandonment. The co-dependent partner acts as a victim, who may fear that they are somehow the cause of the Internet pornography use, asking their partner whether or not they are attractive enough or feeling that they are in competition with the pornographic material. When they look for clues that their partner is still involved in PVB, they are said to be a "co-addict." They compulsively look for evidence that their partner is "sober," or refraining from PVB, much as the partner of an alcoholic becomes overly concerned about drinking.

The difference is that in many relationships, people use pornography as a substitute for sex with their partner. In doing so, they may develop a sexual dysfunction, losing their drive or capacity for sexual arousal with their familiar partner. The impact on the partner who then makes the discovery that the pornography user does have a drive and can get an erection or ejaculate when using pornography can be devastating. The partner may react to the pornography use similarly to infidelity, with initial shock, followed by disgust and rage. Trust is eroded, especially if the partner repeatedly finds evidence of Internet pornography use. The partner with problematic sexual behavior may respond in one of two ways: either denying the extent of use or exhibiting a certain level of entitlement (e.g., asking, "What's the big deal?") and having difficulty taking responsibility for the possible harm caused to the relationship, or expressing an enormous sense of shame, guilt, and remorse. As with infidelity, the partner and/or couple may ask what has gone wrong in the relationship, seeking answers to stop the pain of relationship betrayal. The impact on a woman's self-esteem can be enormous; often statements such as the following are made:

> *"I can't compete with the perfect women he's looking at online!"*
> *"Why did he need to go elsewhere for sexual satisfaction? Aren't I enough?"*
> *"I am so disgusted by his behavior, I can't even look at him."*
> *"What if the children came into the room while he is looking at that!"*
> *"It's just a straight out sin to do what he was doing!"*

Partners sometimes adamantly disagree about viewing pornography. The consumer of pornography may view it as a diversion, like watching a sporting event, while the partner views it as the height of sin. The issue of pornography use may be the tip of an iceberg that includes views on religion, morality, and personal freedom within marriage. Many couples look to the therapist to advocate for one view or the other. Ethics aside, if the therapist is upfront in speaking against any form of sexual behavior outside the sanctity of marriage, then by default any couple who comes into that therapist's practice will know that the goal is to stop such behavior. For therapists who are nonjudgmental, sessions become more problematic in that the therapist can become triangulated. The therapy sessions become stuck as the therapist tries to explain each partner's side to the other or begins to take sides.

TREATMENT OF PVB

Inpatient and intensive outpatient treatment for PVB has become an industry unto itself. A perfunctory Google search using the term "sex addiction treatment program" returned 1.47 million results. Such programs are akin to those for drug and alcohol rehabilitation, offering individual therapy and frequent group therapy or support, some modeled after Sex and Love Addicts Anonymous (SLAA) and Sex Addicts Anonymous (SAA) 12-step meetings. However, individuals who are substance dependent may need such intensive treatment because they can have potentially fatal symptoms such as seizures as part of their withdrawal. People with PVB most likely can benefit from outpatient psychotherapy, much as people with other impulsive/compulsive disorders.

In severe cases, for example, when a man has injured himself such as incurring carpal tunnel syndrome from excessive masturbation (which may sound comical, but most assuredly is not), or when there is a comorbid psychiatric disorder, then a medication evaluation is recommended. Antidepressants can not only help the person with PVB cope with negative affect, but potentially the sexual side effect of decreasing libido may help the person gain control over their behavior while they are learning other means of coping with negative affect, escapism, and emotional isolation.

In individual therapy, themes around intimacy, being vulnerable, and the need for control can be explored. In a case study presented by Marcus (personal communication, 2010), the client demonstrated even at the outset of therapy that making a relationship with the therapist will be a challenge. Thus, developing rapport, remaining nonjudgmental, and normalizing that there may be setbacks can all contribute to the increased likelihood of a successful treatment outcome.

While clearing the environment of pornography and any triggers, such as racy scenes on cable television, seems like an appropriate intervention, for some people with PVB it may be unnecessary and create additional feelings of shame. Just as there are alcoholics who can be at a bar or holiday party without getting triggered to drink, there are people who can refrain from watching pornography if they so wish. What can be more effective is for the individual to become aware of and express negative affect that they experience when they experience an urge to engage in PVB. Keeping a thoughts and feelings journal can yield valuable information in this regard.

Since isolation is a major part of PVB, it can also be helpful to have the individual identify other healthier activities that may also get them out of the house and around others. Yoga seems to be a favorite in my community because it helps to relieve physical tension and is calming to the mind. Simply taking a walk or calling a friend to meet socially can make a difference. Volunteering is another way to get out of one's own way and feel a sense of purpose.

Couples therapy when the problem is PVB may not look much different than therapy when the problem is infidelity. As with infidelity, the person with PVB needs to admit openly to their behavior, demonstrate understanding of why their behavior has been hurtful to a partner (e.g., they haven't shown the partner any sexual interest), and be able to identify their emotional and sexual needs rather than hiding them. The partner needs to be permitted to ventilate anger, loss, or hurt, with the eventual goal of forgiving the partner with PVB.

Sexual dissatisfaction is estimated to affect about 25% of marriages (McCarthy & McCarthy, 2003) and is one reason that men report engaging in PSB. Some dissatisfaction may be attributed to the partner's sexual dysfunction, such as low sexual desire or sexual aversion, but often it is a co-created issue. For example, the partner with PSB may have an inability to discuss his sexual wants and needs with his partner, over which he may have experienced shame, or feel uncomfortable about bringing his "dirty" behaviors into the "clean" bedroom with his "pure" partner. Or, he may not discuss his sexual needs because he wants to avoid conflict.

Couples need to learn how to negotiate their needs. Sexual activities may be overly constrained or lack variety. Even if the non-PSB partner expresses disinterest in a particular activity such as performing oral sex, if they can understand the core need, most problems can be worked out. Does the PSB partner want to be dominant? Passive? More passionate? Or experimental?

In terms of sexual healing in the relationship, the most effective approach is to have the couple discuss what constitutes healthy sexuality. Within the discussion, couples can practice communication skills of listening, rather than reacting, to feelings and opinions. Some of the discussion may concern each partner's feelings about pornography.

WHAT CONSTITUTES HEALTHY SEXUALITY? TOPICS TO BE EXPLORED

- Must sexual activity always take place between two people?
- Is there a time or place for solo sex?
- Why is pornography acceptable or unacceptable?
- Are people who are married or in a committed relationship entitled to some private sexual behaviors?
- How open is each partner to satisfying each other's particular sexual needs?

ACTIVITIES

1. Reflect in your journal on your beliefs about looking at pornography. How might they support or be at odds with the experience of mainstream American adults? Are there any times when looking at pornography might be beneficial, or is it always a negative experience?

2. How might you handle the following common clinical situations:
   - A couple that practices a fundamental, conservative religion; the man looks at pornography once or twice a month and the woman wants him to refrain at looking at pornography altogether.
   - A single man who wonders if his constant viewing of pornography is of any consequence.
   - A woman who cannot get aroused for sex with her long-term partner unless she watches pornography while using a vibrator.
   - A teenage boy with Asperger's syndrome who looks at pornography because he is too socially awkward to relate to teenage girls.
   - A man who downloads child pornography "because it's better than getting caught fondling a child."

RESOURCES

Maltz, W., & Maltz, L. (2009). *The porn trap: The essential guide to overcoming problems caused by pornography*. New York, NY: William Morrow Paperbacks.

Skinner, K. B. (2005). *Treating pornography addiction: The essential tools for recovery*. Provo, UT: GrowthClimate.

DEALING WITH PROBLEMATIC
PORNOGRAPHIC VIEWING BEHAVIOR

Problematic pornographic viewing behavior (PVB) can interfere with your self-esteem, your sexual function, and relationships. PVB can be thought of as a *process addiction*, that is, instead of being addicted to a substance, a person becomes addicted to a behavior. A process addiction is like a habit. Like all behaviors, some habits are healthy and some are unhealthy. Watching football can be healthy for relaxation, but unhealthy if it means not spending any time with a partner. Some people think all viewing of pornography is problematic; that will be something that you can decide with your partner and your therapist.

One way to overcome PVB, or any process addiction, is to make a plan. Researchers think that when someone develops a process addiction, the part of the brain that protects that person from engaging in unwanted behavior doesn't work the way it should. If you have a plan, then you can compensate for that part of the brain and do a better job of stopping or avoiding PVB. Examples of planning include:

- Keeping a log of times when you feel like engaging in PVB. This can make you aware of what triggers you to engage in this behavior so you can do something else instead.

- Make a list of things that will relieve whatever feeling you are trying to avoid or fix when you engage in PVB. If you engage in PVB when stressed, what else can relieve stress? If it happens when you are sad, what is making you sad, and what will help make you feel better? If you identify your feelings or needs, you can usually do something about them to make things better.

- Find enjoyable activities that you can plan in order to remind yourself that there are other ways to have fun besides PVB.

- When you have an interest in PVB, ask yourself honestly if you are avoiding dealing with an issue in your relationship. If so, be honest. Communicate your wants and needs openly with your partner. Let your partner reciprocate. In this way you will build real intimacy and find your need for PVB dissipates.

18

Alternate Sexual Practices

Of all the sexual difficulties therapists may face in their clients, perhaps none is as puzzling as alternative sexual practices, or paraphilias. A *paraphilia* is generally defined as sexual arousal to objects, events, or people outside what is considered the norm. The arousal can be created through fantasy or enacted in reality, and the accompanying release of tension through masturbation or sexual activity is highly rewarding, so that the person continues the behavior despite possible legal or other consequences. The rewarding nature of a paraphilia can also create compulsive or hypersexual behavior.

Generally, therapists and lay people alike associate paraphilias with sex offending, especially *pedophilia*, or the exploitation of children in fantasy and activity for sexual gratification. Other serious paraphilias for which people may be legally prosecuted, include:

- *Frotteurism*: rubbing of one's genitals against another nonconsenting person
- *Voyeurism*: looking at nonconsenting people nude or involved in sexual activity
- *Exhibitionism*: displaying one's genitals to a nonconsenting person
- *Bestiality:* engaging in sexual fantasy or acts with an animal
- *Sadism*: deriving sexual pleasure from causing pain to nonconsenting others

Most therapists are familiar with the harm created in trauma survivors abused by pedophiles or other sex offenders, and offenders are generally treated as pariahs not only in our culture as a whole, but also by therapists. It wouldn't be an exaggeration to state that a reason therapists decline to treat sexual problems at all is that they do not wish to treat sex offenders, for whom they may have limited compassion. While an argument can be made that nearly all (or all, depending on one's view) clients are deserving of compassion, there are differences in working with offending clients that make a referral to a specialist who works with offenders in order. Such specialists are familiar with the legal system, reporting laws, and appropriate treatment such as aversion therapy (pairing sexual stimulation with noxious stimulus), covert sensitization (pairing sexual stimulus with negative imagery), or psychotropic and antiandrogen drug therapy used to control sexual urges.

For the purposes of this chapter, the term *alternate sexual practices* (also known as "alt sex") best describes nonnormative, noncriminal behavior and refers to those individuals most likely to become therapy clients. Common nonoffending alt sex practices include:

- *Fetishism*: Sexual gratification from an object or part of the body. Common fetish objects are high-heeled shoes, unique undergarments (e.g., a garter belt), or fabrics like leather or fur; coveted body parts include feet, legs, breasts, etc., often of a particular size or shape. People will sometimes go to great lengths to acquire objects or find a person with their favored attributes.
- *Sadism:* Sexual gratification from causing physical pain to or "power play" with a *consenting* adult. The dominant partner ("dom") may administer mild pain, such as biting, scratching, or spanking, or more extreme forms such as semi-strangulation (asphyxiation, also called "breath play"). When a couple is engaged in consensual *sadomasochism*, they generally create a "scene" or script they will follow to ensure activity stays within certain boundaries, as well as a "safe word" that the submissive partner can use if that person feels overwhelmed or scared.
- *Masochism:* Sexual gratification from being physically hurt or engaged in "power play" in a *consensual* relationship. The masochist (submissive partner, or "sub") may engage in mild activity, such as spanking or light bondage, or may acquiesce or even request whipping, being tied in chains, or being physically overpowered.
- *Transvestism*: Deriving sexual and/or emotional pleasure from dressing in the clothing of the opposite sex; also called *cross-dressing*. Unlike a female impersonator or "drag queen" who dresses for theatrical performance, the male cross-dresser needs to engage in transvestism for sexual and emotional release.
- *Paraphilia NOS*: There are many very unusual paraphilias that cannot be found listed in the *DSM-5*, such as *coprophilia* and *urophilia*, or sexual

gratification from feces and urine, respectively (also known as "scat," for "scatological"), *klismaphilia*, or gratification from the use of enemas, and *apotmenophilia*, which is sexual attraction to bodily amputations.

In terms of developing a tolerant and nonjudgmental stance toward non-offending alt sex practices, consider what harm there is if a man masturbates to pictures of women's feet in stiletto heels—or cross-dresses in women's shoes or other garments? If a couple dresses in leather and studs, then visits a sex dungeon to meet friends for consensual sessions of sadomasochistic bondage and domination ("BDSM"), should they be considered deviants if they enjoy their activity? ("No different a social activity than bowling!" one such individual quipped in my office.) When a woman imagines having sex with a favorite stuffed animal ("plushophilia"), is she a pervert? Are any or all of these individuals mentally ill? Are they sex addicts?

THE DEBATE FOR REMOVING PARAPHILIA FROM THE *DSM*

Clinicians and researchers on the *DSM-5* work committee on paraphilias pondered the question of what constitutes a true disorder. Because paraphilias constitute such a broad spectrum of behaviors, committee members distinguished between a *paraphilia*, a behavior that may not automatically be diagnosed as a psychiatric disorder, and a *paraphilic disorder*, with the latter being "a paraphilia that causes distress or impairment to the individual or harm to others," a distinction which will assist in forensic evaluation. Still, some believe that paraphilias should be removed from the *DSM-5* altogether (Shindel & Moser, 2011), as the term *paraphilia* is pejorative and pathologizes what is, for some, enjoyable and erotic sexual behavior.

Within each type of paraphilia there are varying degrees of practice, from occasional "light bondage" (spanking, tickling, or using a blindfold) to behavior that might be termed hypersexual, such as spending money one needs for living expenses on prostitutes who will administer or submit to a preferred fantasy or behavior.

ALT SEX PRACTICES IN THERAPY

Although people who practice alt sex usually experience their behavior as ego syntonic and report being content with their sexual self-expression, they may enter therapy for the following reasons:

- Their behavior is so compelling that they cannot function sexually without it, for example, they develop erectile dysfunction or anorgasmia.
- They have had difficulty finding a tolerant partner.

- Their partner has discovered their behavior and feels disgusted or threatened.
- Their partner has participated in the behavior, but has tired of it.
- They have another psychiatric disorder, such as depression; these individuals will often seek out a sex therapist to avoid judgment.
- They fear becoming compelled to act out fantasies for which they may be arrested.

Those individuals who are self-motivated for therapy have a more positive prognosis than those who are brought in by a partner or who have been faced with arrest. Even so, alt sex behaviors can be deeply ingrained and difficult to treat.

WHO PRACTICES ALT SEX—AND WHY?

Due to fear of being misunderstood, shame, and stigma, secrecy marks alternative sex; no one is certain how many people are involved. A look at the alt sex site *fetlife.com* ("Facebook for kinksters like you and me") reveals membership of 1.3 million people; 2 million discussions; and 41,000 groups. A perfunctory search of *Google* gave the following numbers of hits:

- Bondage: 188 million*
- Dominatrix: 28.6 million
- Latex fetishism: 20 million
- Shoe fetish: 2 million
- "Cross-dressing guide": 2 million
- Urophilia: 1.9 million
- Plushophilia: 49K
- Object sexuality: 57K
- Autoerotic asphyxiation: 221K

Characteristics and personalities of those who practice alt sex vary widely, with the exception of gender, as it is mainly a male phenomenon. There are, however, some females who practice sexual sadism or masochism.

---

*At the time of this writing, of E. L. James' books (*Fifty Shades of Grey*, *Fifty Shades Darker*, and *Fifty Shades Freed*) were listed as numbers one, two, and three on the *New York Times Bestsellers* list of print, e-book, and paperback books, which may explain inflated numbers for the term *bondage*.

STEP INTO MY OFFICE...

Born in a foreign country, Margaret was indebted to her American husband for teaching her English. However, he often requested that she wear a latex cat suit during sex because he could not tolerate the feeling of any imperfection on her skin. Seeing no harm, she initially went along with it, but now he was demanding that she wear it every time they had sex. Margaret came to feel he was making love to the suit and not to her. When I met with her husband Mort, it appeared that he had Asperger's syndrome (AS); he not only became aroused by the latex cat suit, but like some people with AS he disliked the tactile feel of human skin. Unable to relate to how wearing the cat suit affected Margaret, Mort refused to give up the cat suit. Ultimately Margaret ended the marriage.

No one is certain why some people develop interest in or practice of alternative sexualities. There may be a biological foundation; those who practice sadism, for example, show greater activity in the amygdala and anterior insula when viewing pain pictures (Harenski, Thornton, Harenski, Decety, & Kiehl, 2012), and there is research, though scant, suggesting that male sadists and others who practice alt sex may have higher levels of testosterone (Jordan, Fromberger, Stolpmann, & Muller, 2011), buoying the prescription of antiandrogens to sex offenders.

Also, many alt sex practitioners, particularly cross-dressers, report having experiences when they were as young as 8 or 9. Thus, early development may play a role. In the case of cross-dressers, psychoanalysts point to a person's wish to experience sexual pleasure without fear of castration. Attachment theorists bypass Oedipal urges, pointing instead to an inability to attain and maintain appropriate healthy relationships due to early trauma. Sexual gratification is then sought with objects rather than humans; through pseudorelationships as with exhibitionism or voyeurism; or based on power differentials rather than affection as with sadomasochism (Wiederman, 2003). Or perhaps classical conditioning has occurred, with a person experiencing arousal paired with an object or experience, then strengthening the association with masturbation and fantasy or actual experiences. Another idea is that Western culture is highly sexualized in a way that is directed at males, but some males may not have an appropriate outlet, thus the alt sex practice is a compromise solution.

Personality characteristics may also play a role (Seligman & Hardenburg, 2000), including low self-esteem, little empathy, poor insight, few social skills, and difficulty with impulse control. When confronted by a partner—or a therapist—they may alternate between self-deprecation and feelings of entitlement. Perhaps understandably, people who practice alt sex may also have mood disorders, anxiety disorders, or substance problems. In therapy, they are often guarded, fearing that they will be judged or having too much shame to admit their level of need or involvement with the alt sex behavior. They have difficulty trusting the therapist, making treatment challenging at least and impossible at times.

Even less is understood about the partner of the person who practices alt sex. In clinical practice, partners often feel threatened by unusual sexual behavior. I have observed very different responses in wives of cross-dressers, for example:

- A minister reported that not only was his wife divorcing him, but threatening to report his behavior to the congregation if he did not agree to give up his share of the assets.
- One woman tolerated her partner's cross-dressing, as long as he kept all evidence hidden and only did it when she was away on business.
- Another woman did not participate with her husband when he cross-dressed, but she would buy him clothing and paint his nails for him.

Female partners of cross-dressers may report concern that their partner is gay, that they will not be able to arouse their partner, or that they themselves will be so turned off by their partner's behavior that they, themselves, will not be aroused. They also fear that if they tolerate a certain level of behavior that their partner will push the boundary. Thus, some partners will choose to terminate the relationship rather than live with the ambivalence created by staying.

STEP INTO MY OFFICE...

Leon and Amy both appeared shell shocked. Amy had discovered that her husband was involved in several affairs with women who were "subs" to Leon, their dom. Shortly after the discovery, Leon revealed to Amy that he was a survivor of a long history of incest. By way of explanation for what triggered his current behavior, Leon reported that when his business failed, he tried without success to get the reassurance he needed from Amy, who was distracted with taking care of their family. Under duress, he began having sadomasochistic dreams and fantasies that he eventually acted out.

Leon stated in therapy that after carrying out his consensual alt sex practices, he could not see himself being entirely happy in his somewhat "vanilla" or traditional marriage. Amy admitted that she had sometimes consensually engaged in mild scenes with Leon, but now that she learned that he enacted these behaviors with other women, she wasn't enthused about satisfying Leon's needs.

Leon declined psychotherapy to address issues related to sexual trauma and expressed that he did not wish to change his core sexual identity. Since Amy was open to S&M play, therapy focused on forgiveness for the affairs and engendering increased trust in the couple's relationship, as well as helping the couple negotiate how much consensual and scripted sadomasochistic activity they would engage in going forward. Note that in as much as some therapists may have wished for Amy to advocate for herself, her acquiescence to Leon reflected a deep-seated dynamic that would be futile to change unless both parties were agreeable.

ASSESSMENT AND TREATMENT OF ALT SEX PRACTICES

Before conducting any assessment, the therapist needs to adapt a nonshaming, compassionate stance toward the alt sex practitioner as well as the partner. It can be helpful to remember that the alt sex practitioner has perhaps already experienced enough embarrassment, either over their behavior or being discovered. On the other hand, stereotypes can create countertransference. Some people who practice alt sex are happy and even proud of their ability to freely express their favorite sexual practices.

Assessing alt sex practices as a problem for treatment often presents a few dilemmas. Is the person coming in for treatment because they want treatment, or is it a partner who is expecting a change? When the behavior is ego syntonic, there is little motivation and treatment may be futile. However, in many cases the person who practices alt sex wants the benefits of a committed relationship (including whatever normalcy and stability it provides) and may be willing to flex in order to retain it. Conversely, it is often the "vanilla" partner who takes a hard stance that the alt sex partner must give up their fetish or cross-dressing altogether.

In assessing the alt sex practice, consider the following questions:

1. When did the behavior begin? Is it a longstanding behavior, or one that was more recently acquired, perhaps as a result of viewing certain pornographic material on the Internet?
2. How does the alt sex partner explain the behavior?
3. Is the person able to achieve sexual gratification in more normative ways with their partner?
4. Is the partner willing to participate in the alt sex practice in some way?
5. If the alt sex practice does not stop, will there be dire consequences to the relationship?
6. What is it about the alt sex practice that is threatening or disturbing to the non–alt sex partner?
7. Has the alt sex partner tried to stop the behavior? What happened?
8. What positive emotional and sexual feelings does the alt sex practitioner get from the behavior? What negative feelings?
9. What was the partner's response to the alt sex practice?
10. What does the alt sex practitioner consider a realistic goal? What about the partner?
11. Is the person at risk for offending? (If high risk, such as fantasizing about sex with children, consider referral to a specialist in treating sex offenders.)

Additional assessment of mental status and sex and relationship history of both partners is also in order to rule out problems such as bipolar disorder and substance abuse. The therapist cannot assume, however, that there must be a comorbid diagnosis, nor should they overpathologize the behavior.

Depending upon the chronicity, severity, and treatment goals, a referral to a psychiatrist may be appropriate to improve mood and manage anxiety and/or sexual urges of a compulsive nature. If the alt sex practice is more difficult to control, then keeping a log of urges and accompanying feelings can help the client understand and break an unwanted pattern, most likely by helping the client cope with dysphoric mood or anxiety. Substance abuse problems may also need to be addressed, but not without providing supportive treatment and coping skills. I have also made referrals to a urologist when it appears that the alt sex practice started late in life, as this sometimes indicates that a male is attempting to compensate for poor erectile function by involving himself in alt sex rather than through requesting more stimulation from his partner.

Other treatment approaches vary. Often there is a cognitive behavioral component to address irrational ideas about sex such as, "My partner 'must' wear latex if I am going to be aroused," or "Vanilla sex is 'always' boring." Open communication is also essential if the partnership is to survive; various questions can be posed for exploration such as how each partner defines "normal" sex or their theories of how people develop sexually.

Information can be broadly supplied, such as explaining what is known about alt sex practices, the possible relationship to early trauma, or how to achieve arousal with one's partner without alt sex. Suggestions for change include sensate focus techniques as well as finding new practices that both partners can enjoy, for example, introducing toys, body paints, objects like feathers or a fur mitt, and light bondage items such as Velcro™ handcuffs or a soft blindfold. The couple then may negotiate a certain percentage of traditional sexual experiences versus alt sex experiences.

While this chapter has focused on tolerance and acceptance of nonoffending alt sex practices when possible, not every client has the same level of self-compassion. People are often extremely embarrassed and wish for removal of the behavior. In such cases, intensive therapy is recommended, with treatment goals of improving self-esteem, eliminating shame, correcting irrational ideas about sex, as well as exploration of early childhood sexual memories and experiences that may have contributed to nonnormative sexual development. Such therapy is usually long and arduous, and it is the rare client who will be able to let go of behavior that has been so rewarding.

ACTIVITIES

1. If you, yourself, do not have any alternative sex practices, reflect on potential countertransference to those who do. What feelings do you have about working with this population? Are you capable of providing compassionate care? Discuss with a trusted colleague or supervisor who is versed in working with this population.

2. Reflect on what value there might be in facilitating someone's interest in alt sex practices. Might you make recommendations on books (see *Resources*), DVDs, or locales where an isolated person might be able to fulfill sexual wants?

RESOURCES

Blue, V. (2011). *Sweet confessions: Erotic fantasies for couples.* San Francisco, CA: Cleis Press.

Brame, W., Brame, G., & Jacobs, J. (1996). *Different loving: The world of sexual dominance and submission.* New York, NY: Villard.

Kleinplatz, P. J. & Moser, M. (2006). *Sadomasochism: Powerful pleasures.* New York, NY: Routledge.

Valdez, N. (2010). *A little bit kinky: A couples' guide to rediscovering the thrill of sex.* New York, NY: Three Rivers Press.

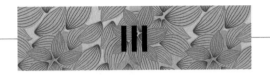

Ethics and Practice
of Sex Therapy

Ethical Management of Sex Therapy Casework

Working with issues surrounding sexuality requires special attention to personal biases and stereotypes; management of transference and countertransference regarding sexual topics; and attaining competence in treating sexual problems. The intention of this chapter is not to provide a complete overview of ethics, but to explore a few select issues that can and do arise in the treatment of sexual problems. Of course, any time questions about ethics arise, it is always wise to consult with a colleague, supervisor, or to seek legal counsel.

MAINTAINING APPROPRIATE BOUNDARIES

The ethical and legal issue in sex therapy that most concerns therapists, supervisors, instructors, and insurance risk managers—as well as psychotherapy clients—is the inappropriate crossing of sexual boundaries. Virtually every ethics code, whether for psychologists, marriage and family therapists, social workers, and counselors, explicitly states that sexual contact between client and therapist must never take place *during* psychotherapy. (*After* psychotherapy terminates is another matter and is discussed later in the chapter.) This is because there exists a natural power differential between therapist and client due to discrepancies in knowledge and authority. The client is dependent on the professional, who is expected to confer not only treatment, but also caring. Clients whose sexuality has been compromised in some way may be more susceptible to imagining special treatment or favor from a therapist who treats sexual concerns.

Sexual misconduct (Plaut, 2008) can consist of any type of inappropriate touch that is intended to create erotic or loving feelings within the relationship. Like the patients of physicians, psychotherapy clients cannot be said to give consent for such instances of touch. Perhaps the most insidious violation occurs when a therapist assures the client that having sex is an important part of treatment, exploiting both the caregiver and client roles for the therapist's own gain. When sexual boundary violations occur, the consequences can be serious for both the perpetrator, who can lose his or her license, and the victim, who may suffer psychological consequences similar to those suffered from sexual abuse, that is, shame, low self-esteem, disruption of trust, and difficulty with current and future intimate relationships. Thus when a therapist takes advantage of the power differential in order to meet sexual or relationship needs, it is looked upon with particular incredulity from ethics and licensing boards as well as colleagues.

The American Association of Sexuality Educators, Counselors, and Therapists (AASECT) has its own *Code of Ethics* that explicitly forbids sexual contact between AASECT members and their clients:

> *The member practicing counseling or therapy shall not engage, attempt to engage or offer to engage a consumer in sexual behavior whether the consumer consents to such behavior or not. Sexual misconduct includes kissing, sexual intercourse and/or the touching by either the member or the consumer of the other's breasts or genitals. Members do not engage in such sexual misconduct with current consumers. Members do not engage in sexual intimacies with individuals they know to be close relatives, guardians, or significant others of a current consumer. Sexual misconduct is also sexual solicitation, physical advances, or verbal or nonverbal conduct that is sexual in nature, that occurs in connection with the member's activities or roles as a counselor or therapist, and that either (1) is unwelcome, is offensive, or creates a hostile workplace or educational environment, and the member knows or is told this or (2) is sufficiently severe or intense to be abusive to a reasonable person in the context. Sexual misconduct can consist of a single intense or severe act, or of multiple persistent or pervasive acts. For purposes of determining the existence of sexual misconduct, the counseling or therapeutic relationship is deemed to continue in perpetuity.*

While the AASECT Code advises that the counseling relationship is said to continue indefinitely, other codes differ. Most notably, the *APA Ethical Principles of Psychologists and Code of Conduct* explicitly states, "Psychologists do not engage in sexual intimacies with former clients/patients for at least two years after cessation or termination of therapy." However, the APA later clarified that such intimacy should not take place "except in the most unusual circumstances." The onus is on the psychologist to determine several factors that create such circumstance, including lack of exploitation;

nature and intensity of the therapy; client's history; client's current mental status; and likelihood of adverse impact on the client.

Additionally, the American Mental Health Counselors Association states that counselors "may not enter into an intimate relationship until five years post termination *or longer as specified by state regulations*" (italics added for emphasis). In point of fact, several states, including Texas and Minnesota, have state laws that supersede such codes and forbid sexual relationships with clients at any point in time, even after the termination of the client–therapist relationship.

TRANSFERENCE AND COUNTERTRANSFERENCE OF ATTRACTION

Transference and countertransference between therapist and client are generally thought to be a constant, even normative experience during the course of therapy (Fisher, 2004b). Self-disclosure of such feelings can be therapeutic, as when the therapist expresses genuine feelings of sadness when a client is grieving, or when a client tells the therapist of his or her gladness for a therapist's help. However, a therapist's self-disclosure in regard to the development of feelings of romantic and sexual attraction is a topic unto itself. On one hand, being open about attraction normalizes that such feelings do develop and can be managed without acting on them. Being open may also allow the client to discuss whether they have sensed any countertransference from the therapist. On the other hand, such disclosure can be a sign of an inappropriate boundary crossing. For example, in an analogue study of therapist ratings of mock scenarios in which therapists either disclosed or kept silent about their sexual feelings, disclosing therapists were seen as less expert and their therapeutic intervention as less effective than those who did not disclose (Goodyear & Shmate, 1996, in Fisher, 2004b).

Aside from issues of professionalism and therapeutic effectiveness, Fisher (2004) reminds therapists that harm to the client can take place without actual sexual touch occurring—harm that can be foreseen and prevented, which makes disclosure of attraction unethical. If the sexual disclosure is unwanted, it may also be perceived as sexual harassment (Fisher, 2004; Plaut, 2008). Unless sexual self-disclosure is part of informed consent (and what therapist would risk stating in their policies that they may disclose feelings of sexual attraction), the client cannot be prepared for such an experience.

Clients, of course, can develop a romantic transference to the therapist. Clients may confuse the open, intimate, and vulnerable nature of the relationship with the therapist as being romantic or as filling emotional needs that may be unmet in other relationships. They may instigate boundary crossings such as requesting to meet for coffee rather than in the office, making frequent contact between sessions, or openly flirting. Therapists have an ethical obligation to maintain appropriate boundaries and act with professional decorum, yet must not be emotionally distant or punitive if the relationship is to be preserved. When romantic disclosures from the client occur, the therapist may want to explore the reason for the transference and assist the client in determining how to get needs met appropriately.

What if the client is overtly sexual rather than simply flirtatious or romantic? If the therapist feels threatened by the client's sexual behavior in any way, then it is appropriate to make referrals so that the client can obtain care with a different provider. If the sexual behavior is harmless or simply unwelcome, then it may be possible to reflect with the client about the incident to understand the meaning of the behavior, what triggered it, and how they might discuss or manage such behaviors in the future.

STEP INTO MY OFFICE...

Kenneth came to my office weekly for depression after having had an embarrassing first try at sex with an older, more experienced woman. Kenneth was still a virgin and had never had a girlfriend. One day, after bitterly complaining about his desire to experience sex before he died, he looked at me with a grin and patted the sofa beside him. "Dr. Buehler, we could close the blinds and lock the door. We could go for it right here, right now!"

I chuckled. "Good try! But listen, if you can say that to me, then you can say it to someone who is closer to you in age and not your therapist!" Kenneth laughed, and then we continued to explore how he could develop his social and dating skills.

There are a variety of solutions when sexual feelings arise in therapy, but the responsibility is on the therapist to manage them, whether they emanate from the therapist or the client. If they emanate from the client, the therapist can help the client understand why they have sexualized a helping relationship and risked putting that potential help into jeopardy. The therapist can also explore what it means to have sexual feelings that cannot be acted on.

If sexual feelings originate with the therapist, then the therapist has several choices. They can silently reflect on their meaning; seek supervision or consultation with a trusted colleague; or enter personal therapy. At such times, the therapist may need to especially ensure good boundaries, such as not permitting appointments after hours when the office space might be more private, or not meeting anywhere outside the office. They may also need to consider whether their objectivity has been compromised and if a referral to another therapist is best for the client's well-being.

OBJECTIVITY AROUND ISSUES OF SEXUALITY

In order to do no harm to the client, therapists who treat sexual issues must be aware of their own biases and refrain from imposing their values on the client. Because sexuality develops in such variable ways, it is sometimes difficult to determine what cultural norms might prevail in any situation. In addition, stereotypes can dash a newly formed therapeutic alliance and must be guarded against. This section will explore three exemplary areas where objectivity is critical: (1) treatment of LGBTQ clients; (2) treatment of clients who engage in alternative sexual practices; and (3) the use of medical interventions in the treatment of sexual concerns.

Homophobia and Treatment of the LGBTQ Population

While attitudes toward the LGBTQ population have shifted over the past 20 years, there still exist cultural misunderstandings and dislike or even hatred of people who engage in homosexual sex. Ahmad and Bhugra (2010) especially note that while media portrayals, law and politics, and medicine have moved to better serve the rights of LGB people, new assumptions have replaced old—but they are still assumptions. In particular, they state that the general population may hold beliefs such as, "Homosexuals are all knowledgeable and open about sex," or "Homosexuals are hedonistic and are not weighed down by responsibilities."

Even well-meaning therapists who consider themselves allies of LGBTQ clients may have developed negative beliefs that are cloaked as beliefs that are positive. Generally, though, people (including therapists) who are politically conservative and belong to a more fundamental religious organization with an authoritarian leader are more likely to have negative attitudes toward lesbian and gay people and less likely to support human rights, while those who are politically liberal and who belong to more open-minded religious organizations tend to have more positive attitudes and to take a position of support for the LGBTQ population (Green, Murphy, & Blumer, 2010).

The case of *Bruff v. North Mississippi Health Services* (2001) demonstrates what can occur when one's conservative religious beliefs collide with laws regarding the rights of LGB people and the tenets of mental health training and services. In brief, Bruff worked as a psychotherapist in an employee assistant program (EAP) and treated a woman who identified as a lesbian. When the client stated that she wanted to work on relationship issues, Bruff told the client that because of her religious beliefs she would only work with the client on other issues. Through a series of lawsuits, the United States Court of Appeals for the Fifth Circuit found that Bruff's stance created a discriminatory environment and could harm a client seeking the help that was wanted or needed.

Using Bowen's theory to analyze dynamics in the *Bruff* case, Priest and Wickel (2011) make the observation that when values differ, therapists may become anxious, causing them to fuse with the group with which they most identify and to assume those values are correct. The result is that therapists may triangulate their values into therapy. Priest and Wickel conclude that therapists must be able to differentiate themselves from such groups and focus on listening to the value of the client without judgment; the therapist's role is not to teach his or her values, but to understand the client's experience. They also advocate that faculty and supervisors involved in training marriage and family therapists (MFTs) in particular engage in "Biblical tolerance" by familiarizing themselves on readings focused on acceptance; emphasizing acceptance and empathy for those who are different; emphasizing secular laws that protect gay rights; and familiarizing trainees with the LGBTQ population by giving them reading assignments on LGBTQ issues, addressing diversity, and working with diverse clientele in all coursework.

Therapists as well as trainees would also do well to heed what Israel, Gorcheva, Walther, Sulzner, and Cohen (2008) labeled as "helpful" and "unhelpful" attitudes and behaviors in the treatment of LGBTQ clients. Helpful interventions included development of gay-affirming attitudes; understanding homophobia, both within themselves and the client; not focusing on the client's orientation unless the client expresses concern; and being aware of community resources for additional support. Unhelpful interventions included seeing homosexuality as a disorder; attributing all the client's concerns to their orientation; lack of knowledge about the process of coming out; and expressing demeaning beliefs about homosexuality.

The Ethics of Treating Clients Practicing Alternative Sex

One factor that prevents therapists from engaging in treatment of sexual problems is fears about working with people who identify as kinky. Although there is not much research on the topic of the ethics of treating this population, there are a variety of professionals who write on the topic, for example, Kolmes, Sock, and Moser, 2006, in Kleinplatz and Moser, 2006., and others. Working with such clients can push therapists to recognize their own limitations and boundaries. If a therapist is to do no harm, then they must not treat someone from the kink community if they do not have appropriate training and supervision. In such cases, referrals may need to be made in a way that does not shame the client, such as transparently disclosing one's limitations, similarly to what one might do if faced with a client who has an eating disorder or other problem that the therapist does not normally treat. A therapist might state something such as the following: "I hope you don't find offense in this, but I don't think I am knowledgeable enough to give you the best help. May I refer you to someone who has better knowledge and training?"

Sufficient training to treat people who practice alt sex does not mean knowing someone who practices bondage, watching kinky porn in one's off hours, or having read *50 Shades of Grey*. It means reading professional literature, taking coursework, and finding an appropriate supervisor with whom to discuss such cases. Kolmes, Sock, and Moser describe "helpful" and "unhelpful" strategies for working with BDSM clients in particular.

Helpful behaviors include being open to reading and learning about BDSM; asking more experienced therapists questions about BDSM; working with the client to overcome internalized stigma of practicing kinky sex; and ensuring the client is practicing "safe, sane, and consensual" BDSM. It is also critical to focus on the behavior and not the objects or details, or as one colleague stated to me, "Poop or shoes, the therapy is the same." Unhelpful strategies include not understanding that BDSM practice requires consent; not maintaining one's own boundaries (e.g., disclosing one's own kinky practices to the client); abandoning clients who engage in such behavior; assuming (and rooting around for evidence of) past abuse; shaming or judging the client; and "expressing a prurient interest" in the client's sexual practices.

SEXUAL MEDICINE: BLESSING OR CURSE?

Before the dawn of Viagra, sexual problems were considered to be largely psychological in nature, treated with behavioral or psychodynamic therapy, or both. The creation of phosphodiesterase type 5 (PDE5) inhibitors generated a flood of direct-to-consumer ads and record sales of prescription medication. Next came the supposition that if older men could now easily have an erection by taking a pill, older women might benefit from medication to generate sexual desire in order to keep up. Thus began research for a low dose testosterone patch for women. This spurred Tiefer (2001) to create a proclamation called the "New View," in which low sexual desire is viewed as being simply a normal variation among people and the pharmaceutical industry is described as disease mongering.

Another concern regarding the medicalization of sexual problems is the currently accepted belief that being sexually active equates with good health (Segal, 2012). Segal especially discusses that cancer survivors are often portrayed as needing to embrace their sexuality even though they are perhaps at their least attractive and energetic. Likewise, Tiefer (2012) points out that a plethora of books by celebrities and self-proclaimed experts depathologize sex, but also make the case that in order for a person to be considered normal, he or she must engage in sexual activity. This creates high expectations leading to sexual discontent, perhaps provoking people to seek various therapies, both medical and nonmedical, which may be unnecessary. Conversely, in an editorial on the need for biological treatments for sexual problems, Kingsberg and Goldstein (2007) assert that "[n]eedless to say, it is wrong to make a woman feel diseased or defective just because she doesn't feel a certain way, but it is just as wrong to discount a woman's distress when she presents with hypoactive sexual desire and wants to be treated."

As the debate regarding the medicalization of sexual problems continues, the ethical, helpful position of the therapist is to listen to the client's complaint and his or her expressed goal, and to explore what has been tried to date. Confronting the client with one's own philosophy regarding disease-mongering or withholding knowledge regarding sexual medicine is likely unhelpful. If medications have proven to be disappointing, then the aim is not to tell the client to stop them, but to explore why the medications did not work and review alternatives to medications if available. Also helpful is to identify whether the client holds realistic expectations about sexuality given their age, circumstances, or health status, and to help the client come to terms with those goals that cannot be achieved. Finally, decisions about the appropriateness of medical treatment are best made in conjunction with a physician, and not by the therapist alone.

MANAGING SECRETS IN CONJOINT THERAPY

The final ethical issue for exploration is coming to terms with the divulgence of secrets in marital therapy. Since much of sex therapy is conducted with couples, therapists need to ensure that they are prepared to handle certain disclosures in order to prevent harm, that is, as when one partner is involved in another relationship without consent of the other. The legal and ethical need to maintain confidentiality sometimes collides with the need keep communication open in couples therapy (Butler, Rodriguez, Roper, & Feinauer, 2010; Kuo, 2009). Butler et al. (2010) make the case that when the therapist holds secrets for one partner, it shifts power and control to that partner, and prevents the betrayed partner from making an "empowered decision." Additionally, the therapist needs to consider the effect if he or she chooses to keep secret a disclosed affair, but the client later tells the partner that the therapist knew about the affair all along. On the other hand, learning about an affair has been known to create PTSD-like symptoms for the betrayed partner (Lusterman, 2005). Pittman (1989), in Butler et al. (2010) and Abrahms-Spring (1996, in Butler et al., 2010) maintain that disclosing an affair may lead to divorce, which is by many therapists considered to be an antithetical goal of couples therapy and which may cause more harm than good.

What is the ethical approach to maintaining confidentiality? Kuo (2009) observes that therapists differ in their approaches to holding secrets and identifies four basic models, including (1) no secrets held; (2) secrets held unless there is an explicit release of information; (3) secrets held with identified exceptions, for example, extramarital affairs, contagious diseases, and terminal illness; and (4) secrets held at the therapist's discretion. Each model has its drawbacks. For example, if the therapist will not hold any secrets, one or both clients may feel inhibited from sharing material that is essential to healing. If the therapist takes it upon him- or herself to determine which secrets to disclose, then the balance of power may shift to the therapist and make therapy less effective. Finally, if the therapist determines that a secret needs to be shared, who has the responsibility to share the information, and what might its effect be, depending on the party who is chosen to disclose?

Therapists sometimes choose to conduct what Butler et al. (2010) terms "facilitated disclosure," helping the client who disclosed the secret to the therapist to talk about it with their partner in the next conjoint session. Therapists may also choose to give the client who disclosed time to stop the behavior in question. Alternatively, the therapist can tell the individual who disclosed that if he or she doesn't share the information, the therapist will disclose and refer the couple out. Finally, the therapist may not share the information but make the referral nonetheless because they believe the therapy has been compromised and rendered ineffective.

STEP INTO MY OFFICE...

One of my initial sex therapy cases turned sour quickly because I had not developed a policy regarding disclosure of secrets. I met with a conservative Egyptian couple who had not consummated their marriage because he had erectile dysfunction (ED). I determined to split the second session to get more history and met with the male partner first. He immediately disclosed that he was gay but that I could not, under any circumstances, tell his wife.

I realized that I had created an ethical conundrum for myself and took a minute to reflect. Since I could no longer be objective, nor truthful to the wife, I told the client that unless he disclosed, I could not continue couples therapy. He declined. I called his wife back into the treatment office and stated, "I have some critical reasons that I will not be able to treat your case. I am going to give you three referrals to other therapists who may—or may not—be able to help." After that, I developed a "no secrets" policy that I modify under some circumstances, for example, if someone has a sexual behavior their partner knows about but doesn't want to hear details, or if a partner once engaged in sexual behavior that has no bearing on the present relationship.

ACTIVITIES

1. Reflect on times in your practice when you may have been sexually attracted to a client. Are you satisfied with how you handled the situation? What changes might you make to how you approach your countertransference? Have you identified a trusted colleague, supervisor, or therapist with whom you can process your feelings?
2. Reflect in the same way on times a client expressed or you sensed a client's attraction to you.

3. What kinds of biases do you hold regarding working with people who are LGBTQ, practice alt sex, or regarding sexual medicine? How might you work through these biases?
4. If you have not done so already, develop a policy regarding secrets in couples therapy.

RESOURCES

Kleinplatz, P. (Ed.). (2012). *New directions in sex therapy: Innovations and alternatives* (2nd ed.). New York, NY: Routledge.

Pope, K. S., Sonne, J. L., & Holroyd, J. (1993). *Sexual feelings in psychotherapy: Explorations for therapists and therapists-in-training.* Washington, DC: American Psychological Association.

Sex Therapy:
Now and in the Future

Sex therapy is often distinguished from other types of psychotherapy as being specialized strictly in the treatment of sexual issues. This is unfortunate, because sex therapy covers a much broader spectrum of human problems. Our sexuality can touch almost any aspect of life, with minor or profound effects. Our self-esteem, our relationships with others, our perception of life as being joyful or dismal, can all depend on our sexuality. Thus, it is erroneous to think of sex therapy as being limited. The therapist who does sex therapy needs to be a good diagnostician, excel at quickly developing rapport, and have adequate training in treating couples as well as individuals.

Therapists who include treatment of sexual problems must also be adept at several different theoretical approaches. When Masters and Johnson conceived of sex therapy, it was mainly a behavioral approach to treating distinct sexual problems. Later, Kaplan added a psychodynamic perspective. Weeks (1987) furthered treatment possibilities by combining sex therapy with family systems theory, encouraging therapists to examine underlying relationship dynamics to expose contributing factors. Most recently, with the advent of medications such as phosphodiesterase type 5 (PDE5) inhibitors, sex therapists must understand the biology of sexual dysfunction in order to stay abreast of pharmaceutical and other therapeutic treatments. In short, sex therapy is a broad, evolving field, changing not only in theoretical outlook, but also with the evolution of society and its mores.

As it currently stands, for most clinicians the path to becoming a sex therapist is long and complicated; each therapist comes into the field by following a unique path. Though a handful of schools have degree programs specialized in sexuality that lead to a master's or doctorate degree and licensure (e.g., Widener University), nearly all those who want to be a sex therapist will need to avail themselves of a more general degree. The choice of whether that degree is in marriage and family therapy, professional counseling, social work, or psychology is an individual one, as is whether one wants to practice at the master's level or go the distance of getting a doctorate.

My own path may inform some readers. I earned a Master of Arts in psychology, then applied to earn a doctorate in psychology (PsyD) with an emphasis on family therapy. Within that emphasis, I chose to concentrate on medical family therapy. At that time, I had no thought of specializing in sex therapy, but I ensured that I trained and was employed in settings where I would work not only with children, but with adult couples. I am glad that I did; although I was certain I wanted to work with children, once I was in private practice I changed my mind for the simple fact that I wanted to save all of my "kid energy" for home, with my own child.

My specialization in medical family therapy lead me to work with an endocrinologist, and together we formed a wellness center that included a physical therapist, dietitian, and acupuncturist. Endocrinologists are physicians who specialize in diseases and conditions affected by hormones, which naturally include those concerning sexual health. It was the endocrinologist who suggested that I learn about sex therapy, because while people frequently came to her complaining of low libido, it was rarely because of hormone imbalance.

This piqued my interest! Sex therapy perfectly combined my interest in medical conditions and family systems. But I was at a loss as to how to acquire the education and training I needed to practice ethically. Through an Internet search, I found the American Association of Sexuality Educators, Counselors and Therapists and attended my first conference in Portland, Oregon. I felt electrified by the atmosphere, the camaraderie, and the workshops, and a sense that I had found my "tribe." At some point I determined that I wanted to acquire certification and found a mentor, supervisor, and friend in Stephen Braveman, a marriage and family therapist in private practice, to help me. I have been on the path of sex therapy practice for almost a decade and have never had a moment of regret. Sexuality is infinitely interesting, and there is much work to be done.

PROBLEMS IN THE FIELD

Conducting sex therapy, however, also carries stigma. As discussed in Part I, whenever sex is the topic of conversation, red flags may be raised.

There are other less obvious reasons for concern, however. Sex therapists have been asked to or may seek to be in the limelight. Often they are sincere in their wish to educate the public, but even when well intended, their media appearances may seem self-serving or gratuitous, making the profession appear lightweight or frivolous. Sex therapists also put a great deal of emphasis on the importance of sex, rather than correctly locating it as but one aspect of overall mental health and well-being. Through their own doing, or through the manipulation of the media, talking about sex becomes just another form of entertainment, part of the noise in the background rather than focusing on the message that "good enough sex" (Metz & McCarthy, 2010) is just that—good enough.

Another problem facing the practice of sex therapy is the dilution of the field by nonlicensed professionals, particularly sex educators. Sex educators originally were individuals who created learning materials and lectures for organizations with a need to inform their students, clients, or patients, such as universities, public school districts, and family planning centers. Currently, there are sex educators who have turned their skills into an industry known as "sex coaching" and parlay their knowledge to a public that doesn't know the difference between a psychiatrist and a psychologist, let alone a therapist and a coach. Often, sex coaching comes down to a list of suggestions to increase sexual confidence and expand sexual repertoire—a sort of living *Cosmopolitan* magazine. Putting aside the lack of protection for the consumer who seeks treatment from an unlicensed educator or coach, the issue may be that sex becomes sexualized. That is, rather than treating sexual problems from the core or root of the client's being with psychotherapy, the client or consumer is taught how to be sexy, which may or may not be an appropriate goal. As you can see from having read this book, sexual problems may run deep; telling a woman how to masturbate with the latest gizmo is quite different from addressing sexual abuse and shame that may prevent a woman from looking at her own body, let alone touching it.

As Binik and Meana (2009) point out, certification of sex therapists by organizations such as the American Association of Educators, Counselors, and Therapists may not be the answer to ensuring professional competence to the consumer. American Association for Sexuality Educators, Counselors, and Therapists (AASECT), though well-meaning, through its certification of educators and counselors (who are not licensed professional counselors, but individuals licensed in an allied field such as nutrition or physical therapy) has elevated the competence status of non-psychotherapists and diluted the credibility of psychotherapists. It should be up to licensing boards to determine who is and who is not competent to practice sex therapy. However, as things currently stand it is only the state of Florida that requires psychotherapists to obtain a requisite amount of training before they can call themselves a sex therapist.

Thus, it is my belief that every therapist needs to be able to treat sexual problems. Sexuality should not be viewed as a frill, but as a legitimate aspect of mental, emotional, physical, and relationship health. Nor should sexuality be marginalized as a side issue to be dealt with at the end of therapy, as if a dollop of healing is all that is needed for remedy. Therapists need to proudly embrace their ability, among all other professionals, to help people repair the places where they may be the most deeply and privately broken. Therapists alone have the skills, the time, and hopefully, the compassion to treat sexual problems.

THE PRACTICE OF SEX THERAPY

One decision to make is whether doing sex therapy will be a major or minor part of your practice. It is truly up to you to decide how far you want to treat people's sexual concerns when they arise. The point of asking about sexual concerns is to identify any confounds that may inhibit the treatment of the presenting or identified problem. If clients endorse such concerns, then you can follow the Permission, Limited Information, Specific Suggestions, and Intensive Therapy (PLISSIT) model to provide information and suggestions; in the case of complex cases, refer out for intensive therapy.

If you wish to stay within the information and suggestions part of the PLISSIT framework, then you will need to have lists of resources for your clients. Such resources may include handouts from this book and others, as well as from the Internet; titles of self-help books; names of physicians who treat sexual problems of various types; and community resources, for example, a contact at the nearest LGBTQ center.

You will also want to acquaint yourself with nearby clinicians who identify as sex therapists. You may find that some only work with couples, some only with women, and some only with the LGBTQ population. Be sure to let them know your specialty, whether it is treating substance abuse, eating disorders, chronic illness, etc. so that you can cross-refer.

If you are intrigued enough to make sex therapy a bigger part of your practice, venturing into doing intensive therapy, then I am going to transparently state that reading this book is not enough to put out your shingle. Unless you are one of the very, very few individuals who are completely comfortable with the topic of sex, you are going to need support.

"Support" does not refer only to a consultant or supervisor. It also refers to emotional and collegial support. Many therapists who practice sex therapy report feeling marginalized, misunderstood, or isolated. Discomfort with sex is so great that sex therapy is stigmatized, especially in smaller, more conservative communities. That is why belonging to an organization that serves sex therapists can be a critical part of one's development. A list of such organizations appears at the end of this chapter.

Will you keep the fact that you do sex therapy something you share only with colleagues in order to get referrals, or will you market yourself to the public as such? Marketing to professionals has the advantage that stigmatization may be minimized and your colleagues in essence are prescreening some of your clients as being appropriate for sex therapy. A disadvantage is that your community may benefit from marketing your services. There are several states, such as Montana and Wyoming, where there are no AASECT-certified sex therapists. People who truly need services may not get the therapy they need or may travel long distances for help.

MARKETING YOURSELF AS A SEX THERAPIST

If you decide to take the steps to be able to conduct intensive therapy, and if you wish to market your services to the community, then you will need to market yourself. Some therapists are nearly as afraid of marketing as they are of sex! They may see marketing as cheapening their profession or as being counterproductive to one's aim of helping people. Marketing is not a bad word! Marketing allows people to identify you as someone who can give them the help they need.

Aside from the common ways therapists currently market, for example, with a website and through directory listings, there are a few other means to get the word out that you do sex therapy. One of the most critical is making referral connections with physicians. Not only do they need you, but also you need them so that you can appropriately refer your clients for medical evaluation. Were I to begin this type of marketing, I would follow these steps:

1. Identify various types of physicians who provide services your clients need, especially urologists and gynecologists.
2. Send out three to five letters at a time to physicians introducing yourself and your practice.
3. Follow up your letter with a phone call and, potentially, a visit. Ask to speak to the practice manager, who may either meet with you or facilitate a meeting with the physician.
4. When and if you do meet with the physician or someone else in the office, ask how you can help them with their clients who have sexual complaints.
5. After the meeting, follow up with a thank-you letter. Be sure to ask for some of the physician's cards, too.

It really isn't that difficult. Remember, you are not asking for referrals— you are offering a service to a busy physician.

A second way is through appearances in the media. It isn't as hard as you might imagine. Start by making a list of local or cable television and radio programs that invite live guests. Make a list also of journalists at the local paper who write about science and health. You can include college media as well. Let them know who you are and some topics you are able to cover. You may not hear anything right away, but it is perfectly acceptable to follow up when you have a quote on a relevant story. For example, it was recently the 10th anniversary of Viagra; local media might have been interested in interviewing you on how this medication has changed the public's view of sexuality.

CONTINUING EDUCATION

Sexuality is a fluid topic. New ideas and information are constantly being discovered. How we understand sexual development, behavior, and function both expands and deepens. Any mental health professional who works with sexual concerns needs to stay current in the field. There are multiple conferences and journals to serve that purpose. They are listed in the *Resources* section as well. Ongoing consultation is also an important part of being able to competently treat clients' sexual concerns. Because sexual problems develop in private, they can be particularly difficult to understand or off-putting. Consultation can help the therapist maintain an appropriately nonjudgmental and compassionate stance.

IN CLOSING

For the past 10 or so years, I have devoted my career to treating people with sexual concerns. I have never been bored. Sex can be sad, funny, perplexing, disturbing, endearing, loving, and enraging. Sex can bond two people like nothing else. It can be a form of entertainment and stress relief. Sex can become a journey of self-knowledge, an understanding of one's body and capacity for pleasure that can be achieved in no other way. It can be self-affirming, life-affirming, and life-giving. Sex is a beautiful thing.

By reading this book, I hope I have inspired you to become a therapist who "does sex." I hope that in 10 years' time, people will no longer be referred to me because their therapist refused to help them with a sexual problem. It has been my pleasure to fulfill part of my mission to help every therapist be comfortable with sexual concerns by writing this book. May you embark on a journey to your own sexual wellness, as well as the sexual wellness of your clients.

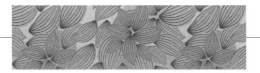

Bibliography

Abbey, R. D., Clopton, J. R., & Humphreys, J. D. (2007). Obsessive-compulsive disorder and romantic functioning. *Journal of Clinical Psychology, 63*, 118–192.

Abdul, Z. R., Thakar, R., & Sultan, A. H. (2009). Postpartum female sexual function. *European Journal of Obstetrics, Gynecology, & Reproductive Biology, 145*, 133–137.

Abrahms-Spring, J. (1996). *After the affair.* New York, NY: Harper Collins.

Acele, E. Ö., & Karaçam, Z. (2012, June). Sexual problems in women during the first postpartum year and related conditions. *Journal of Clinical Nursing, 41*(3), 929–937.

Ackard, D. M., Kearney-Cooke, A., & Peterson, C. B. (2000). Effect of body image and self-image on women's sexual behaviors. *International Journal of Eating Disorders, 28*, 422–429.

Ahmad, S., & Bhugra, D. (2010). Homophobia: An updated review of the literature. *Sexual and Relationship Therapy, 25*(4), 447–455.

Ahrold, T. K., Farmer, M., Trapnell, P. D., & Meston, C. M. (2011). The relationship among sexual attitudes, sexual fantasy, and religiosity. *Archives of Sexual Behavior, 40*, 619–630.

Aksaray, G., Berkant, Y., Kaptanoglue, C., Oflu, S., & Ozaltin, M. (2001). Sexuality in women with obsessive-compulsive disorder. *Journal of Sex & Marital Therapy, 72*, 273–277.

Albersen, M., Orabi, H., & Lue, T. F. (2012). Evaluation and treatment of erectile dysfunction in the aging male: A mini-review. *Gerontology, 58*(1), 3–14.

Alder, E. M. (1989). Sexual behavior in pregnancy, after childbirth, and during breastfeeding. *Clinical Obstetrics and Gynaecology, 3*(4), 805–821.

Al-Juraifani, R. (2012, October). Physical therapist as sex therapist: Challenges and opportunities. *IOPTWH Newsletter*, 5–6.

Althof, S. E. (2006, March). Prevalence, characteristics and implications of premature ejaculation/rapid ejaculation. *The Journal of Urology, 175*, 842–848.

Althof, S. E., Abdo, C. H., Dean, J., Hackett, G., McCabe, M., McMahon, C. G., … Tan, H. M. (2010). International Society for Sexual Medicine's guidelines for the diagnosis and treatment of early ejaculation. *Journal of Sexual Medicine, 7*(9), 2947–2969.

American Association of Sexuality Educators, Counselors, and Therapists. (2008). *Code of ethics, revised.* Washington, DC: Author.

American Mental Health Counselors Association. (2010). *Code of ethics, revised.*

American Psychiatric Association. (2013). *Diagnostic and statistical manual of mental disorders* (5th ed.). Washington, DC: Author.

American Psychiatric Association. (2000). *Diagnostic and statistical manual of mental disorders* (4th ed., text rev.). Washington, DC: Author.

American Psychological Association. (2002). *Ethical principles of psychologists and code of conduct.* Washington, DC: Author.

Anand, M. (1990). *The art of sexual ecstasy: The path of sacred sexuality for western lovers.* Santa Barbara, CA: Jeremy P. Tarcher.

Anderson, R. U., Wise, D., Sawyer, T., & Chan, C. A. (2006). Sexual dysfunction in men with chronic prostatitis/chronic pelvic pain syndrome: Improvement after trigger point release and paradoxical relaxation training. *The Journal of Urology, 176*, 1534–1539.

Angel, K. (2010). The history of 'Female Sexual Dysfunction' as a mental disorder in the 20th century. *Current Opinions in Psychiatry, 23*(6), 536–541.

Annon, J. S. (1976). The PLISSIT model: A proposed conceptual scheme for the behavioral treatment of sexual problems. *Journal of Sex Education and Therapy, 2*(1), 1–15.

Atjamasoados, L. (2003). Alcoholism, marital problems, and sexual dysfunction. *Annals of General Hospital Psychiatry, 2*(Suppl. 1), S40.

Attwood, T. (2007). *Asperger disorder: A complete guide.* Jessica Kingsley.

Baldwin, D. (2001). Depression and sexual dysfunction. *British Medical Bulletin, 57*, 88–99.

Baldwin, D., & Mayers, A. (2003). Sexual side-effects of antidepressant and antipsychotic drugs. *Advances in Psychiatric treatment, 9*, 202–210.

Balon, R., Segraves, R. T., & Clayton, A. (2007). Issues for DSM-V: Sexual dysfunction, disorder, or variation along normal distribution: Toward rethinking DSM criteria of sexual dysfunctions. *American Journal of Psychiatry, 164*(2), 198–200.

Bancroft, J., & Graham, C. A. (2011). The varied nature of women's sexuality: Unresolved issues and a theoretical approach. *Hormones and Behavior Journal, 59*(5), 717–729.

Bancroft, J., Loftus, J., & Long, J. S. (2003). Distress about sex: A national survey of women in heterosexual relationships. *Archives of Sexual Behavior, 32*(3), 193–208.

Bancroft, J., & Vukadinovic, Z. (2004). Sexual addiction, sexual compulsivity, sexual impulsivity or what? Toward a theoretical model. *The Journal of Sex Research, 41*(3), 225–234.

Bang-Ping, J. (2009). Sexual dysfunction in men who abuse illicit drugs: A preliminary report. *Journal of Sexual Medicine, 6*, 1072–1078.

Bargiota, A., Dimitropoulos, K., Tzortzis, V., & Kourkoulis, G. N. (2011). Sexual dysfuncion in diabetic women. *Hormones, 10*(3), 196–206.

Barker, M. (2005). This is my partner: Constructing a polyamorous identity in a monogamous world. *Journal of Constructivist Psychology, 18*, 75–88.

Barker, M., & Langridge, D. (2010). Whatever happened to non-monogamies? Critical reflections on recent research and theory. *Sexualities, 13*(6), 748–772.

Bartoi, M. G., & Kinder, B. N. (1998). Effects of child and adult sexual abuse on adult sexuality. *Journal of Sex and Marital Therapy, 24,* 75–90.

Basson, R. (2005, May 10). Women's sexual dysfunction: Revised and expanded definitions. *Canadian Medical Association Journal, 172*(1), 1327–1333.

Bell, R. (1999). ABC of sexual health: Homosexual men and women. *British Medical Journal, 318*(7181), 452–455.

Bella, A. J., Perelman, M., Brant, W. O., & Lue, T. F. (2007). Peyronie's disease. *Journal of Sexual Medicine, 4,* 1527–1538.

Betchen, S. J. (2003). Suggestions for improving intimacy in couples in which one partner has attention-deficit/hyperactivity disorder. *Journal of Sex & Marital Therapy, 29,* 103–124.

Betschneider, J. G., & McCoy, N. L. (1988). Sexual interest and behavior in healthy 80- to 102-year-olds. *Archives of Sexual Behavior, 17*(2), 109–129.

Bhasin, S. (2007) Approach to the infertile man. *Journal of Clinical Endocrinology and Metabolism, 92*(6), 1995–2004.

Berman, J. R., Berman, L. A., Tolder, S. M. Gill, J., & Haughie, S. (2003). Safety and efficacy of sildenafil citrate for the treatment of female sexual arousal disorder: A double-blind, placebo controlled study. *Journal of Urology, 170*(6 Pt 1), 2333–2338.

Bhugra, D., & Wright, B. (2007). Sexual dysfunction in gay men and lesbians. *Psychiatry, 6*(3), 125–129.

Billups, K. L. (2002). The role of mechanical devices in treating female sexual dysfunction and enhancing the female sexual response. *World Journal of Urology, 20,* 137–141.

Binik, Y. M., & Meana, M. (2009). The future of sex therapy: Specialization or marginalization? *Archives of Sexual Behavior, 38,* 1016–1027.

Bitzer, J., Platano, G., Tschudin, S., & Alder, J. (2008). Sexual counseling in elderly couples. *Journal of Sexual Medicine, 5*(9), 2027–2043.

Blazquez, A., Alegre, J., & Ruiz, E. (2009). Women with chronic fatigue syndrome and sexual dysfunction: Past, present, and future. *Journal of Sex & Marital Therapy, 35*(5), 347–359.

Bockting, W., Benner, A., & Coleman, E. (2009). Gay and bisexual identity development among female to male transsexuals in North America: Emergences of a trangender sexuality. *Archives of Sexual Behaviors, 38*(5), 688–701.

Bogren, L. Y. (1991). Changes in sexuality in women and men during pregnancy. *Archives of Sexual Behavior, 20*(1), 35–45.

Borg, C., Peters, M. L., Schultz, W. W., & de Jong, P. J. (2012). Vaginismus: Heightened harm avoidance and pain catastrophizing cognitions. *Journal of Sexual Medicine, 9*(2), 558–567.

Bouchard, S., Sabourin, S., Lussier, Y., & Villeneuve, E. (2009). Relationship quality and stability in couples where one partner suffers from borderline personality disorder. *Journal of Marital and Family Therapy, 35,* 446–455.

Bowen, M. (1974). Toward the differentiation of self in one's family of origin. In F. Andres & J. Lorio (Eds.), *Georgetown Family Symposium* (Vol.1).

Bradford, A., & Meston, C. M. (2006). The impact of anxiety of sexual arousal in women. *Behavior Research and Therapy, 44*(8), 1067–1077.

Bronfenbrenner, U. (1977). Toward an experimental ecology of human development. *American Psychologist, 32*, 513–531.

Bronner, G., Royter, V., Korczyn, A. D., & Giladi, N. (2004). Sexual dysfunction in Parkinson's disease. *Journal of Sex and Marital Therapy, 30*(2), 95–105.

Bronner, G., & Vodusek, D. B. (2011). Management of sexual dysfunction in Parkinson's disease. *Therapeutic Advances in Neurological Disorders, 4*(6), 375–383.

Brotto, L. (2011, August). Non-judgmental, present-moment, sex … as if your life depended on it. *Sexual and Relationship Therapy, 26*(3), 215–216.

Brotto, L. A. (2010). The DSM diagnostic criteria for sexual aversion disorder. *Archives of Sexual Behavior, 39*(2), 271–277.

Brotto, L. A., Basson, M., & Luria, M. (2008). A mindfulness-based group psychoeducation intervention targeting Sexual Arousal Disorder in women. *Journal of Sexual Medicine, 5*, 1646–1659.

Brown, J. D., Keller, S., & Stern, S. (2009). Sex, sexuality, sexting, and sexed: Adolescents and the media. *The Prevention Researcher, 16*(4), 12–16.

Browning, C. R., & Laumann, E. O. (1997). Sexual contact between children and adults: A life course perspective. *American Sociology Review, 62*, 540–560.

Buckwalter, K. C. (1982). The influence of skin disorders on sexual expression. *Sexuality and Disability, 5*(2), 98–107.

Bruff v. North Mississippi Health Services, 244 F.3d 495 (5th Cir. 2001).

Buehler, S. (1999). *Ecosystemic systemic assessment of families of children with cancer returning to school*. Doctoral dissertation, California School of Professional Psychology, San Diego, CA.

Buehler, S. (2008). Childhood sexual abuse: Effects on female sexual function and its treatment. *Current Reports in Sexual Health, 5*, 154–158.

Buehler, S. (2011). *Sex, love, and mental illness: A couples' guide to staying connected*. Santa Barbara, CA: Praeger/ABC-Clio.

Burgess, E. O. (2004). Sexuality in midlife and later life couples. In J. Harvey, A. Wenzel, & S. Sprecher (Eds.), *The handbook of sexuality in close relationships* (pp. 437–454). Mahwah, NJ: Lawrence Erlbaum Associates, Inc.

Burr, W. (2011). Sexuality of the disabled often overlooked. *Canadian Medical Association Journal, 183*(5), E259–E260.

Butler, M. H., Rodriguez, M. A., Roper, S. O., & Feinauer, L. L. (2010). Infidelity secrets in couple therapy: Therapists' views on the collision of competing ethics around relationship-relevant secrets. *Sexual Addiction & Compulsivity, 17*, 82–105.

Cairns, K. V. (1997). Counseling the partners of heterosexual male cross-dressers. *Canadian Journal of Human Sexuality, 6*(4), 297–306.

Calabros, R. S., Gali, A., Marino, S., & Brmanti, P. (2012). Compulsive masturbation and chronic penile lymphedema. *Archive of Sexual Behavior, 41*(3), 737–739.

Calzo, J. P., Antonucci, T. C., Mays, V. M., & Cochran, S. D. (2011). Retrospective recall of sexual orientation identity among gay, lesbian, and bisexual adults. *Developmental Psychology, 47*(6), 1658–1673.

Canada, A. L., Neese, L. E., Sui, D., & Schover, L. R. (2005, December 15). Pilot intervention to enhance sexual rehabilitation for couples after treatment for localized prostate carcinoma. *Cancer, 104*(12), 2689–2700.

Cantor, C. (2012). "Do Pedophiles Deserve Sympathy?" CNN. Retrieved from http://www.cnn.com/2012/06/21/opinion/cantor-pedophila-sandusky

Caplan, A. L. (2012, September 5). Clinicians should promote sex among nursing home residents. Retrieved from Medscape at http://www.medscape.com/viewarticle/769523_print

Carnes, P. (2001). *Out of the shadows: Understanding sexual addiction.* Center City, MN: Hazelden.

Carpentier, M. Y., & Fortenberry, J. D. (2010). Romantic and sexual relationships, body image, and fertility in adolescent and young adult testicular cancer survivors: a review of the literature. *Journal of Adolescent Health, 47*(2), 115–125.

Carvalho, J., & Nobre, P. (2011). Biopsychosocial determinants of men's sexual desire: Testing an integrative model. *Journal of Sexual Medicine, 8*(3) 754–763.

Cass, V. C. (1979). Homosexual identity formation: A theoretical model. *Journal of Homosexuality, 4*(3), 219–235.

Centers for Disease Control and Prevention. (2011). STD Trends in the United States: 2010 national data for gonorrhea, chlamydia, and syphilis. Retrieved October 26, 2012 from http://www.cdc.gov/std/stats10/trends.htm

Chartier, M. J., Walker, J. R., Naimark, B. (2007). Childhood abusive, adult health, and health care utilization: Results from a representative community sample. *American Journal of Epidemiology, 165*, 1031–1038.

Cherng-Jye, J. (2004). The pathophysiology and etiology of vaginismus. *Taiwanese Journal of Obstetrics and Gynecology, 43*(1), 10–15.

Chivers, M. L., Pittini, R., Grigoriadis, S., Villegas, L., & Ross, L. E. (2011). The relationship between sexual functioning and depressive symptomatology in postpartum women: A pilot study. *Journal of Sexual Medicine, 8*(3), 792–799.

Clayton, A., Keller, A., & McGarvey, E. L. (2006). Burden of phase-specific sexual dysfunction with SSRIs. *Journal of Affective Disorders, 91*(1), 27–32.

Cobia, D. C., & Harper, A. J. (2005). Perimenopause and sexual functioning: Implications for therapists. *The Family Journal: Counseling and Therapy for Couples and Families, 13*(2), 226–231.

Cohn, R. (2011). *Coming home to passion: Restoring loving sexuality in couples with histories of childhood trauma and neglect.* Santa Barbara, CA: Praeger.

Coleman, H., & Charles, G. (2001). Adolescent sexuality: A matter of condom sense. *Journal of Child and Youth Care, 14*(4), 17–18.

Comfort, A. (1972) *The joy of sex.* New York, NY: Simon & Schuster.

Connan, S. (2010). A kink in the process. *Therapy Today, 21*(6), 10–15.

Conner, M., Charlotte, J., & Grogan, S. (2004). Gender, sexuality, body image, and eating behaviors. *Journal of Health Psychology, 9*, 505–515.

Conroy, M. (2010). Treating transgendered children: Clinical methods and religious mythology. *Zygon, 45*(2), 301–316.

Cooper, A., Galbreath, N., & Becker, M. A. (2004). Sex on the internet: Furthering our understanding of men with online sexual problems. *Psychology of Addictive Behaviors, 18*(3), 223–230.

Courtois, C. A., & Ford, J. (Eds.). (2009). *Treating complex traumatic stress disorders [Adults]: An evidence-based guide.* New York, NY: Guilford Press.

Crenshaw, T. L., Goldberg, J. P., & Stern, W. C. (1987). Pharmacologic modification of psychosexual dysfunction. *Journal of Sex & Marital Therapy, 13*(4), 239–252.

Crowe, M. (2006). Managing couple relationship and individual psychological problems in psychosexual therapy. *Psychiatry, 6*(3), 95–98.

Culbert, K. M., & Klump, K. L. (2005). Impulsivity as an underlying factor in the relationship between disordered eating and sexual behavior. *International Journal of Eating Disorders, 38,* 361–366.

Damon, W., & Simon Rosser, B. W. (2005). Anodyspareunia in men who have sex with men: Prevalence, predictors, consequences and the development of DSM diagnostic criteria. *Journal of Sex and Marital Therapy, 31,* 129–141.

Dandona, P., & Rosenberg, M. T. (2010, May). A practical guide to male hypogonadism in the primary care setting. *International Journal of Clinical Practice, 64*(6), 682–696.

Dankoski, M. E., & Pais, S. (2007). What's love got to do with it? Couples, illness, and MFT. *Journal of Couples and Relationship Therapy, 6*(1), 31–43.

Davis, S. N. P., Binik, Y. M., & Carrier, S. (2009). Sexual dysfunction and pelvic pain in men: A male sexual pain disorder? *Journal of Sex & Marital Therapy, 35,* 182–205.

Davis, S. R., & Jane, F. (2011). Sex and perimenopause. *Australian Family Physician, 40*(5), 274–278.

Dean, J., Rubio-Aurioles, E., McCabe, M., Eardley, I., Speakman, M., Buvat, J., … Fisher, W. (2008). Integrating partners into erectile dysfunction treatment: Improving the sexual experience for the couple. *International Journal of Clinical Practice, 62*(1), 127–133.

Dean, L., Meyer, I. H., Robinson, K., Sell, R. L., Sember, R., Silenzio, V. M. B., … Xavier, J. (2000). Lesbian, gay, bisexual, and transgender health: Findings and concerns. *Journal of the Gay and Lesbian Medical Association, 4*(3), 102–151.

DeLamater, J. (2012). Sexual expression in later life: A review and synthesis. *Journal of Sex Research, 49*(2–3), 125–141.

DeLamater, J., & Friedrich, W. N. (2002). Human sexual development. *Journal of Sex Research, 39*(1), 10–14.

DeLamater, J., Hyde, J. S., & Fong, M. C. (2008). Sexual satisfaction in the seventh decade of life. *Journal of Sex and Marital Therapy, 34*(5), 439–454.

DeLamater, J., & Karraker, A. (2009) Sexual functioning in older adults. *Current Psychiatry Reports, 11*(1), 6–11.

DeRogatis, L., Rosen, R. C., Goldstein, I., Werneburg, B., Kempthorne-Rawson, J., & Sand, M. (2012). Chracterization of hypoactive sexual desire disorder (HSDD) in men. *Journal of Sexual Medicine, 9*(3), 812–820.

De Villers, L., & Turgeon, H. (2005). The uses and benefits of "sensate focus" exercises. *Contemporary Sexuality,* i–iv.

Diamond, L. (2009). *Sexual fluidity: Understanding women's love and desire.* Boston, MA: Harvard University Press.

Donaldson, R. L., & Meana, M. (2011). Early dyspareunia experience in young women: Confusion, consequences, and help-seeking barriers. *Journal of Sexual Medicine, 8,* 814–823.

Dzelme, K., & Jones, R. A. (2001). Male cross-dressers in therapy: A solution focused perspective for marriage and family therapists. *The American Journal of Family Therapy, 29,* 293–305.

Easton, S. D., Coohey, C., O'leary, P., Zhang, Y., & Hua, L. (2011). The effect of childhood sexual abuse on psychosexual functioning during adulthood. *Journal of Family Violence, 26,* 41–50.

Edwards, W. M., & Coleman, E. (2004). Defining sexual health: A descriptive overview. *Archives of Sexual Behavior, 33*(3), 189–195.

Eisenberg, M. E., Ackard, D. M., Resnick, M. S., & Neumark-Sztainer, D. (2009). Casual sex and psychological health among adults: Is having "friends with benefits" emotionally damaging? *Perspectives on Sexual and Reproductive Health, 41*(4), 231–237.

Elliott, A., & O'Donohue, T. (1997). The effects of anxiety and distraction on sexual arousal in a nonclinical sample of heterosexual women. *Archives of Sexual Behavior, 26*, 607–625.

Ellis, E. M. (2012). What are the confidentiality rights of collaterals in family therapy? *The American Journal of Family Therapy, 40*, 369–384.

Emlet, C. A. (2006). "You're awfully old to have this disease": Experiences of stigma and ageism in adults 50 years and older living with HIV/AIDS. *Gerontologist, 46*(6), 781–790.

Estellon, V., & Mouras, H. (2012). Sexual addiction: insights from psychoanalysis and functional neuroimaging. *Socioaffective Neuroscience & Psychology, 2*, 118–114.

Facelle, T. M., Sadeghi-Nejad, H., & Goldmeier, D. (2013). Persistent genital arousal disorder: Characterization, etiology, and management. *Journal of Sexual Medicine, 10*, 439–450.

Fahrner, E. (1987). Sexual dysfunction in male alcohol addicts: Prevalence and treatment. *Archives of Sexual Behavior, 16*, 247–257.

Farley, M., & Keaney, J. C. (1997). Physical symptoms, somatization, and dissociation in women survivors of childhood sexual assault. *Women's Health, 25*(3), 33–45.

Farrell, J., & Cacchioni, T. (2012). The medicalization of women's sexual pain. *Journal of Sex Research, 49*(4), 328–336.

Feldman, H. A., Goldstein, I., Harzichristou, D. G., Krane, R. J., & McKinlay, J. B. (1994). Impotence and its medical and psychosocial correlates: Results of the Massachusetts male aging study. *Journal of Urology, 151*(1), 54–61.

Figueira, I., Possidente, E., Marques, C., & Hayes, K. (2001) Sexual dysfunction: A neglected complication of panic disorder and social phobia. *Archives of Sexual Behavior, 30*(4), 369–377.

Finger, B. (2006). Sexuality and chronic illness. Personal collection, lecture handout, American Association of Physician's Assistants.

Finkelhor, D., & Browne, A. (1985). The traumatic impact of child sexual abuse: A conceptualization. *American Journal of Orthopsychiatry, 66*, 530–541.

First, M., & Zucker, Z. (2013, June) DSM-5: Implications for the field of sexuality. Plenary Lecture, American Association of Sexuality Educators, Counselors, and Therapists, Miami, FL.

Fisher, H. E. (2004a). *Why we love: The nature and chemistry of romantic love.* New York, NY: Henry Holt.

Fisher, S. (2004b). Ethical issues in therapy: Therapist self-disclosure of sexual feelings. *Ethics & Behavior, 14*(2), 105–121.

Foley, S., Kope, S. A., & Sugrue, D. P. (2011). *Sex matters for women: A complete guide for taking care of your sexual self.* New York, NY: Guilford Press.

Foley, S., Wittmann, D., & Balon, R. (2010). A multidisciplinary approach to sexual dysfunction in medical education. *Academic Psychiatry, 34*(5), 386–389.

Fontanelle, L. F., Wanderson, F., de Menezes, G. B., & Menlowicz, M. V. (2007). Sexual function and dysfunction in Brazilian patients with Obsessive-Compulsive Disorder and Social Anxiety Disorder. *Journal of Social and Personal Relationships, 23*, 367–386.

Fooladi, E., & Davis, S. R. (2012). An update on the pharmacological management of female sexual dysfunction. *Expert Opinions in Pharmacotherapy, 13*(15), 2131–2142.

Ford, M. P., & Hendrick, S. S. (2003). Therapists' sexual values for self and clients: Implications for practice and training. *Professional Psychology, Research and Practice, 34*(1), 80–87.

Ford, J. J., Jared, A., & Franklin, D. L. (2012). Structural therapy with a couple battling pornography addiction. *The American Journal of Family Therapy, 40,* 336–348.

Fourcroy, J. L. (2006). Customs, culture, and tradition—What role do they play in a woman's sexuality? *Journal of Sexual Medicine, 3*(6), 954–959.

Francoeur, R. T., & Noonan, R. J. (Eds.). (2004). *The continuum complete Encyclopedia of sexuality.* New York, NY. Retrieved from http://www.kinseyinstitute.org/ccies/

Freeman, N. K. (2007, April). Preschoolers' perceptions of gender appropriate toys and their parents' beliefs about genderized behaviors: Miscommunication, mixed messages, or hidden truths? *Early Childhood Education Journal, 34*(5).

Friedman, M. J., Jalowiec., J., McHugo, G., Wang, S., & McDonagh, A. (2007, August). Adult sexual abuse is associated with elevated neurohormone levels among women with PTSD due to childhood sexual abuse. *Journal of Traumatic Stress, 20*(4), 611–617.

Furukawa, A., Patton, P., Amato, P., Li, H., & Leclair, C. (2012). Dyspareunia and sexual dysfunction in women seeking fertility treatment. *Fertility and Sterility, 98*(6), 1544–1548.

Fyfe, B. (1980). Counseling and human sexuality: A training model. *The Personnel and Guidance Journal, 59*(3), 147–150.

Galbraith, M. E., Fink, R., & Wilkins, G. G. (2011). Couples surviving prostate cancer: Challenges in their lives and relationships. *Seminars in Oncology Nursing, 27*(4), 300–308.

Galst, J. P. (1986). Stress and stress management for the infertile couples: A cognitive–behavioral approach to the psychological sequelae of infertility. *Infertility, 9,* 171–179.

Gambescia, N. (2009). The treatment of erectile dysfunction. *Journal of Family Psychotherapy, 20,* 220–240.

Garcia, F. D., & Thibaut, F. (2011). Current concepts in the pharmacotherapy of paraphilia. *Drugs, 71*(6), 771–790.

Giannotten, W. L. (2007). Sexuality in the palliative-terminal phase of cancer. *Sexologies, 16,* 299–303.

Giannotten, W. L. (2008a). Pregnancy and sexuality, part two. *Women's Sexual Health Journal, XV,* 2–7.

Giannotten, W. L. (2008b). Pregnancy and sexuality, part three. *Women's Sexual Health Journal, XVI,* 2–9.

Gilbert, E., Ussher, J. M., & Perz, J. (2011). Sexuality after gynaecological cancer: A review of the material, intrapsychic, and discursive aspects of treatment on women's sexual-wellbeing. *Maturitas, 70*(1), 42–57.

Giraldi, A., & Kristensen, E. (2010). Sexual dysfunction in women with diabetes mellitus. *Journal of Sex Research, 47*(2), 199–211.

Giugliano, J. R. (2009). Sexual addiction: Diagnostic problems. *International Journal of Mental Health and Addiction, 7,* 283–294.

Goldberg, P. D., Peterson, B. D., Rosen, K. H., & Sara, M. L. (2008). Cybersex: The impact of a contemporary problem on the practices of marriage and family therapists. *Journal of Marital and Family Therapy, 34*(4), 469–480.

Gooren, L. (2006). The biology of human psychosexual differentiation. *Hormones and Behavior, 50*(4), 589–601.

Gordon, W. M. (2002). Sexual obsessions and obsessive-compulsive disorder. *Sexual and Relationship Therapy, 17*(4), 343–354.

Gottman, J. M., & Levenson, R. W. (1992). Marital processes predictive of later dissolution: Behavior, physiology, and health. *Journal of Personality and Social Psychology, 63*(2), 221–233.

Graziottin, A. (2010). Menopause and sexuality: Key issues in premature menopause and beyond. *Annals of the New York Academy of Sciences, 1205,* 254–261.

Green, M. S., Murphy, M. J., & Blumer, M. L. C. (2010). Marriage and family therapists' comfort working with lesbian and gay male clients: The influence of religious practices and support for lesbian and gay male human rights. *Journal of Homosexuality, 57,* 1258–1273.

Greil, A., Slauson-Bevins, K., & McQuillan, J. (2010). The experience of infertility: A review of recent literature. In *Sociology Commons at University of Nebraska,* Paper 102, Lincoln, NB: University of Nebraska.

Groopman, J. (2012, October 1). Sex and the superbug. *New Yorker, 88*(30), 26.

Guay, D. R. (2009). Drug treatment of paraphilic and nonparaphilic sexual disorders. *Clinical Therapy, 31*(1), 1–31.

Gunger, S., Baser, I., Cyhan, T., Karasahin, E., & Kilic, S. (2008). Does mode of delivery affect sexual functioning of the man partner? *Journal of Sexual Medicine, 5*(1), 155–163.

Gurkan, L., Raynor, M. C., & Hellstrom, W. J. (2009). Sex and the infertile male. *Seminars in Reproductive Medicine, 27*(2), 186–190.

Hall, J. H., Fals-Stewart, W., & Fincham, F. D. (2008). Risky sexual behavior among married alcoholic men. *Journal of Family Psychology, 22,* 287–292.

Hall, K. (2008). Childhood sexual abuse and adult sexual problems: A new view of assessment and treatment. *Feminism & Psychology, 18,* 546–556.

Hall, K. (2009). Sexual dysfunction and childhood sexual abuse: Gender differences and treatment implications. In S. Leiblum (Ed.), *Principles and practice of sex therapy* (4th ed., pp. 379–415). New York, NY: Guilford Press.

Halpern, C. T., & Haydon, A. A. (2012). Sexual timetables for oral-genital, vaginal, and anal intercourse: Sociodemographic comparisons in a nationally representative sample of adolescents. *American Journal of Public Health, 102*(6), 1222–1228.

Hanh, T. N. (2012). Mindful living: Thich Nhat Hanh on the practice of meditation. *Shambhala Sun.* Retrieved October 24, 2012 from http://www.shambhalasun.com

Halverstadt, J. (1998). *A.D.D. and Romance.* Lanham, MA: Taylor Trade Publishing.

Harenski, C. L., Thornton, D. M., Harenski, K. A., Decety, J., & Kiehl, K. A. (2012). Increased frontotemporal activation during pain observation in sexual sadism: Preliminary findings. *Archive of General Psychiatry, 69*(3), 283–292.

Harris, S. M., & Hays, K. W. (2008). Family therapist comfort with and willingness to discuss client sexuality. *Journal of Marital and Family Therapy, 34,* 239–250.

Hayes, R. D. (2011). Circular and linear modeling of female sexual desire and arousal. *Journal of Sex Research, 48*(2/3), 130–141.

Heaphy, B. (2007). Sexualities, gender, and ageing: Resources and social change. *Current Sociology, 55*(2), 193–210.

Heiman, J. R. (2002). Sexual dysfunction: Overview of prevalence, etiological factors, and treatments. *Journal of Sex Research, 39*(1), 73–78.

Hertlein, K. M. (2011). Therapeutic dilemmas in treating internet infidelity. *The American Journal of Family Therapy, 39,* 162–173.

Hickey, D., Carr, A., Dooley, B., Guerin, S., Butler, E., & Fitzpatrick, L. (2005). Family and marital profiles of couples in which one partner has depression or anxiety. *Journal of Psychiatric and Mental Health Nursing, 12,* 439–446.

Hicks, T. L., Goodall, S. F., Quattrone, E. M., & Lydon-Rochelle, M. T. (2004). Postpartum sexual functioning and method of delivery: Summary of the evidence. *Journal of Midwifery & Women's Health, 49,* 430–436.

Higgins, A., Barker, P., & Begley, C. M. (2005). Neuroleptic medication and sexuality: The forgotten aspect of education and care. *Journal of Psychiatric and Mental Health Nursing, 12*(4), 439–446.

Higgins, A., Barker, P., & Begley, C. M. (2006). Sexual health education for people with mental health problems: What can we learn from the literature? *Journal of Psychiatric and Mental Health Nursing, 13*(6), 687–697.

Hillman, J. (2011). A call for an integrated biopsychosocial model to address fundamental disconnect in an emergency field: An introduction to the special issue on "Sexuality and Aging." *Aging International, 36,* 303–312.

Hinchliff, S., Gott, M., & Galena, E. (2005). 'I daresay I might find it embarrassing: General practitioners' perspectives on discussing sexual health issues with lesbian and gay patients. *Health and Social Care in the Community, 13*(4), 345–353.

Hirschfeld, R. M. A., Bowden, C. L., Gitlin, M. J., Keck, P. E., Perlis, R. H., Suppes, T., … Wagner, K. D. (2002). Practice guideline for the treatment of patients with Bipolar Disorder (Revision). *American Journal of Psychiatry, 159*(Suppl. 4), 64–110.

Hollows, K. (2007). Anodyspareunia: A novel sexual dysfunction? An exploration into anal sexuality. *Sexual and Relationship Therapy, 22*(4), 429–442.

Huddart, R. A., Norman, A., Moynihan, C., Horwich, A., Parker, C., Nicholls, E., & Dearnaley, D. P. (2005). Fertility, gonadal, and sexual function in survivors of testicular cancer. *British Journal of Cancer, 93*(2), 200–207.

Hughes, A., Hertlein, K. M., & Hagey, D. W. (2011). A MedMFT-informed sex therapy for treating sexual problems associated with chronic illness. *Journal of Family Psychotherapy, 22*(2), 114–127.

Humphrey, K. M. (2000). Sexuality counseling in counselor preparation programs. *The Family Journal: Counseling and Therapy for Couples and Families, 8*(3), 305–308.

Irwig, M. S., & Kolukula, S. (2011). Persistent sexual side effects of finasteride for male pattern hair loss. *Journal of Sexual Medicine, 8*(6), 1747–1753.

IsHak, W. W., Mikhail, A., Amiri, S. R., Berman, L. A., & Vasa, M. (2005). Sexual dysfunction. *Focus: The Journal of Lifelong Learning in Psychiatry, III*(4), 520–525.

IsHak, W. W., Bokarius, A., Jeffrey, J. K., Davis, M. C., & Bakhta, Y. (2010). Disorders of orgasm in women: A literature review of etiology and current treatments. *Journal of Sexual Medicine, 7*(10), 3254–3268.

Israel, T., Gorcheva, R., Walther, W. A., Sulzner, J. M., & Cohen, J. (2008). Therapists' helpful and unhelpful situations with LGBT clients: An exploratory study. *Professional Psychology: Research and Practice, 39*(3), 361–368.

Jack, L. (2005). A candid conversation about men, sexual health, and diabetes. *The Diabetes Educator, 31*(6), 810–817.

Jain, K., Radhakrishnan, G., & Agrawal, P. (2000). Infertility and psychosexual disorders: Relationship in infertile couples. *Indian Journal of Medical Science, 54*(1), 1–7.

James, S. D. (2011, June 9). Honeymoon with Viagra could be over, say doctors. Retrieved from http://abcnews.go.com/Health/viagra-prescription-sales-sexual-expectations/story?id=13794726#.UbaepetQ1f4

Jannini, E. A., & Porst, H. (2011). Case studies: A practical approach to early ejaculation. *Journal of Sexual Medicine, 8*(Suppl. 4), 360–367.

Jeng, C. (2004). The pathophysiology and etiology of vaginismus. *Taiwanese Journal of Obstetrics and Gynecology, 43*(1), 10–15.

Ji, P. (2007). Being a heterosexual ally to the lesbian, gay, bisexual, and transgendered community: Reflections and development. *Journal of Gay and Lesbian Psychotherapy, 11*(3/4), 173–185.

Joannides, P. (2012). *Guide to getting it on: A book about the wonders of sex.* Waldport, OR: GoofyFoot Press.

Jodoin, M., Bergeron, S., Khalifé, S., Dupuis, M. J., Desrochers, G., & Leclerc, B. (2011). Attributions about pain as predictors of psychological symptomatology, sexual function, and dyadic adjustment in women with vestibulodynia. *Archives of Sexual Behavior, 40*(1), 87–97.

Johnson, C. E. (2011). Sexual health during pregnancy and the postpartum. *Journal of Sexual Medicine, 8*(5), 1285–1286.

Johnson, S., & Zuccarini, D. (2010, October). Integrating sex and attachment in emotionally focused couple therapy. *Journal of Marital and Family Therapy, 36*(4), 431–445.

Johnson, S. D., Phelps, D. L., & Cottler, L. B. (2004). The association of sexual dysfunction and substance use among a community epidemiological sample. *Archives of Sexual Behavior, 33*(1), 55–63.

Jones, K. E. (2011). Sexological Systems Theory: an ecological model and assessment approach for sex therapy. *Sexual & Relationship Therapy, 26*(2), 127–144.

Jordan, K., Fromberger, P., Stolpmann, G., & Müller, J. L. (2011, November). The role of testosterone in sexuality and paraphilia: A neurobiological approach. Part II: Testosterone and paraphilia. *Journal of Sexual Medicine, 8,* 3008–3029.

Kainz, K. (2001). The role of the psychologist in the evaluation and treatment of infertility. *Women's Health Issues, 11*(6), 481–485.

Kalichman, L. (2009). Association between fibromyalgia and sexual dysfunction in women. *Clinical Rheumatology, 28,* 365–369.

Kalmuss, D. (2004). Nonvolitional sex and sexual health. *Archives of Sexual Behavior, 33*(3), 189–195.

Kao, A., Binik, Y. M., Kapuscinski, B. A., & Khalifé, S. (2008). Dyspareunia in postmenopausal women: A critical review. *Pain Research & Management, 13*(3), 243–254.

Kaplan, H. S. (1983). *The evaluation of sexual disorders: Psychological and medical aspects.* New York, NY: Routledge.

Kaplan, H. S. (1988). *The illustrated manual of sex therapy.* Levittown, PA: Brunner/Mazel.

Karim, R., & Chaudhri, P. (2012). Behavioral addictions: An overview. *Journal of Psychoactive Drugs, 44*(1), 5–17.

Katz, A. (2007). *Sex when you're sick: Reclaiming sexual health after illness or injury.* Westport, CT: Praeger Publishers.

Katz, A. (2009). *Woman cancer sex.* Pittsburgh, PA: Hygeia Media.

Kendurkar, A., & Brinder, K. (2008). Major depressive disorder, obsessive-compulsive disorder, and generalized anxiety disorder: Do the sexual dysfunctions differ? *Primary Care Companion to the Journal of Clinical Psychiatry, 10,* 299–305.

King, J. A., Mandinsky, D., King, S., Fletcher, K. W., & Brewer, J. (2001, February). Early sexual abuse and low cortisol. *Psychiatry and Clinical Neurosciences, 55*(1), 71–74.

Kingsberg, S., & Althof, S. E. (2009). Evaluation and treatment of female sexual disorders. *International Journal of Urogynecology, 20*(Suppl. 1), S33–S43.

Kingsberg, S., & Goldstein, I. (2007). The *Journal of Sexual Medicine* supports research and choice in women's sexual health management. *Journal of Sexual Medicine, 4*(Suppl. 3), 209–210.

Kleinman, A. (1989). *The Illness Narratives: Suffering, Healing, and the Human Condition.* New York, NY: Basic Books.

Kleinplatz, P. J. (1996). The erotic encounter. *Journal of Humanistic Psychology, 35*(3), 105–123.

Kleinplatz, P. J. (1998). Sex therapy for vaginismus: A review, critique, and humanistic alternative. *Journal of Humanistic Psychology, 38*(2), 51–81.

Kleinplatz, P. J. (2007). Building blocks toward optimal sexuality: Constructing a conceptual model. *The Family Journal: Counseling and Therapy for Couples and Families, 15*(1), 72–78.

Kleinplatz, P. J., & Moser, C. (Eds.). (2006). *Sadomasochism: Powerful pleasures.* Binghamton, NY: Haworth Press.

Kolmes, K. (2010, November). Don't get caught in the web: Avoiding sticky ethical issues on the Internet. *Division I Briefings: The Journal of the California Psychological Association Division of Professional Practice, 172,* 9–11.

Kolmes, K., Sock, W., & Moser, C. (2006). Investigating bias in psychotherapy with BDSM client. In P. Kleinplatz & C. Moser (Eds.), *Sadomasochism: Powerful pleasures.* Binghamton, NY: Haworth Press.

Kort, J. (2007). *Gay affirmative therapy for the straight therapist: The essential guide.* New York, NY: W. W. Norton & Company.

Kosciw, J. G., Greytak, E. A., & Diaz, E. M. (2008). Who what, where, when, and why: Demographic and ecological factors contributing to hostile school climate for lesbian, gay, bisexual, and transgender youth. *Journal of Youth & Adolescence, 38,* 976–988.

Kost, K., & Henshaw, S. (2012, February). *U.S. teenage pregnancies, births and abortions, 2008: National trends by age, race and ethnicity.* Washington, D.C.: Guttmacher Institute.

Krafchick, J., & Biringen, Z. (2002). Parents as sexuality educators: The role of family therapists in coaching parents. *Journal of Feminist Family Therapy, 14*(3/4), 57–71.

Kralik, D., Koch, T., & Telford, K. (2001). Constructions of sexuality for midlife women living with chronic illness. *Journal of Advanced Nursing, 35*(2), 180–187.

Kreider, R. M., & Ellis, R. (2011). *Number, timing, and duration of marriages and divorces: 2009*(Current Population Reports, pp. 70–125). Washington, DC: U.S. Census Bureau.

Kriston, L., Günzler, C., Agyemang, A., Bengel, J., & Berner, M. M. (2010). Effect of sexual function on health related quality of life mediated by depressive symptoms in cardiac rehabilitation findings of the SPARK project in 493 patients. *Journal of Sexual Medicine, 7*(6), 2044–2055.

Krychman, M. (2007). *100 Questions and answers for women living with cancer: A practical guide for survivorship*. Burlington, MA: Jones and Bartlett Publishers, Inc.

Kuo, F. (2009). Secrets or no secrets: Confidentiality in couple therapy. *The American Journal of Family Therapy, 37,* 351–354.

Kuper, L. E., Nussbaum, R., & Mustanski, B. (2012). Exploring the diversity of gender and sexual orientation identities in an online sample of transgender individuals. *49,* 2–3.

Ladsen, D., & Welton, R. (2007). Recognizing and managing erotic and eroticized transference. *Psychiatry, 4*(4): 47–50.

La Pera, G., Carderi, A., Zelinda, M., Peris, F., Lentini, M., & Taggi, F. (2008). Sexual dysfunction prior to first drug use among former drug addicts and its possible causal meaning on drug addiction: Preliminary results. *Journal of Sexual Medicine, 5,* 164–172.

Lau, J. T., Kim, J. H., & Tsui, H. Y. (2008). Prevalence and sociocultural predictors of sexual dysfunction among Chinese men who have sex with men in Hong Kong. *Journal of Sexual Medicine, 5*(12), 2766–2779.

Laumann, E. O., Paik, A., & Rosen, R. C. (1999). Sexual dysfunction in the United States: Prevalence and predictors. *Journal of the American Medical Association, 281*(6), 537–544.

Laumann, E. O., Paik, A., Glasser, D. B., Kang, J. H., Wang, T., Levinson, B., … Gingell, C. (2006, April). A cross-national study of subjective sexual well-being among older women and men: Findings from the Global Study of Sexual Attitudes and Behaviors. *Archives of Sexual Behavior, 35*(2), 145–161.

La Vignera, S., Condorelli, R., Vicari, E., D'Agata, R., & Calogero, A. E. (2012). Physical activity and erectile dysfunction in middle-age men. *Journal of Andrology, 33*(2), 154–161.

Lawrence, A. A., & Love-Crowell, J. (2008). Psychotherapists' experience with client who engage in consensual sadomasochism: A qualitative study. *Journal of Sex & Marital Therapy, 24,* 67–85.

Leclerc, B., Bergeron, S., Binik, Y. M., & Khalifí, S. (2010, February). History of sexual and physical abuse in women with dyspareunia: Association with pain, psychosocial adjustment, and sexual functioning. *Journal of Sexual Medicine, 7*(2 Pt. 2), 971–980.

Leeman, L. M., & Rogers, R. G. (2012). Sex after childbirth: Postpartum sexual function. *Obstretrics & Gynecology, 119*(3), 647–655.

Leeners, B., Stiller, R., Block, E., Görres, G., Imthurn, B., & Rath, W. (2007, October). Effect of childhood sexual abuse on gynecologic care as an adult. *Psychosomatics, 48*(5), 385–393.

Leiblum, S., & Brezsnyak, M. (2006). Sexual chemistry: Theoretical elaboration and clinical implications. *Sexual and Relationship Therapy, 21*(1), 55–69.

Leiblum, S. R. (2007). *Principles and practice of sex therapy*. New York, NY: Guilford Press.

Leiblum, S., Seehuus, M., & Brown, C. (2007). Persistent genital arousal disorder: Disordered or normative aspect of female sexual response? *Journal of Sexual Medicine, 4,* 680–689.

Liebschutz, J., Savetsky, J., Saitz, R., Horton, N., Lloyd-Travaglini, C., & Samet, J. (2002). The relationship between sexual and physical abuse and substance abuse consequences. *Journal of Substance Abuse Treatment, 22,* 121–128.

Lemieux, S. R., & Byers, E. S. (2008). The sexual well-being of women who have experienced child sexual abuse. *Psychology of Women Quarterly, 32*, 126–144.

Lester, R. J. (1997). The (dis)embodied self in anorexia nervosa. *Social Science & Medicine, 44*, 479–489.

Levine, S. B. (2010) What is sexual addiction? *Journal of Sex and Marital Therapy, 36*(3), 261–275.

Lewis, L. J. (2004). Examining sexual health discourses in a racial/ethnic context. *Archives of Sexual Behavior, 33*(3), 223–234.

Lewis, R. W., Fugl-Meyer, K. S., Corona, G., Hayes, R. D., Laumann, E. O., Moreira, E. D., … Segraves, T. (2010). Definitions/epidemiology/risk factors for sexual dysfunction. *Journal of Sexual Medicine, 7*, 1598–1607.

Lin, I. F., & Brown, S. L. (2012. April). Unmarried Boomers confront old age: A national portrait. *Gerontologist, 52*(2), 153–165.

Lindau, S. T., & Gavrilova, N. (2010). Sex, health, and years of sexually active life gained due to good health: Evidence from two US population based cross sectional surveys of ageing. *British Medical Journal*, 1–11. Retrieved from http://www.bmj.com/content/340/bmj.c810.pdf%2Bhtml..

Lockwood-Rayermann, S. (2006). Survivorship issues in ovarian cancer: A review. *Oncology Nursing Forum, 33*(3), 553–562.

LoFrisco, B. M. (2011). Female sexual pain disorders and cognitive behavioral therapy. *Journal of Sex Research, 48*(6), 573–579.

Lowenstein, L. F. (2002). Fetishes and their associated behavior. *Sexuality and Disability, 20*(2), 135–147.

Lue, T. F., Giuliano, F., Montorosi, F., Rosen, R. C., Andersson, K., Althof, S., … Wagner, G. (2004). Summary of the recommendations on sexual dysfunctions in men. *Journal of Sexual Medicine, 1*, 6–23.

Lustermann, D. D. (2005). Marital infidelity: The effects of delayed traumatic reaction. *Journal of Couple & Relationship Therapy, 4*(2/3), 71–81.

Luzz, G. A., & Law, L. A. (2006). The male sexual pain syndromes. *International Journal of STD & AIDS, 17*, 720–726.

Magon, N., & Kalra, S. (2011). The orgasmic history of oxytocin: Love, lust, and labor. *Indian Journal of Endocrinology and Metabolism, 15*(Suppl. 3), S156–S161.

Malatesta, V. J. (2007). Sexual problems, women and aging: An overview. *Journal of Women & Aging, 19*(1/1), 139–154.

Malpas, J. (2011). Between pink and blue: A multi-dimensional family approach to gender nonconforming children and their families. *Family Process, 50*(4), 453–457.

Maltz, W. (2003). Treating the sexual intimacy concerns of sexual abuse survivors. *Contemporary Sexuality, 37*(7), i–vii.

Maltz, W. (2012). *The sexual healing journey: A guide for survivors of sexual abuse* (3rd ed.). New York, NY: William Morrow Paperbacks.

Maltz, W., & Boss, S. (2012). *Private thoughts: Exploring the nature of women's sexual fantasies*. Novato, CA: New World Library.

Mao, A., & Raguram, A. (2009). Online infidelity: The new challenge to marriages. *Indian Journal of Psychiatry, 51*(4), 302–304.

Marshall, W. L., Marshall, L. E., & Serran, G. A. (2006). Strategies in the treatment of paraphilias: A critical review. *Annual Review of Sex Research, 17*, 162–182.

Martin, C., Godfrey, M., Meekums, B., & Madill, A. (2010). Staying on the straight and narrow. *Therapy Today, 21*(5), 10–14.

Mason, M. (2006, September 3). Thailand's sex change industry. *The Seattle Times*. Retrieved from http://seattletimes.com/html/health/2003237830_healthsexchannel

Masters, W. H. & Johnson, V. E. (1976). An interdisciplinary approach to sexuality. *The Personnel and Guidance Journal, 54*(7), 368–369.

May, K., & Riley, A. (2002). Sexual function after 60. *Journal of the British Menopause Society*, 112–115.

Mayo Clinic Staff. Birth control options: Things to consider. Retrieved October 23, 2012 from http://www.mayoclinic.com/health/birth-control-options/MY01084

McCabe, M. P. (1999). The interrelationship between intimacy, relationship functioning, and sexuality among men and women in committed relationships. *The Canadian Journal of Human Sexuality, 8*, 31–38.

McCabe, M. P. (2009). Anorgasmia in women. *Journal of Family Psychotherapy, 20*, 177–197.

McCabe, M. P., & Delaney, S. M. (1992). An evaluation of therapeutic programs for the treatment of secondary inorgasmia in women. *Archives of Sexual Behavior, 21*(1), 69–89.

McCandless, F., & Sladen, C. (2003). Sexual health and women with Bipolar Disorder. *Journal of Advanced Nursing, 44*, 42–48.

McCarthy, B., & McCarthy, E. (2003). *Rekindling desire: A step by step program to help low-sex and no-sex marriages.* New York, NY: Routledge.

McCarthy, B., & Thestrup, M. (2008). Integrating sex therapy interventions with couple therapy. *Journal of Contemporary Psychotherapy, 38*, 139–149.

Meana, M. (2010). Elucidating women's (hetero) sexual desire: Definitional challenges and content expansion. *Journal of Sex Research, 47*(2–3), 104–122.

Meeuwis, K. A., de Hullu, J. A., van de Nieuwenhof, H. P., Evers, A. W., Massuger, L. F., van de Kerkhof, P. C., & van Rossum, M. M. (2011). Quality of life and sexual health in patients with genital psoriasis. *British Journal of Dermatology, 164*(6), 1247–1255.

Melisko, M. E., Goldman, M., & Rugo, H. S. (2010). Amelioration of sexual adverse effects in the early breast cancer patient. *Journal of Cancer Survivorship, 4*(3), 247–255.

Melnik, T., Althof, S., Atallah, A. N., Puga, M. E., Glina, S., & Riera, R. (2011). Psychosocial interventions for early ejaculation (Review). *Cochrane Database of Systematic Reviews*, 1–22. New York, NY: John Wiley & Sons, Ltd.

Melton, S. T. (2012). How is antidepressant-associated sexual dysfunction managed? *Medscape*. Retrieved October 27, 2012 from http://www.medscape.com/viewarticle/769813/print

Mercer, B. (2008). Interviewing people with chronic illness about sexuality: an adaptation of the PLISSIT model. *Journal of Nursing and Healthcare of Chronic Illness*, in association with *Journal of Clinical Nursing, 17*, 341–351.

Meston, C. M., Heiman, J. R., & Trapnell, P. D. (1999). The relation between early abuse and adult sexuality. *Journal of Sex Research, 36*, 385–395.

Metz, M. E., & Epstein, N. (2002). Assessing the role of relationship conflict in sexual dysfunction. *Journal of Sex and Marital Therapy, 28*(2), 139–164.

Metz, M. E., & McCarthy, B. W. (2004). *Coping with erectile dysfunction: How to regain confidence and enjoy great sex.* Oakland, CA: New Harbinger.

Metz, M. E., & McCarthy, B. W. (2010). The "Good Enough Sex" model for couple sexual satisfaction. *Sexual and Relationship Therapy, 22*(3), 351–362.

Mick, T. M., & Hollander, E. (2006). Impulsive-compulsive sexual behavior. *CNS Spectrum, 11*(12), 944–955.

Miller, S. A., & Byers, E. S. (2009). Psychologists' continuing education and training in sexuality. *Journal of Sex & Marital Therapy, 35*(3), 206–219.

Millheiser, L. S., Helmer, A. E., Quintero, R. B., Westphal, L. M., Milki, A. A., & Lathi, R. B. (2010). Is infertility a risk factors for female sexual dysfunction. A case-control study. *Fertility & Sterility, 94*(6), 2022–2025.

Millon, M., Millon, C. M., Meagher, S., Grossman, S., & Ramnath, R. (2004). *Personality disorders in modern life* (2nd ed.). Hoboken, NJ: Wiley.

Minter, S. P. (2012). Supporting transgender children: New legal, social, and medical approaches. *Journal of Homosexuality, 59*, 422–433.

Mintz, L. B. (2009). *A tired woman's guide to passionate sex: Reclaim your desire and reignite your relationship.* Avon, MA: Adams Media.

Monga, T. N., Tan, G., Ostermann, H. J., Monga, U., & Grabois, M. Sexuality and sexual adjustment of patients with chronic pain. *Disability Rehabilitation, 29*, 317–329.

Montgomery, K. A. (2008, June). Sexual desire disorders. *Psychiatry, 5*(6), 50–55.

Moore, K. L. (2010). Sexuality and sense of self in later life: Japanese men's and women's reflections on sex and aging. *Journal of Cross Cultural Gerontology, 24*, 149–163.

Moretz, C. (2011). An application of the quantum model to improve sexual intimacy for a sexagenarian couple with erectile dysfunction. *Ageing International, 36*, 418–422.

Mosher, W. D., Chandra, A., & Jones, J. (2005). Sexual behavior and selected health measures: Men and women 15–44 years of age, United States, 2002. *Advance data from vital and health statistics*; no 362. Hyattsville, MD: National Center for Health Statistics.

Mullen, P. E., Martin, J. L., Anderson, J. C., Romans, S. E., & Herbison, G. P. (1994). The effect of child sexual abuse on social, interpersonal and sexual function in adult life. *British Journal of Psychiatry, 165*(2), 35–47.

Murtagh, J. (2010). Female sexual function, dysfunction, and pregnancy: Implications for practice. *Journal of Midwifery & Women's Health, 55*(5), 438–446.

Murthy, S., & Wylie, K. R. (2007). Sexual problems in patients on antipsychotic medication. *Sexual and Relationship Therapy, 22*(1), 97–107.

Mustanski, B. S., Garofalo, R., & Emerson, E. M. (2010). Mental health disorders, psychological distress, and suicidality in a diverse sample of lesbian, gay, bisexual, and transgender youths. *American Journal of Public Health, 100*(12), 2426–2431.

Naeinian, M. R., Shaeiri, M. R., & Hosseini, F. S. (2011). General health and quality of life in patients with sexual dysfunction. *Journal of Urology, 8*(2), 127–131.

Nappi, R. E., Martini, E., Terreno, E., Albani, F., Santamaria, V., Tonani, S., … Polatti, F. (2010). Management of hypoactive sexual desire disorder in women: Current and emerging therapies. *International Journal of Womens Health, 2*, 167–175.

National Institute for Mental Health. *The Numbers Count: Mental Disorders in America.* Retrieved from http://www.nimh.nih.gov/health/publications/the-numbers-count-mental-disorders-in-america/index.shtml

Neel, A. B. (2012). 7 meds that can wreck your sex life. AARP. Retrieved October 27, 2012 from http://www.aarp.org/health/drugs-supplemental.

Nelson, C. J. (2008). The role of psychological treatment strategies in ejaculatory dysfunction. *Current Sexual Health Reports, 5*, 90–104.

Nelson, S. (2002). Physical symptoms in sexually abused women: Somatization or undetected injury? *Child Abuse Review, 11*, 51–64.

Neumann, D. A. and Gamble, S. J. (1995). Issues in the professional development of psychotherapists: Countertransference and vicarious traumatization in the new trauma therapist. *Psychotherapy: Theory, Research, Practice, Training, 32*(2), 341–347.

Newman, A. G., Clayton, L., & Zuellig, A. (2000). The relationship of childhood sexual abuse and depression with somatic symptoms and medical utilization. *Psychological Medicine, 30*, 1063–1077.

Nguyen, N., & Holodniy, M. (2008). HIV infection in the elderly. *Clinical Interventions in Aging, 3*(3), 453–472.

Nhat Hanh, T. (1999). *The miracle of mindfulness: An introduction to the practice of meditation.* Boston, MA: Beacon Press.

Nichols, M. (2004). Rethinking lesbian bed death. *Journal of the British Association for Sexual and Relationship Therapy, 19*(4), 101–114.

Nichols, M. (2005). Sexual function in lesbians and lesbian relationships. In I. Goldstein, C. M. Meston, S. Davis, & M. Traish (Eds.), *Women's sexual function and dysfunction: Study, diagnosis, and treatment.* New York, NY: Taylor & Francis.

Nichols, M. (2006). Psychotherapeutic issues with "kinky" clients: Clinical problems, yours and theirs. *Journal of Homosexuality, 50*(2–3), 281–300.

Nichols, M., & Shernoff, M. (2007). Therapy with sexual minorities: Queering practice. In S. Leiblum (Ed.), *Principles and practice of sex therapy.* New York, NY: Guilford Press.

Nutall, R., & Jackson, H. (1994). Personal history of childhood abuse among clinicians. *Child Abuse and Neglect, 18*(5), 455–472.

O'Brien, R., Rose, P., Campbell, C., Weller, D., Neal, R. D., Wilkinson, C., … Watson, E. (2011, August). "I wish I'd told them": A qualitative study of the unmet psychosocial needs of prostate cancer patients during follow-up after treatment." *Patient Education and Counseling, 84*(2), 200–207.

O'Connor, D. B., Corona, G., Forti, G., Abdelouahid, T., Lee, D. M., Finn, J. D., … Wu, F. C. (2008). Assessment of sexual health in aging men in europe: Development and validation of the European male ageing study sexual function questionnaire. *Journal of Sexual Medicine, 5*(6), 1374–1385.

Ogden, G. (2006). *The heart and soul of sex: Making the ISIS connection.* Boston, MA: Trumpeter.

Onat, G., & Beji, N. K. (2012). Marital relationship and quality of life among couples with infertility. *Sexuality and Disability, 30*, 39–52.

Ostrander, N. (2009). Sexual pursuits of pleasure among men and women with spinal cord injuries. *Sex and Disabilities, 27*, 11–19.

Palacios, S. (2011). Hypoactive sexual desire disorder and current pharmacotherapeutic options in women. *Women's Health, 7*(1), 95–107.

Palha, A. P., & Esteves, M. (2008). Drugs of abuse and sexual functioning. In R. Balon (Ed.), *Sexual dysfunction: The brain-body connection. Advanced Psychosomatic Medicine* (vol. 29., pp. 131–149).

Palmer, N. R., & Stuckey, B. G. (2008). early ejaculation: A clinical update. *Medical Journal of Australia, 188*(11), 662–666.

Parets, N., & Schmerzler, A. J. (2008). Neurologic disability and its effect on sexual functioning. *Medical Management of Adults with Neurologic Disabilities*, 353–362.

Parker, M. G., & Yau, MK. (2012). Sexuality, identity and women with spinal cord injury. *Sex and Disabilities, 30*, 15–27.

Pauleta, J. R., Pereira, N. M., & Graça, L. M. (2010). Sexuality during pregnancy. *Journal of Sexual Medicine, 7*(1 Pt 1), 136–142.

Pauls, R. N., Occhino, J. A., & Dryfhout, V. L. (2008). Effects of pregnancy on female sexual function and body image: A prospective study. *Journal of Sexual Medicine, 5*(8), 1015–1922.

Pearlman, J. (2010, January/February). Hypochondria: The impossible illness. *Psychology Today*, 28–31.

Penner, C. L., & Penner, J. L. (2003). *The gift of sex: A guide to sexual fulfillment.* Nashville, TN: Thomas Nelson.

Perel, E. (2007). *Mating in captivity: Unlocking erotic intelligence.* New York, NY: Harper Perennial.

Perelman, M. A., & Rowland, D. L. (2006). Retarded ejaculation. *World Journal of Urology, 24*(6), 645–652.

Peterson, B. D., Gold, L., & Feingold, T. (2007). The experience and influence of infertility: Considerations for couple counselors. *The Family Journal: Counseling and Therapy for Couples and Families, 15*(3), 251–257.

Peterson, B., Boivin, J., Norré, J., Smith, C., Thorn, P., & Wischmann, T. (2012). An introduction to infertility counseling: A guide for mental health and medical professionals. *Journal of Assistive Reproduction & Genetics, 29*(3), 243–248.

Pines, A. (2011). Male menopause: Is it a real clinical syndrome? *Climacteric, 14*(1), 15–17.

Pittman, F. (1989). *Private lies: Infidelity and the betrayal of intimacy.* New York, NY: Norton.

Plaut, S. M. (2008). Sexual and nonsexual boundaries in professional relationships: Principles and teaching guidelines. *Sex and Relationship Therapy, 23*(1), 85–94.

Pope, K. S. (1986). Research and laws regarding therapist-patient sexual involvement: Implications for therapists. *American Journal of Psychotherapy, XL*(4), 564–571.

Pope, K. S., & Feldman-Summers, S. (1992). National survey of psychologists' sexual and physical abuse history and their evaluation of training and competence in these areas. *Professional Psychology and Research, 23*(5), 353–361.

Popovic, M. (2011). Pornography use and closeness with others in men. *Archives of Sexual Behavior, 40*, 449–456.

Polomeno, V. (2000). Sex and pregnancy: A perinatal educator's guide. *Journal of Perinatal Education, 9*(4), 15–27.

Priest, J. B., & Wickel, K. (2011). Religious therapists and clients in same-sex relationships: Lessons from the court case of Bruff v. North Mississippi Health Service, Inc. *The American Journal of Family Therapy, 39*, 139–148.

Quadflieg, N., & Manfred, M. F. (2003). The course and outcome of Bulimia Nervosa. *European Child & Adolescent Psychiatry, 12*(Suppl. 1), 99–109.

Quattrini, F., Ciccarone, M., Tatoni, F., & Vittori, G. (2010). Psychological and sexological assessment of the infertile couple. *Sexologies, 19*, 15–19.

Quartana, P. J., Campbell, C. M., & Edwards, R. R. (2009). Pain catastrophizing: A critical review. *Expert Review of Neurotherapeutics, 9*(5), 745–758.

Quinn, C., & Browne, G. (2009). Sexuality of people living with a mental illness: A collaborative challenge for mental health nurses. *International Journal of Mental Health Nursing, 18*(3), 195–203.

Ralph, D. J., & Wylie, K. R. (2005). Ejaculatory disorders and sexual function. *British Journal of Urology International, 95*(9), 1181–1186.

Ralph, D., Gonzales-Cadavid, N., Milrone, V., Perovic, S., Sohn, M., Usta, M., & Levine, L. (2010). The management of Peyronie's disease: Evidence-based 2010 guidelines. *Journal of Sexual Medicine, 7,* 2359–2374.

Ramage, M. (2006). Female sexual dysfunction. *Psychiatry, 6*(3), 105–110.

Ramezanzadeh, F., Aghssa, M. M., Jafarabadi, M., & Zayeri, F. (2006). Alterations of sexual desire and satisfaction in male partners of infertile couples. *Fertility & Sterility, 85*(1), 139–143.

Reef, K., & Chaudhri, P. (2012). Behavioral addictions: An Overview. *Journal of Psychoactive Drugs, 44*(1), 5–17.

Rellini, A., & Meston, C. (2007). Sexual function and satisfaction in adults based on the definitions of child sexual abuse. *Journal of Sexual Medicine, 4*(5), 1312–1321.

Rellini, A. H., & Meston, C. M. (2011). Sexual self-schemas, sexual dysfunction, and the sexual responses of women with a history of childhood sexual abuse. *Archives of Sexual Behavior, 40*(2), 351–362.

Resnick, S. (2012). *The heart of desire: Keys to the Pleasures of love.* Hoboken, NJ: Wiley.

Reuben, D. (1966/1999). *Everything you ever wanted to know about sex* but were afraid to ask.* New York, NY: Harper Collins.

Reynolds, A. L., & Caren, S. L. (2000). How intimate relationships are impacted when heterosexual men cross dress. *Journal of Psychology and Human Sexuality, 12*(3), 63–79.

Ribner, D. S. (2009). Editorial: Vanilla is also a flavor. *Sexual and Relationship Therapy, 24*(3–4), 233–234.

Richardson, D. (2003). *The heart of tantric sex: A unique guide to love and sexual fulfillment.* Self-published through Mantra Books.

Richardson, D., Nalabanda, A., & Goldmeier, D. (2006). Retarded ejaculation: A review. *International Journal of STD & AIDS, 17*(3), 143–150.

Riese, S. P., & Wright, T. M. (1996). Brief report: Personality traits, cluster B personality disorders, and sociosexuality. *Journal of Research in Personality, 30,* 128–136.

Robinson, B., Bockting, W., Rosser, B., Miner, M., & Coleman, E. (2002). The Sexual Health Model: Application of a sexological approach to HIV prevention. *Health Education Research, 17,* 43–57.

Robinson, B. B., Munns, R. A., Weber-Main, A. M., Lowe, M. A., & Raymond, N. C. (2011). Application of the sexual health model in the long-term treatment of hypoactive sexual desire and female orgasmic disorder. *Archives of Sexual Behavior, 40*(2), 469–478.

Robinson, F. (2011). Addressing sexual problems. *Practical Nurse, 41*(5), 10–11.

Rodriguez, S. J., Mata, L., Lameiras, M., Fernandex, M. C., & Vila, J. (2007). Dyscontrol evolked by erotic and food images in women with bulimia nervosa. *European Eating Disorders Review, 15,* 231–239.

Rolland, J. (1994). *Families, illness, and disability: An integrative treatment model.* New York, NY: Basic Books.

Rosen, C. (2005, July 16–22). Reproductive health problems in ageing men. *Lancet, 366*(9481), 183–185.

Rosenbaum, T. (2010). Physical therapy for sexual pain. *Journal of Sexual Medicine, 7*(12), 4025–4026.

Rosenbaum, T. (2013). An integrated mindfulness-based approach to the treatment of women with sexual pain and anxiety: Promoting autonomy and mind/body connection. *Sex and Relationship Therapy.* Retrieved from DOI:10.1080/14681994. 2013.764981

Ross, C. A. (2009). Ethics of gender identity disorder. *Ethical Human Psychology and Psychiatry, 11*(3), 165–170.

Rossen, P., Pedersen, A. F., Zachariae, R., & von der Maase, H. (2012). Sexuality and body image in long-term survivors of testicular cancer. *European Journal of Cancer, 48,* 571–578.

Rowland, D., & Cooper, S. (2011). Practical tips for sexual counseling and psychotherapy in early ejaculation. *Journal of Sexual Medicine, 8*(Suppl. 4), 360–367.

Rowland, D., McMahon, C. G., Abdo., C., Chen, J., Jannini, E., Waldinger, M. D., & Ahn, T. Y. (2010). Disorders of orgasm and ejaculation in men. *Journal of Sexual Medicine, 7,* 1668–1686.

Rowland, D., van Diest, S., Incrocci, L., & Slob, A. K. (2005). Psychosexual factors that differentiate men with inhibited ejaculation from men with no dysfunction or another sexual dysfunction. *Journal of Sexual Medicine, 2*(3), 383–389.

Rowland, D. L., Keeney, C., & Slob, A. K. (2004). Sexual response in men with inhibited or retarded ejaculation. *International Journal of Impotence Research, 16*(3), 270–274.

Rutter, P. A. (2011). Sex therapy with gay male couples using affirmative therapy. *Sex and Relationship Therapy, 27*(1), 35–45.

Ryan, S., Hill, J., Thwaites, C., & Dawes, P. (2008). Assessing the effect of fibromyalgia on patients' sexual activity. *Nursing Standards, 23*(2), 35–41.

Saakvitne, K. W., & Pearlman, L. A. (1996). *Transforming the pain: A workbook on vicarious traumatization.* New York, NY: W. W. Norton & Company.

Sachs-Ericsson, N., Cromer, K., Hernandez, A., & Kendall-Tackett, K. (2009). A review of childhood abuse, health, and pain-related problems: The role of psychiatric disorders and current life stress. *Journal of Trauma and Dissociation, 10*(2), 170–188.

Sacomori, C., & Cardoso, F. L. (2008). Variations in sexual frequency among pregnant women. *Women's Sexual Health Journal, XVII,* 2–6.

Sadovsky, R., Basson, R., Krychman, M., Morales, A. M., Schover, L., Wang, R., & Incrocci, L. (2010). Cancer and sexual problems. *Journal of Sexual Medicine, 7*(1 Pt 2), 349–373.

Salonia, A., Giraldi, A., Chivers, M., Georgidis, J., Levine, R., Maravilla, K. R., & McCarthy, M. M. (2007). Physiology of women's sexual function: Basic knowledge and new findings. *Journal of Sexual Medicine, 7,* 2637–2660.

Sanchez, D. T., & Kiefer, A. K. (2007). Body concerns in and out of the bedroom: Implications for sexual pleasure and problems. *Archives of Sexual Behavior, 7, 36,* 808–820.

Sandfort, T. G., & de Keizer, M. (2001). Sexual problems in gay men: An overview of empirical research. *Annual Review of Sex Research, 12,* 93–120.

Sandfort, T. G., & Ehrhardt, A. A. (2004). Sexual health: A useful public health paradigm or a moral imperative? *Archives of Sexual Behavior, 33*(3), 181–187.

Sarwer, D. B., & Durlak, J. A. (1996). Childhood sexual abuse as a predictor of adult female sexual dysfunction: A study of couples seeking sex therapy. *Child Abuse and Neglect, 20*(10), 963–972.

Satcher, D. (2001). *The Surgeon General's call to action to promote sexual health and responsible sexual behavior,* Washington, D.C: U. S. Department of Health and Human Services.

Savin-Williams, R. C., & Ream, G. L. (2007). Prevalence and stability of sexual orientation components during adolescence and young adulthood. *Archives of Sexual Behavior, 36,* 385–394.

Sayin, H. Ü. (2012). Doors of female orgasmic consciousness: New theories on the peak experience and mechanisms of female orgasm and expanded sexual response. *NeuroQuantology, 10*(4), 692–714.

Schnarch, D. (1991). *Constructing the sexual crucible: An integration of sexual and marital therapy.* New York, NY: Norton Professional Books.

Schnarch, D. (2011). *Intimacy & desire: Awaken the passion in your relationship.* New York, NY: Beaufort Books.

Schope, R. D. (2005). Who's afraid of growing old? Gay and lesbian perceptions of aging. *Journal of Gerontological Social Work, 45*(4), 23–39.

Schover, L. R. (1981). Male and female therapists' responses to male and female client sexual material: An analogue study. *Archives of Sexual Behavior, 10*(6), 477–492.

Segal, J. Z. (2012). The sexualization of the medical. *Journal of Sex Research, 49*(4), 369–378.

Seligman L., & Hardenburg, S. A. (2000). Assessment and treatment of paraphilias. *Journal of Counseling and Development, 78,* 107–113.

Serati, M., Salvatore, S., Siesto, G., Cattoni, E., Zanirato, M., Khullar, V., … Bolis, P. (2010). Female sexual function during pregnancy and after childbirth. *Journal of Sexual Medicine, 7*(8), 2782–2790.

Shafer, A. (2001). The big five and sexuality trait terms as predictors of relationships and sex. *Journal of Research in Personality, 35,* 313–338.

Shaw., J. A., Lewis, J. E., Loeb, A., Rosado, J., & Rodriguez, R. A. (2000). Child on child sexual abuse: Psychological perspectives. *Child Abuse & Neglect, 24*(12), 1591–1600.

Shernoff, M. (2006). Negotiated nonmonogamy and male couples. *Family Process, 45*(4), 407–418.

Shilo, G., & Savaya, R. (2012). Mental health of lesbian, gay, and bisexual youth and young adults: Differential effects of age, gender, religiosity, and sexual orientation. *Journal of Research on Adolescence, 22*(2), 310–325.

Shindel, A. W., & Moser, C. A. (2011, March). Why are the paraphilias mental disorders? *The Journal of Sexual Medicine, 8*(3), 927–929.

Sitron, J. A., & Dyson, D. A. (2012, March 13). Validation of sexological worldview: A construct for the use in the training of sexologists in sexual diversity. *Sage Open.* doi:10.1177/2158244012439072.

Slowinski, J. (2001). Multimodal sex therapy for the treatment of vulvodynia: A clinician's view. *Journal of Sex and Marital Therapy, 27*(5), 607–613.

Smith, J. F., Walsh, T. J., Conti, S. L., Turek, P., & Lue, T. (2008). Risk factors for emotional and relationship problems in Peyronie's disease. *Journal of Sexual Medicine, 5*(9), 2179–2184.

Smith, J. F., Walsh, T. J., Shindel, A. W., Turek, P. J., Wing, H., Pasch, L., & Katz, P. P. (2009). Sexual, marital, and social impact of a man's perceived infertility diagnosis. *Journal of Sexual Medicine, 6*(9), 2505–2515.

Smith, S. (2007). Drugs that cause sexual dysfunction. *Psychiatry, 6*(3), 111–114.

Sobsczak, J. A. (2009). Struggling to reconnect: Women's perspectives on alcohol dependence, violence, and sexual function. *Journal of the American Psychiatric Nurses Association, 14*, 421–428.

Sommer, F., Goldstein, I., & Korda, J. B. (2010). Bicycle riding and erectile dysfunction: A review. *Journal of Sexual Medicine, 7*, 2346–2358.

South, S. C., Turkheimer, E., & Oltmanns, T. F. (2008). Personality disorder symptoms and marital functioning. *Journal of the Consulting and Clinical Psychology, 76*, 769–780.

Southern, S., & Cade, R. (2011). Sexuality: A professional specialization comes of age. *The Family Journal: Counseling and Therapy for Couples and Families, 19*(30), 246–262.

Sperry, L., & Carlson, J. (2000). Couples therapy with a personality-disordered couple. *The Family Journal: Counseling and Therapy for Couples and Families, 8*, 118–123.

Stanford, A. (2002). *Asperger syndrome and long-term relationships*. London, UK: Jessica Kingsley.

Steffens, B. A., & Rennie, R. L. (2006). The traumatic nature of disclosure of wives of sexual addicts. *Sexual Addiction & Compulsivity, 12*, 247–267.

Stephenson, K. R., & Meston, C. M. (2010). When are sexual difficulties distressing for women? The selective protective value of intimate relationships. *Journal of Sexual Medicine, 7*(11), 3683–3694.

Stewart, S. E., Stack, D. E., & Wilhelm, S. (2008). Severe obsessive-compulsive disorder with and without body dysmorphic disorder: Clinical correlates and implications. *Journal of Clinical Psychiatry, 201*, 33–38.

Stimmel, G. L., & Gutierrez, M. A. (2007). Counseling patients about sexual issues. Retrieved October 27, 2012 from http://www.medscape.com/viewarticle/549253_print

Stinson, R. D. (2009). The behavioral and cognitive-behavioral treatment of female sexual dysfunction: How far we have come and the path left to go. *Sexual and Relationship Therapy, 24*(3 and 4), 271–285.

Stout, H. (2011, June 5). Cultural studies; Viagra: The thrill that was. *New York Times*.

Symonds, T., Roblin, D., Hart, K., & Althof, S. (2003, October–December). How does early ejaculation impact a man's life? *Journal of Sex & Marital Therapy, 29*(5), 361–370.

Tan, H. M, Tong, S. F., & Ho, C. C.K. (2012). Men's health: Sexual dysfunction, physical, and psychological health—Is there a link? *Journal of Sexual Medicine, 9*, 663–671.

Tan, Y., & Zhong, Y. (2001). Chinese style psychoanalysis—assessment and treatment of paraphilias: Exhibitionism, frotteurism, voyeurism, and fetishism. *International Journal of Psychotherapy, 6*(3), 297–314.

Taverner, W., & McKee, R. (2011). *Taking sides: Clashing views in human sexuality*. New York, NY: McGraw Hill/Dushkin.

Tayebi, N., Mojtaba, S., & Arkadani, Y. (2009). Incidence and prevalence of the sexual dysfunctions in infertile couples. *European Journal of General Medicine, 6*(2), 74–77.

Taylor, B., & Davis, S. (2006). Using the extended PLISSIT model to address sexual healthcare needs. *Nursing Standards, 21*(11), 35–40.

Taylor, H. A., Jr. (1999). Sexual activity and the cardiovascular patient: Guidelines. *American Journal of Cardiology, 84*(5B), 6N–10N.

Tiefer, L. (2001, May). A new view of women's sexual problems: Why new? Why now? *The Journal of Sex Research. 38*(2), 88–96.

Tiefer, L. (2012). Medicalizations and demedicalizations of sexuality therapies. *Journal of Sex Research, 49*(4), 311–318.

Tiefer, L., Hall, M., & Tavris, C. (2002). Beyond dysfunction: A new view of women's sexual problems. *Journal of Sex and Marital Therapy, 28*(Suppl 1), 225–232.

Thomas, S. G. (2012, March 3). The gray divorcee. *The Wall Street Journal.*

Thompson, W. K., Charo, L., Vahia, I. V., Depp, C., Allison, M., & Jeste, D. V. (2011, August). Association between higher levels of sexual function, activity, and satisfaction and self-rated successful aging in older postmenopausal women. *Journal of the American Geriatric Society, 59*(8), 1503–1508.

Turner, D. S., & Dudek, F. A. (1982). An analysis of alcoholism and its effects on sexual functioning. *Sexuality and Disability, 5*, 143–157.

Twenge, J. M., Campbell, W., & Foster, C. A. (2003). Parenthood and marital satisfaction: A meta-analytic review. *Journal Of Marriage & Family, 65*(3), 574–583.

Valadares, A. L., Pinto-Neto, A. M., de Suuza, M. H., Osis, M. J., & da Costa Paiva, L. H. (2011). The prevalence of components of low sexual function and associated factors in middle-aged women. *Journal of Sexual Medicine, 8*(10), 2851–2858.

Van Dernoot Lipsky, L., & Burk, C. (2009). *Trauma stewardship: An every day guide to caring for self while caring for others.* San Francisco, CA: Berrett-Koehler.

van Lankveld, J. J. D. M., Granot, M., Willibrord, C. M., Schultz, W., Binik, Y. M., Wesselmann, U., … Achtrari, C. (2010). Women's sexual pain disorders. *Journal of Sexual Medicine, 7*, 615–631.

Van Minnen, A., & Kampman, M. (2000). The interaction between anxiety and sexual functioning: A controlled study of sexual functioning in women with anxiety disorders. *Sexual and Relationship Therapy, 15*, 47–57.

Vasquez, M. J. T. (1991). Sexual intimacies with clients after termination: Should a prohibition be explicit? *Ethics and Behavior, 1*(1), 45–61.

Ventolini, G. (2011). Measuring treatment outcomes in women with vulvodynia. *Journal of Clinical and Medical Research, 3*(2), 59–64.

Vercellini, P., Somigliana, E., Buggio, L., Barbara, G., Frattaruolo, M., & Fedele, L. (2012). "I Can't Get No Satisfaction": Deep dyspareunia and sexual functioning in women with rectovaginal endometriosis. *Fertility and Sterility, 98*(6), 1503–1511.

Wade, L. D., Kremer, E. C., & Brown, J. (2005). The incidental orgasm: The presence of clitoral knowledge and the absence of orgasm for women. *Women's Health, 42*(1), 117–138.

Waite, L. J., Laumann, E. O., Das, A., & Schumm, L. P. (2009). Sexuality: Measures of partnerships, practices, attitudes, and problems in the National Social Life, Health, and Aging Study. *The Journals of Gerontology, Series B, 64*(Suppl. 1), i56–i66.

Waldinger, M. D., & Schweitzer, D. H. (2005). Retarded ejaculation in men: An overview of psychological and neurobiological insights. *World Journal of Urology, 32*(2), 76–81.

Walsh, K. E., & Berman, J. R. (2004). Sexual dysfunction in the older woman: An overview of the current understanding and management. *Drugs and Aging, 21*(1), 665–675.

Weaver, J. B., 3rd, Weaver, S. S., Mays, D., Hopkins, G. L., Kannenberg, W., & McBride, D. (2011). Mental- and physical-health indicators and sexually explicit media use behavior by adults. *Journal of Sexual Medicine, 8*(3), 764–772.

Weeks, G. R. (1987). *Integrating sex and marital therapy: A clinical guide*. New York, NY: Routledge.

Weeks, G. R. (2005). The emergence of a new paradigm in sex therapy: Integration. *Sexual and Relationship Therapy, 20*(1), 89–105.

Weeks, G. R., Hertlein, K. M., & Gambescia, N. (2009). The treatment of hypoactive sexual desire disorder. *Journal of Family Psychotherapy, 20*, 129–149.

Weiss, S. J. (2007). Neurobiological alterations associated with traumatic stress. *Perspectives in Psychiatric Care, 43*, 114–122.

Wetterneck, C. T., Burgess, A. J., Short, M. B., Smith, A. H., & Cervantes, M. E. (2012). The role of sexuality compulsivity, impulsivity, and experiential avoidance in internet pornography use. *The Psychological Record, 62*, 3–18.

Whisman, M. A., & Wagers, T. P. (2005). Assessing relationship betrayals. *JCLP/In Session, 61*(11), 1383–1391.

Wiederman, M. W., & Pryor, T. (1997). Body dissatisfaction and sexuality among women with Bulimia Nervosa. *International Journal of Eating Disorders, 21*, 361–365.

Wiederman, M. W. (1998). The state of theory in sex therapy. *Journal of Sex Research, 35*(1), 88–99.

Wiederman, M. W. (2001) Gender differences in sexuality: Perceptions, myths, and realities. *The Family Journal: Counseling and Therapy for Couples and Families, 9*(4), 468–471.

Wiederman, M. W. (2003). Paraphilias and fetishism. *The Family Journal: Counseling and Therapy for Couples and Families, 11*(3), 315–321.

Wierman, M. W., Nappi, R. E., Avis, N., Davis, S. R., Labrie, F., Rosner, W., & Shifren, J. L. (2010). Endocrine aspects of women's sexual function. *Journal of Sexual Medicine, 7*(1 Pt 2), 561–585.

Williams, M. W., & Farris, S. G. (2011). Sexual orientation in obsessive-compulsive disorder: Prevalence and correlates. *Psychiatry Research, 187*, 156–159.

Wilson, D. R. (2010). Health consequences of childhood sexual abuse. *Perspectives in Psychiatric Care, 46*(1), 56–64.

Wilson, J. E., & Wilson, K. M. (2008). Amelioration of sexual fantasies to sexual abuse cues in an adult survivor of childhood sexual abuse: A case study. *Journal of Behavioral Therapy and Experimental Psychiatry, 39*(4), 417–423.

Wilson, S. K., Delk, J. R., 2nd., & Billups, K. L. (2001). Treating symptoms of female sexual arousal disorder with the eros-clitoral therapy device. *The Journal of Gender-Specific Medicine, 4*(2), 54–58.

Winters, J., Christoff, K., & Gorzalka, B. B. (2010). Dysregulated sexuality and high sexual desire: Distinct constructs? *Archives of Sexual Behavior, 39*, 1029–1043.

Wischman, T. H. (2010). Sexual disorders in infertile couples. *Journal of Sexual Medicine, 7*(5), 1868–1876.

Wolak, J., Mitchell, K., & Finkelhor, D. (2007). Unwanted and wanted exposure to online pornography in a national sample of youth internet users. *Pediatrics, 119*(2), 247–257.

World Health Organization. (2006). *Gender and reproductive rights, glossary, sexual health*. Retrieved June 10, 2013 from http://www.who.int/reproductivehealth/topics/sexual_health/sh_definitions/en/.

Wylie, K., & Froggatt, N. (2010). Late onset hypogonadism, sexuality and fertility. *Human Fertility, 13*(3), 126–133.

Wylie, K., & Kenney, G. (2010). Sexual dysfunction and the ageing male. *Maturitas, 65*(1), 23–27.

Yan, E., Wu, A. M., Ho, P., & Pearson, V. (2011). Older Chinese men and women's experiences and understanding of sexuality. *Culture, Health and Sexuality, 13*(9), 983–999.

Yee, L. (2010). Aging and sexuality. *Australian Family Physician, 39*(10), 718–721.

Younggren, J., & Harris, E. (2011, January/February). Risk management: When marital therapy is. *The National Psychologist, 9,* 26.

Zamboni, B. D., & Crawfod, I. (2007). Minority stress and sexual problems among African-American gay and bisexual men. *Archives of Sexual Behavior, 36*(4), 569–578.

Zimmerman, K. J. (2012). Clients in sexually open relationships: Considerations for therapists. *Journal of Feminist Family Therapy, 24*(3), 272–289.

Zitzman, S. T., & Butler, M. H. (2005). Attachment, addiction, and recovery: Conjoint marital therapy for recovery from a sexual addiction. *Sexual Addiction & Compulsivity, 12,* 311–337.

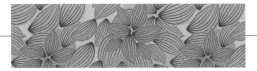

Index

MUSE™. *See* medicated urethral systems for erections.
Myths, 94, 218–220
  male sexual problems, 86

Narcissistic personality disorder (NPD), 157
National Vulvodynia Association, 183
Nerve-sparing procedures, 206
Neurological disorders, 94, 208–209
  Parkinson's disease, 208
  sexual dysfunction, 208
    early ejaculation, 208
    erectile dysfunction, 208
    vaginal atrophy, 208
  spinal cord lesion, 208
  stroke, 208
New View, sexual dysfunction, 66
Nonsteroidal anti-inflammatory drugs, 180
Normalization, 211
NPD. *See* narcissistic personality disorder.
Neurontin™, 160

Obsessive compulsive disorder (OCD), 53, 67, 79, 148, 149–150, 157
Oedipal complex, 35
Olanzapine, 158
Online Slang Dictionary, 16
Opioids, 152
  codeine, 152
  heroin, 152
  morphine, 152
  oxycodone, 152
Oral contraceptive, 37
Oral vasodilators, 223
Orgasm
  capacity for, 69–70
  definition of, 69
  experiencing of, 83
  per Freud, 36
Outercourse, 187
Ovaries, 19
Oxycodone, 152

Pain catastrophizing, 178
Pain
  management, 186
  understanding of, 176
    acute, 176
    chronic, 176
Paraphilia NOS, 234, 241, 242
  bestiality, 241
  exhibitionism, 241
  frotteurism, 241
  pedophilia, 241
  sadism, 241
  voyeurism, 241
Parental concerns re sex, 126–131
  abuse, 130–131
  exposure to pornography, 129
  family discussions, 133
  gay siblings, 128–129
  gender confusion, 127
  masturbation, 127
  menstrual cycles, 130
  premarital activities, 129
  sex education classes, 129
  sexual abuse by another child, 128
  sexual values, 134
Parents, children and sex, 121–134
  masturbation, 124
  early education, 123–126
    infant, 123
    toddlers, 123
  parental concerns, 126–131
  pornography, 126
  safe sex discussions, 125
Parkinson's Disease, 67, 87, 96, 208, 209
  treatment of, 209
    antidepressant, 209
    antihypertensive, 209
    dopamine agonist, 209
    PDE5 inhibitors, 209
    vacuum pump, 209
Paroxetine (Paxil™), 92
Passion vs. domesticity, couples and, 107–109
Passionate love, 108
Paxil™. *See* paroxetine.